C000194723

Fashion and Orie

Fashion and Orientalism

Dress, Textiles and Culture from the 17th to the 21st Century

Adam Geczy

B L O O M S B U R Y

LONDON • NEW DELHI • NEW YORK • SYDNEY

Bloomsbury Academic
An imprint of Bloomsbury Publishing Plc

50 Bedford Square
London
WC1B 3DP
UK

175 Fifth Avenue
New York
NY 10010
USA

www.bloomsbury.com

First published 2013

British Library Cataloguing-in-Publication Data
A catalogue record for this book is available from the British Library.

ISBN: 978 1 84788 600 2 (Cloth)
       978 1 84788 599 9 (Paper)
e-ISBN 978 0 85785 427 8 (epub)
        978 0 85785 426 1 (ePDF)

Library of Congress Cataloging-in-Publication Data
A catalogue record for this book is available from the Library of Congress.

Typeset by Apex CoVantage, LLC, Madison, WI, USA
Printed and bound in Great Britain

To my son Marcel; to his
imagination and venturesome spirit

Contents

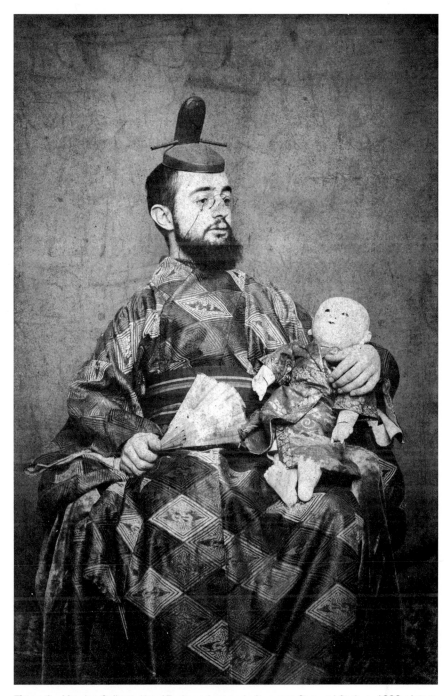

Figure 1 Maurice Guibert, *Henri Toulouse-Lautrec in Japanese Samurai Garb*, c. 1892, vintage albumen proof print © Richard and Ellen Sandor Family Collection.

List of Illustrations

Introduction

Thou by the Indian Ganges' side
Shouldst rubies find.

—Andrew Marvell, 'To His Coy Mistress'

We arrived at the opulent bazaars that form the centre of Istanbul, a solidly constructed stone labyrinth in the Byzantine style which served as a vast shelter from the daytime heat. Its huge galleries of arched and vaulted ceilings supported by sculpted pillars were in colonnades, each dedicated to particular kinds of merchandise. Most remarkable were the clothes and the female slippers [*babouches*], fabrics embroidered or in lamé, cashmeres, carpets, gold, silver or opal-encrusted furniture, the silverware, and most of all the brilliant weaponry assembled in the part of the bazaar known as Bésastain.

—Gérard de Nerval, *Voyage to the Orient*[1]

While in my early teens at an island resort in Australia's Barrier Reef, I was introduced to the sarong. A generous swathe of coarse, thin cotton batik of Malay and Indonesian origin, it could either be tied at the waist, much like a towel, or wrapped to make bulbous, floppy, low-lying shorts. It was worn by both men and women and seemed to me an altogether sensible piece of clothing given the balmy climate and casual living conditions. Airy and cool, here was something that could be used as a towel surrogate for lying on the sand and then as an item of clothing after leaving the beach. True enough, I found the design exotically appealing, but I was in no way aware that I was adopting orientalism in dress, per se. The use of this item was adventitious: I wore the sarong because it was practical. In retrospect, now armed, or straddled, depending on how you see it, with a stock of cultural theory, I could level at myself the charge of cultural tokenism. But that would be pressing the matter, since the sarong was worn without self-consciousness. Ignorance perhaps—yet far from the affectation of cross-cultural masquerade that was so rife since the sixteenth century.

And it has now been surpassed with a new inclination that repudiates difference in its apparent embrace of it. Were I that age today, I would, perhaps, through the reminding of my friends made over digital networks, be partaking in 'world' fashion, as I might listen to 'world' music. The new term is 'cultural borrowing', a palliative phrase, unlike 'cultural plunder', because it has had the guilt and the opprobrium drained from it. 'Borrowing' is particularly felicitous (insidious) because it implies that something can always be returned to its rightful origin. When the origin is deemed lost, or displaced, the onus of any moral imperative is lifted altogether. These euphemistic revisions and what they reflect of our understanding of the world make the topic of the relationship between fashion and orientalism timely. No less so is the extent to which global power is wagered according to 'East' and 'West'. In this book I argue that the study of dress—the site in which politics, identity and subjectivity encounter one another—is perhaps the best way of understanding the superficiality of this opposition. For East and West are not contraries, but they require the fallacy that they are, for the sake of their own self-image and illusion of autonomy. Differences abound, but opposites are few. Orientalism in fashion and dress is a series of overlaps, codependencies and shared redefinitions hiding behind a simplistic binary.

We might start with the astonishing fact that almost every name for pre-synthetic textiles derives from Middle Eastern or Asiatic roots. To anyone with a passing interest in the topic of orientalism of fashion, the list is staggering. We might begin with the most common of all, cotton, which is from the Old French *cotton*, which is taken from the Arabic, *ḳutn*. Satin can also be traced back to the Arabic *zaytūnī* meaning 'of Tsinkiang', a town in China. Then there's silk: the Old English *sioloc*, *seolec*, comes from late Latin *sericum*, neuter of *sericus*, itself coming from the Greek *Sēres*, which was the name for the merchants from the Far East who first brought the coveted cloth to Europe. Taffeta evolved from the Old French *taffetas* or medieval Latin *taffata*, based on the Persian *tāftan*, 'to shine'. Damask comes from Damascus, where it was first made; the light silk material *surah* takes its name from the textile centre of Surat, angora drives from Ankara, cashmere from Kashmir, and calico is from Calicut, the seaport on the Malabar coast in south-west India. Muslin was first produced in *Mosul*, a town in Iraq, and since the Venetians were among the most prolific traders of it, they dubbed it *mussolina*. Gingham arrives to us via the Dutch *gingang*, from the Malayan adjective *genggang*, which means 'striped'. Fustian, a twilled cloth with a nap texture like suede, is a modification of the Old French *fustaigne*, itself from medieval Latin *fustaneum*, a truncation of *pannus fustaneus*, '*cloth from Fostat'*, a suburb of Cairo. Gabardine, from the Old French, *gawardine*, was associated with Jewish men and pilgrims, so the relationship to the East is not far off, especially since Jewish people were long conflated with 'orientals'. Chintz, originally a painted or stained calico imported from India, is from *chints*, the plural of *chint*, hailing from the Hindi *hīmṭ*, which means 'spattering' or 'stain'. Jute comes to us from the Bengali *jhūṭo*, a variant of the Prakrit *jhṣṭi*, The exceptions are preciously few. Only velvet, cambric, chiffon, felt, flax, tulle and linen have

European–Latinate etymologies. Albeit not exhaustive, this litany helps to anchor the premise of this book—that Western fashion and dress is unthinkable without engaging with the role of Eastern influences.

Although most if not all accounts of orientalism and the arts touch on aspects of fashion, it is largely in passing in order to describe the passages of influence and obsession. Yet fashion—used here as the portmanteau term that includes clothing, dress and costume—occupies a position different both from art and of design objects, while constantly borrowing from and impinging upon both. As opposed to painting, film or music, which are heard or beheld and are therefore physically separate experiences, clothing is worn and therefore by degrees involves and implicates the subject wearing it. Rare if not nonexistent are the instances when a painter is an object of the gaze. As Joanne Eicher puts it in the introduction to her volume on ethnicity and dress, 'Dress is a coded sensory system of non-verbal communication that aids human interaction in space and time. The codes of dress include visual as well as other sensory modifications (taste, smell, sound, and feel) and supplements (garments, jewellery, and accessories) to the body'.[2] There is a degree of lived, performative intent to clothing's role in asserting personality and identity that is potentially odious to art, which claims to make statements that not only epitomize the moment but also transcend it. With clothing, the fact that it is inhabited as well as seen means that the positioning of gaze, the locus of power, is potentially skewed. The ambiguities belonging to certain pictorial images are made different when brought into the realm of fashion, since fashion involves use, being and action. The subject–object relations belonging to pictorial representation are rendered multivalent and uncertain. Making a picture about a particular condition, as the oriental painters were apt to do, is different from attempting to inhabit that condition when one dresses up in clothes that announce themselves as foreign. Moreover, depending on the era and the person, oriental styling also follows more than one line of effect and intent. As suggested earlier, the degree to which oriental motifs, styles and materials have permeated Western fashion and dress is so immeasurable that to name one dominant dynamic of power is untenable.

The aims of this book are roughly threefold. The first is to trace where orientalist styles and motifs have featured in Western culture since the late seventeenth to early-eighteenth century and how orientalism, or orientalisms, have influenced and shaped the modern concept of Western dress. The second is to canvass key debates, subtleties and blind-spots within the field. The term *oriental* has changes more than once over the last four hundred years, due to socio-economic changes, shifts in taste and, of course, more recently, owing to the seminal postcolonial theory of Edward Said, his followers and challengers. For the sake of coherence, the organization of this book is roughly chronological. But chronology is the most fragile of armatures to handle a topic rife with the vicissitudes of whim and personal invention. This is above all a book about a style which is considered rooted in a culture, a culture which is far more a mutating cluster of cultures and whose characteristics are generally more at the behest of the other culture—the West, itself a mutating and complex body—that consumes them. But it is also too reductive to say that this is a subject confined to the Western vision. An underlying feature is the way in which East and West influenced one another. Another is the way in which styles within the much larger (and nebulous) ambit of orientalism have enjoyed re-emergence, recrudescence and recreation, for it is remarkable the extent to which the West configured orientalism for itself as a set of variations on a foreign theme. The conception could be independent, and frequently ignorant, of the countries and histories that once nourished such themes. The third aim of this book is to introduce a new way of thinking about orientalist fashion and dress—for which I coin the term *transorientalism*—that has come to light in the last century or so.

By highlighting the variety of coordinates of orientalism in fashion, this study contributes in no small way to the growing cohort of scholarship that either seeks to challenge if not cast a wider net than Said's. One of the drawbacks of a canonic theory is that it must continue to be used as a dialectical touchstone for its successors. But we have travelled a great deal since then. An important aspect of recent scholarship has been to emphasize the two-sidedness of the cultural encounter and to consider it as one of imbrication and exchange rather than in terms of a dominant party sucking the life and dignity out of another.[3] Such scholarship is by no means dismissive of postcolonial abuses, but it also draws out the subtlety and complexity of how different cultures disclosed themselves to others. For cultural identity is by no means autochthonous or essential or natural. It is imagined and manufactured and then transacted either willingly or by force. These are the dynamics of influence on one hand and repression on the other.

Thus, I make the audacious claim that, for the reasons cited above, fashion and dress are the very best loci by which to understand the various spaces by which the signs of nation, identity and novelty have become transacted, adapted and owned. This book contends that these exchanges are nowhere more evident than in fashion and dress, so much so that the changes, exchanges, renamings and reacculturations in this field are so diverse and paradoxical that they can scarcely fit within a Saidian framework. In a most vivid and tangible way, the history of orientalism in fashion and dress shows the close networks of reliance of East and West that exist beneath the spectacle of opposition between Christianity and Islam. The dichotomy of East–West, oriental–western is simplistic and to many objectionable, but it is tenacious nonetheless: in academic discourse, in the media, and in both fashion theory and practice.

This leads me again to third trajectory of this book and the term *transorientalism*. Transorientalism in fashion and dress—and also other aspects of design and art, but that is the subject of a later study—identifies three planes of experience. The first is the less mediated circumstances of the developed world, before it gets transformed into the 'oriental' exotic 'other' from which the Westerner draws aesthetic and economic sustenance. These are the lived, 'real' spaces. It is not a dream-space or a place of possibility, for unlike the West it has no other as its beneficiary. These circumstances connect to the second level of transorientalism, which is the extent to which the cultural other has adopted and moulded its own particular types of orientalism for economic benefit or national rebadging. While contemporary Indian, Korean or even Senegalese fashions and dress are by degrees still beholden to the dominant signs emanating from Paris, London and New York, it is also true that they have internalized orientalist ideas. Here the transient and the hazy of the European Bohemian's opium dream blend furtively into the solemn words about cultural self-determination through language and dress.

In her lecture 'Nationalism and the Imagination', Gayatri Chakravorty Spivak speaks about the conflicts arising from a country's commitment to 'cultural' nationalism while maintaining 'civic' nationalism committed to a Group of Eight state, the group of the eight most powerful economies in the world. A country must traverse independent aims whilst being compliant with the aims of dominant powers. This leads to a social justice that could compromise the internal aims and interests of a subjected state.[4] In fashion and dress, however, we see a far different dynamic that does not reflect the problems facing non-G8 economies (which include two of the great oriental states, China and Japan). For more than a century we have seen the Orient market its own self-conscious orientalism to Europe and America while internally adopting more Western forms of dress. More interesting still is the way that countries have taken possession of a particular style of dress (such as Korea and the *hanbok* in the 1990s) whose origins are hybrid to wage their case on a national identity. The oriental sign as it is trafficked in fashion and dress is therefore fluid and dodges, although not entirely eludes, the critical warnings of Said, Spivak and other postcolonial theorists. Thus, transorientalism, like transgender, is a space that has not renounced the base realities but at the same time commands another, independent space. Transorientalism openly claims for itself the space of fantasy and freedom which had always been inscribed in the orientalist construct. On the simplest level, orientalism is practiced by oriental and nonoriental designers, and when a collection arrives it does not court a colonialist or postcolonialist critique. This does not mean that as an uncritical space it cannot be immune to theory. On the contrary, it gives one much to think about.

In its third and most pervasive incarnation, transorientalism denotes a self-conscious use of the Orient as a geographically uncircumscribed zone, whose cultural specifics are secondary to the imaginative uses to which it can be put. It is manifested initially in a diversity of modernist eclecticisms, from Paul Poiret and Sonia Delaunay to the costumes of the Ballets Russes, in which oriental influences from Chinese to Turkish to Persian are used with open abandon, heedless of any connective thread between inspiration and actuality. Not that this thread had necessarily been there in the earlier centuries, but earlier the cultural liberties within orientalist styling were attended by tenuous links to authenticity. Before the twentieth century, cultural 'isms' had epochal prominence as symptoms of foreign policy, be it trade, threat of war or the removal of that threat: chinoiserie belongs to the seventeenth century in a way that turquerie belongs to the eighteenth century and *Japonisme* belongs to the latter half of the nineteenth century. To couch transorientalism in a psychoanalytic parlance, one might say that it is a loosening of the super-ego of empirical social frameworks and anthropological accuracy. It is making peace with an expectation which, in fashion, was either falsely affirmed or subverted.

* * *

Fashion, as Georg Simmel presciently observed, is the primary locus of the way in which people both register their belonging to a group and simultaneously assert their independence from it. And as Stéphane Mallarmé was aware, through his writing for the periodical *La Dernière Mode*, it was the most stable way of showing publicly that one belongs to change. Although neither writer was terribly interested in orientalism in fashion or dress, orientalism has long been the most consistent and most locatable device by which Western fashion has sought to remake itself. It is the sign of belonging to a nameless cult, but a cult in the name of difference, which is alternative, free and therefore pregnant with potentialities that the opposite term, the staid West, is less able to offer. This is how the West enlisted the Orient for itself—and time and again we hear this refrain—that as distant promise, it afforded an antidote to local strictures. In a symbolic or sublimated way, orientalist fashion is an avatar of the erotic. Elizabeth Wilson does not mean sex as such, yet this is particularly poignant if we consider the gnomic statement by her that fashion is 'obsessed with gender',[5] because it places orientalism within a slippery terrain in which sexual stereotypes are both affirmed, such as embodied in the harem, and challenged, as we find in cross-dressing and masquerade. As writers such as Richard Berstein and Ronald Hyams have shown, the Orient was a rich resource for mass sexual exploitation, and military colonialism cannot be seen in isolation from sexual colonialism. The vague promise of forbidden pleasures not only increased its attraction but added to its imaginative allure—and the complicity was not one-sided.[6] If opulence and sensuality were components of the orientalist myth, other concepts that were at odds with this were grafted to it as well. In the seventeenth century, the oriental despot was held as a paragon of stately authority—particularly by rulers of divine right, such as Louis XIV—and viewed against the historical relief of the way Prophet Muhammad was remembered as the great unifier of the Arab state.

In the more secular age of the nineteenth century, orientalism was enlisted to a cause that came close to the polar opposite of this. Mixing the sensuous and the sensual, in the hands of Bohemians it carried the air of flamboyant anti-establishment. Some simple parallels are still with us. Where blacks and earth tones belonged to the sober, cerebral West, bright reds and vivid yellows belonged to the hallucinatory orient. The Romantic poet Théophile Gautier's famous vest of 'Chinese vermilion' that he wore to the opening of Victor Hugo's play *Hernani*—in which the Bohemians confronted their nemesis, the bourgeoisie—must be seen in this light. It was intended literally as a sensualist red rag to the bourgeois bull. In his words, it was a 'symbolic protest against the grayness of modern life'.[7] Whether Gautier knew it or not, the oriental association of the colour red in clothing came from the much-desired dye 'Turkey Red', a secret formula made from Anatolian madder. With both textiles and fashion, the immaterial dreamscapes in orientalist painting, music and literature are made flesh, brought into the bodily frame. For having fewer of the aspirations of the higher and permanent arts, fashion can be a rich repository of signs for the ways in which a culture asserts itself and for how it tries to compensate for what it thinks it lacks.

We might start by delineating two ways in which orientalism enters into Western fashion and dress: consciously and unconsciously. The unconscious abounds us, and the strata of influence are so many that the real origin is either symbolic or lost; today's floral designs associated with chintz and wallpaper are an example. Having flooded into Europe from both India and China since the sixteenth century, they are now a common international language in art and design whose attribution is as remote as their origins. For instance, the silk scarf designed for Princess Grace of Monaco in 1966, the Gucci Flora print, has subsequently be used and reused on clothing and handbags (and has recently lent its idea to a fragrance). Recognized as originating with Gucci via Princess Grace, it is 'essentially' orientalist: the exuberant intricacy of its design—not to mention the abundance of flowers depicted there that were imported long ago from Asia and the Middle East. The scarf also shows an unmistakable debt to Indian silks and Persian carpets from at least the twelfth century. Appearances and historical lines of provenance are deceptive, for tulips are about as Dutch as paprika is Hungarian. The list of flowers, not to say plant types, that were introduced into Europe, from the Middle Ages to the eighteenth century, are too many to enumerate. Species such as the camellia, magnolia, wisteria, azalea, anemone japonica and rhododendron all came from the region of Cathay, now China. The ubiquitous floral scarf, no less than the English garden, owes the Orient an inestimable debt.

In other cases the evolution of a motif is expedient. Paisley, a leaf or teardrop design with intricate curlicues, is a motif taken from India, named after the Scottish town that produced textiles in quantities and variations that has made it accessible and popular. We are therefore faced with a rather postmodern paradox in which our acquaintance with paisley is of Scottish variations on the theme. Another example is Liberty prints. Founded by Sir Arthur Lazenby Liberty in 1875, when the firm was called the 'East India House', the firm was a hub of influences that flowed in via orientalist designers such as Thomas Wardle and writers such as Christopher Dresser (who was also a superb designer), stocking imports ranging from woollens to muslins from all over the Middle and Far East. Although standards from Middle Eastern suppliers had begun to slump to meet demand, Liberty rallied local firms to improve their own dyeing techniques to Moorish designs. Persian silks were imported and then dyed and printed with oriental motifs designed in London. In many ways, Liberty was improving upon what could be found in the East, while contributing the popular perception that oriental textiles were the best. As we shall also see, art nouveau, an avowedly European style, had a similar genesis with an accountable debt to oriental influences, and not solely to Japan (Siegfried Bing, who is credited with coining the term, sold Japanese objets d'art in his shop on the Rue de Provence). Such patterns of repossession, which displace a design of motif and also make it more desirable and enduring through re-elaboration, away from its indigenous context, are recurring themes of this book.

Despite the lines of demarcation being never clear, the more conscious use of orientalism can be understood by asking whether orientalism within art, fashion and design is matched by an obverse quality in the East. The fact that the elite of Saudi Arabia, Kuwait and Jordan are among the most avid consumers of haute couture exposes the imbalance in notions of prosperity and power, for in fashion, in the strictest sense of the term, one never just wears a garment, one attires oneself with a wish which can be lavish or covert. The designs of what mostly French designers have come to symbolize are the links between beauty, wealth and sophistication, attributes which since ancient times have been perceived to belong to culture at its highest. While Western style is very much part of the East's consumption, it is the embodiment of a very different kind of imaginary, which is more about present and future, tied to real material gain and palpable comfort and security. This was the impetus behind the drive in Turkey under Atatürk (1923–38) and in Japan, first in the Meiji period (1868–1912) and then under Hara Takashi (1919–21), to foster

Western modes of dress to help guide the populace's minds to a more forward, Western way of thinking.

Adopting Western dress was seen as a constructive, necessary component to their own industrial development, a sign to their neighbours that they were progressive and modern. A noteworthy distinguishing feature of such mass cultural reorientation is that the newly assumed style is used as a sign of superior development, whereas orientalism is prone to use culturally specific signs in a capricious way that, philosophically, at least, does not tamper with the ideal core (such as it is) of Western identity and power. In ways that are at root economic, it is convenient for the West to cling to orientalist clichés, like the belly dancer or the geisha (Puccini's *Madame Butterfly* continues to be one of the most popular in the opera repertoire). A recent example from couture is John Galliano's 2007 collection, which followed an origami-like idiom that was wholly recognizable as Japanese in flavour but wholly alien to Japanese traditions of either fashion or dress.

But this kind of arbitrariness need not be cited for blanket condemnation, for when we turn to dress as opposed to fashion, from the ready-to-wear range of clothing to the vernacular adoption of design motifs and cuts of clothing, we see in such influences a level of cultural exchange that is impossible to place into firm contours. A contemporary sign of this fluidity is in the current debate in India that suggests that it can sell itself as exotic to the West while having absorbed this notion within its own domestic market. Viewed critically, one might say that Indian designers are selling a caricature of India to their fellow Indians (a widespread example is in the association of the *swadeshi* with Gandhi). Or as Ann Marie Leshkowich and Carla Jones so pithily ask: 'What happens when Asian Chic becomes Asian Chic in Asia?'[8]

Such twists and about-faces within oriental cultures since the twentieth century are to be contrasted with the tendency in Western fashion to galvanize or, to use a loaded metaphor, to spice up a fashion ensemble. More so than in dress, fashion is under constant pressure to announce its revitalization in all sorts of ways, and it is to orientalist idioms that it constantly turns. In the seminal *European Vision and the South Pacific*, a book that many see as ushering in postcolonial discourse, Bernard Smith educes the thesis that the new landscapes of the South Pacific were one of the prime enablers of the burgeoning Romantic vision. His radical insight lies in revealing that the foreign and the exotic, by virtue of their foreignness, showed up the limitations of the imperialist European way of seeing things. More importantly, he suggests, it was places like Australia that allowed Europe to see itself with fresh eyes. In other words, Europe, especially Britain and France, relied on their colonies for the ways in which they viewed themselves and the manner in which they revived and nourished their own national self-image.[9] This is one of the main trajectories of this book. It is in fashion where this condition was most commonly available and most amply visible. And to this day it is in fashion that the Orient, understood as a shapeless yet conveniently identifiable set of signs and values, continues to foster such an illusion.

Orientalism is in myriad cases the sine qua non of this illusion of newness—newness seen as transgression which carries immediate connotations of breaking with the status quo—that is the mainstay of fashion and the fashion industry that began in the early-twentieth century. In the way that fashion can bring together personal intimacy and public spectacle, the orientalism in fashion has long been used to register dislocation from the habitual status quo. But as the many histories and stray accounts of Western encounters with the Orient reveal, it is questionable whether such acts are in the interests of those from whom the clothing, styles or motifs are taken. Wearing orientalist clothing is rarely an act of assimilation or complete conciliation, it is rather the obverse. Since clothes become part of the individual, they are the very avatars of that individual's power. As Reina Lewis and Gail Low have pointed out, a Westerner dressing in non-Western clothing is a kind of play-acting, whose titillation is augmented by the knowledge of the white skin underneath. As Lewis states, 'Cross-dressing offers both the pleasures of consumption—the Orient as a space full of enticing goods to be bought, savoured and worn—and the deeper thrill of passing as a native'.[10]

Yet as we will see, there are whole sets of cultural circumstances that provide exceptions to the rule. A central term within the whole of the history and debates surrounding orientalism and fashion is *identification*. Orientalism in theory as in practice survives off the selective, fanciful way in which it is understood and in the way it traduces the identities of others. But the cultural solecisms are only the most extreme cases. In others, orientalist fashion, when worn in Western contexts, is highly cathartic. The wearing of Indian-style clothes by the hippies and yippies of the 1960s and 1970s for example differs from the kind of cross-dressing described above. When we look at Bohemianism, orientalism is used to pique bourgeois conservatism. Given that 'orientals' were free to adopt any form of Western dress, it is therefore tenuous to seek out such areas of influence for too-swift condemnation. In this light it is also profitable to look at the most culturally and semantically innocent yet physically penetrating sense, the olfactory (after all, perfume is part of dress no less than millinery and jewellery). The theoretical discourse of orientalism in perfume is meagre and bears considerable mention. Yves Saint Laurent's *Opium* was so commercially popular in the 1980s as to make it known to all users of perfumes; it is now a classic, and so are several fragrances by Guerlain, notably *Shalimar*, *Mitsouko*, and *Habit Rouge*, putatively the first male 'oriental' cologne.

Let us draw together some of these seams to say that there are three basic, albeit convergent, kinds of orientalist styling and influence within fashion and dress.

1. Assimilation, improvement, adoption and influence: this relates to anything from the adoption of an oriental designs, such as chintz for wallpaper, dresses or upholstery to the introduction of flowing clothing, thin cottons or beading which have been so readily melded into Western dress over the last century as to be very much part of it. Here orientalism tends to be more unselfconscious and is often practical, or expedient, and thus more appropriate of the term *dress* rather than *fashion*.

2. Masquerade, repatriation or re-identification: this is simpler to identify and argue through because the use of clothing can read more as fancy dress; the body of one is recognizably in the sheath of the other. Here it is largely oriental *costume*, defined as static and archetypical, such as the kimono, which is employed as a sheath for the purpose of some form of escape. For the subsumption of identity through dressing as someone else—frequently as an 'other' that courted fascination or fear—afforded temporary release from social restrictions. In the case of the French aristocrats it was a way of signalling their access to exclusive rarities; in the case of upper-class females, such as Mary Montagu, in the eighteenth century, it was a way of resisting the constricting mores provided by the male-dominated West. This paradigm also applies to the case of someone who is repatriated or, in the case of Turkey, to when Western clothes were the index of modernization. Here orientalism is thus strategic and/or socio-linguistic.

3. Inflection, inspiration, tokenism and galvanization: the main vectors are economics and politics. When it is political, orientalism in dress is called upon to register difference from a purportedly unimaginative status quo (Bohemians, hippies). The economy of orientalist influence can be defined in two ways: first as to economies of scale, namely the degree to which something identifiably oriental is used, whether implied or exaggerated, and second within the realm of monetary exchange and the extent to which orientalist styling can help this along. Clothes as commodities, from mass-produced articles to couture, equally avail themselves of orientalism as a sign in order to divert the suspicion away from the article of clothing being generic—quite a conundrum since orientalism is used as a generic sign of difference. An example of this in everyday wear might be a raised tapered toe *à la turque* in a shoe, or a miniskirt made from kimono fabric (the cheongsam-like dress from Cavalli's 2003 collection springs to mind). When we turn to couture, orientalism is typically called upon to 'spice up' a single ensemble or a collection. (Precouture examples of this include the

silken shawls and turbans that women liked to wear in the early-nineteenth century; present examples include that of Galliano, earlier.) Fictive itself, the construct of orientalism, although integrated and crucial to the meaning of Western fashion, hovers in a fictive space that is outside the West, or outside Western fashion. This self-conscious awareness of the subliminal hovering since the twentieth century I call transorientalism. The mythic space that it occupies ensures that orientalism remains what designers call 'inspiration', always making the mythic journey from an elsewhere as external attribute into the substance of Western fashion. In turn, Western fashion survives on orientalism never receiving full admission into that substance. Seen from the perspective of fashion, orientalism is thence always *structural*.[11]

Ethically speaking, the third kind of orientalism is the most complex and delicate. While the example of couture makes us aware of how fondly and unquestioningly we cling to the myth of the flamboyant East, the history is a long one. At the end of the eighteenth century, for instance, Egyptianizing within architecture and furniture was associated with progressive, even revolutionary mentality.[12] As Jennifer Craik emphasizes, 'because fashion systems are built on the inter-relationship and tension between exotic and familiar codes, exotic looks are all the more effective as techniques of display'.[13] Her emphasis on the clothing's role in 'power and prestige' is of a piece with the suggestion that fashion is about staking a claim.[14] Orientalism's deployment within this paramount sphere of claim is crucial, since it is an indirect and unapologetically specious claim to dominion, a presumption of conquest.

But the dignity and monumentality that make cultural pilfering palatable (perhaps)—hence politenesses like 'homage' and 'borrowing'—are less available to the modality of fashion and dress, which has the potential to play havoc with complex issues arising when ritual and personal identity are inseparable. Here is where the greatest insensitivities of decontextualizing non-Western designs occur: when sacred or highly specific motifs are arbitrarily appropriated. The more recent misuses of Australian Aboriginal designs in textiles is an excellent example of this and illustrates a sacred–secular divide that is at the root of the tension between Western and Middle Eastern society. The most immediate corollary in clothing in the Middle East is the burqa, hijab and the chador, which, as it is often phrased, is an attitude, a state of mind, and not a fashion. They are not fashion choices but embrace a different category altogether of religious and cultural mores; they are seamless with some interpretations of Muslim womanhood and worn like a second skin. It is the perception of promiscuous eclecticism that has hardened the more devout Muslims of the Middle East and Indonesia against the West, and it is in codes of dress where these variances are often expressed. While such discrepancies in use and signification are cause for misunderstanding and antagonism, it must also be admitted that, for the Western experience at least, fashion and dress are among the principal vectors in the demystification and popularization of the Islamic (Middle) East. We are faced with a paradox here: Orientalism, by definition a mystification suited to the Western mind (if we admit this binarism), is also a source of demystification.

What is clear is that the finer issues on which this book touches have ethical complications, many of which involve convolutions of discourse and cultural measure. Much of this has to do with the way things are defined. This is evident on a daily basis with regard to class and race, but there are also the divisions within fashion theory itself. In *The Fashioned Body*, Joanne Entwistle locates what she sees as the two main strands of fashion theory. Although she is not alone, her observation is usefully concise: anthropology, preoccupied with 'dress' and 'adornment' and sociology, concerned with 'fashion' in modern societies. Anthropology is primarily interested in the ethnographic richness of their subject, whereas authors of fashion literature prioritize the so-called fashion system 'which they treat in a historical or theoretical rather than ethnographic or empirical way'.[15] She does allow for the many ways in which the two disciplines interpenetrate. However, it is my contention that with orientalism the two fields are constantly, intricately, vertiginously overlapping. Orientalism and fashion encompasses fabric—*étoffe* in French evokes the sense of material stuff—motifs, accoutrements, hairstyles and makeup, whole styles of clothing down to an overall look, an 'air'—and then we ought not to discount the presence of intangibles such as perfume.

The analysis of textiles and fabrics alone, for which there exists an entire literature, traverses its economic transaction as well as the meanings of the designs upon the woven cloth. Most crucially with orientalism, anthropological characteristics can be used with passing reference to their original meaning, like Ankh earrings, which have been popular since the Napoleonic Empire, or they need not; they need only pass off as Egyptian–oriental, that is, they are just different enough from something identifiably Western (even though the registration of this difference is part of Western fashion—and other forms of discourse). Simplifications of Eastern dress abound. Outside of Iran and Egypt, for instance, it is little known that veiling is a fairly complex affair and is practiced differently by each country.[16] To say it is a mechanism of female subjugation is simplistic and contentious, as Mary Wortley Montagu found— to be discussed in detail in Chapter 2—stepping into the mould at the beginning of the eighteenth century. Her newly found veiled anonymity granted her a freedom in public spaces unknown to her in Europe.

Orientalist fashion has a long lineage of extracting an item of clothing that has experienced very little change over centuries, such as Chinese court dress from the eleventh to fifteenth centuries, and placing it into a milieu of social mobility in which change is imminent and necessary. The former is an anthropological context; the latter is oriented to the fashion system. The ingrown Western prejudice equates change with progress. As Veblen has shown, fashion is inexorably inscribed as the most visible system within this perception of change, in which economic and social superiority are inextricably linked. J. C. Flügel is well known in fashion theory for making the distinction between 'fixed' dress, such as a sari, as opposed to 'modish' dress, which is germane to modern civilization.[17] But how change announces itself is for non-Western countries, such as India or Turkey, a moot point. In their own passages to modernization, their reprising of tradition is often strongly mediated by Western appropriations.

A point of definition needs to be made before going to the first chapter. Up until now I have presumed to use 'East' almost interchangeably with 'the Orient'. Inconveniently, 'West' and 'East' are only loosely geographic. The West of course implies the two imperial nations to the west of Europe—France and Britain—which are the prime focus of this book—and onward to North America. It is also loaded with a bias evinced in Hegel's observation that as culture develops, it moves West. In *The Philosophy of History*, he speaks about a 'determinate East', despite the generality of the spherical globe. The diaphanousness of the idea of the Orient spreads inevitably to its definition. In common French parlance, rife by the end of the eighteenth century, *orientale* has been used to refer to anything that does not denote Western traits or habits. One accepted circumscription, applied by Said, is that of the former Ottoman Empire at its height during the reign (1520–66) of Suleiman the Magnificent, which incorporated North Africa and stretched to Mongolia. But it also encompassed Anatolia, Hungary and southern Spain. They are not the most prominent states within the orientalist's imagination, but they call for some peripheral comment. Africa Japan, most of China or South East Asia, on the other hand, feature strongly as they should, as they are now the most active producers in clothing production and still active in the ongoing recreations of their own image and sartorial identities. As this book progresses, there will be subtle change in the meaning of orient and oriental, which reflects the transition from colonialism to postcolonialism and which is analogous to the change from primitive to 'primitive', for which the use of scare quotes sanitizes the negative undertones of the term. But *orient* and *oriental* are not as pejorative and have quite routine uses—particularly in fashion. So as to minimize caveats and scare quotes, I have remained liberal in my use of the term *orient*. There is more than enough information here to suggest the multilayered and often contradictory use of the term.

−1−

Early Orientalism and the Barbaresque

And say, besides,—that in Aleppo once,
Where a malignant and turban'd Turk
Beat a Venetian and traduc'd the state

—Shakespeare, *Othello* (V: 2)

Hee had a faire companion of his way,
A goodly Lady clad in scarlet red,
Purfled with gold and pearle of rich assay;
And like a Persian mitre on her hed
Shee wore, with crowns and owches garnished,
The which he lavish lovers gave.

—Spenser, *The Faerie Queene* (2: XIII)

The notion of a pre- or early orientalism derives from the presumption, held by the majority of orientalist scholars, that orientalism begins with a deliberate, qualitative and self-conscious separation between cultures. This begins to take shape with the age of exploration in the sixteenth and seventeenth centuries and is well and truly in place by the eighteenth century with Enlightenment ideals of self-determination and national identity. Nourished by free thinkers like Rousseau and Herder, individuals came to believe that they were bound by more than defensiveness to states or by fealty to a local liege, but rather were bound by a series of identifiers of place and belonging with those around them. To share beliefs and a common history with others was therefore more than incidental; it had to do with a shared nature and a common destiny. The Orient is the unspecific frontier to this consciousness, the region beyond the neighbourly realm, where people and their ways are, in a characteristically unqualified fashion, very, very different. The transformations of attitude that amounted to the orient–occident divide are coterminous with industrial and imperial growth as well as with the development of the idea of comfort and luxury, conditions from which oriental fabrics and styles are never far away.

To this web of relationships we must also add the rise of taxonomic science in the more sharply defined natural sciences of anthropology and entomology. With the discovery of new materials and food types came the discovery of new races, with different facial characteristics and unfamiliar customs. By the beginning of the eighteenth century, the Orient becomes more than an-ecdotal discovery and an ever-greater accumulation of facts, albeit facts that are ordered according to a Western credo. Moreover, the age of science was also the age of imperial claim. From the late-sixteenth century, the empirical to the hyperbolic to the apocryphal arrived on domestic shores with a rapidity that, by the eighteenth century, could not meet with demand. Here the basic association of human desire for danger with excitement becomes woven into the very semantics of orientalism, lovingly preserved to this day. Finally, it is only in the eighteenth century that fashion emerges as something resembling a rounded concept that resembles today's fashion system. To be sure, the Orient enjoyed currency as a term well before this, and there had always been talk of what was fashionable or not. Hand in glove with the quickly burgeon-ing principles of individual agency and social mobility—the latter an essen-tial condition under which fashion 'thrives', according to Entwistle[1]—arose a whole new consciousness of competition and image. With this, dress codes were perforce more manipulable, deceptive and persuasive, as opposed to the coercive sumptuary protocols of the seventeenth century. To be seen became an integral part of social intercourse; the sombre austerity of Span-ish fashion was abandoned for newly available motley silks and chintzes of oriental flavour.[2] Through the daily circulation of information generated out of newspapers and their earlier incarnation, the *affiches*, through bona fide journals devoted to fashion, such as the popular *Galerie des modes*, through industrial mass-production and the idea of modern commerce fuelled by the middle classes, we can identify a language of difference, advantage, pres-tige and novelty. It is then that we might begin to speak of 'orientalist fash-ion' as such. This chapter briefly surveys the vast prelude to this period. It maps out salient lines of influence and makes special note of the ways in which Europe and its trading partners, from China to India and the Otto-man Empire, made reciprocal use of one another, in a tangle of adaptation and influence.

The conquests of Alexander the Great (334–335 BC) expanded the possi-bilities for trade. East and West were not yet divided but mutually reliant con-cepts, and cultural fascination was less important than military and economic opportunities. Ancient Greece, which is commonly the divider between the Orient and the West, was in fact deeply indebted to the clothing of the em-pires of Bactria and Gandhara, in which we see an early version of the dhoti, a loincloth known as the *paridhana*. This was commonly covered by a free-flowing expanse of cloth, like a shawl (*uttariya*) or a cloak (*chadar*). From the region that is now India, spreading to Greece and Albania, both sexes would typically wear a large piece of cloth bound around the hips and optionally brought under the legs to resemble pants, much in the manner of a sarong.

Usually very long, it could also be slung over the torso, as it is still done in India to this day. Around the same period, in 325 BC, the Gauls were wearing something akin to breeches, pants with an opening in the front and bound at or above the ankle, which they referred to as a *paison*, a relative of Persian trousers. In this period the Gauls also acquired knowledge of felting, probably from their distant Asian neighbours.

As we know, Byzantine costume, like its culture, was a meeting point of numerous influences. The basic line of court costume was classical, but it was Eastern in its chromatic brilliance. Emperor Justinian himself is known to have worn a combination that brought together the Roman toga with a *trabea*, a scarf crossed at the chest, and a *paragaudion*, a Persian tunic with sleeves embroidered with gold. His belt was dyed the royal purple. When Europe began to be invaded in around the fourth century, Byzantium was a crucial point of trade for unusual and luxury items. Traders from all over Europe travelled there to obtain wares from Africa, the Middle East and Asia. It was indeed thanks to Byzantine trade that Alexandrian and Syrian merchants set up offices in ports north and south of the Mediterranean, thus enabling the easier dissemination of Eastern garments and textiles. Byzantium took liberally from the Huns, as they did the Persians, who themselves had taken from the Assyrians and Medeans. It was Justinian who was responsible for the first known sumptuary laws in textiles, because of his apprehensiveness that too much of his realm's available money went into buying Persian textiles, while the Persians had nothing like the same demand for anything the Byzantines were producing. As a measure to stem the flow, or to choke it, in 540 he proclaimed a ceiling on the prices to be paid for silk, which caused the Persians to retreat en masse in protest. As is often recounted, his courtiers were forced to chafe with coarser underclothes made of linen or wool. The trade block created from Justinian's proscription eventuated in silkworms being smuggled into Byzantium by a group of missionary monks in 552. But neither the price ceiling nor the import of silkworms broke the monopoly; the oriental textile industry and trade continued to flourish, including from Egypt, Chaldea and further east.

LUXURY TEXTILES AND THE BEGINNINGS OF THE SILK TRADE

Just to what extent Justinian was instrumental in the demystification of silk within Europe is debatable, because the fibres of the highest quality still emanated from elsewhere: the Middle East and Cathay. Silks had always been the commodity of choice for the Roman citizenry and aristocracy. Although the earliest dates of trade with Asia and the Middle East are uncertain, they can be traced to as far back as the fourth century BC, when the commerce was predominately with India and Persia. China became part of the arteries of trade when the silk roads became established by the first century AD.

Before the crusades, luxury textiles had already made their entry into the West, mostly brought by pilgrims. But they were still rarities, confined to the wealthy. The enormous amount of travel occasioned by the crusades from the twelfth century onwards made the refinements of Eastern dress more the norm. For instance, Western invaders increasingly wore the tunic, which began to appear in Syria in the second century and which had gained popularity amongst Christians as liturgical vestments. The crusaders were known to have worn tunics with wide sleeves of Arab origin which could be decorated with beads or golden braiding. Luxurious goods included pelisses lined with ermine (known as 'skin of Babylon'), dark marten, squirrel or white fox that was indigenous to the area around the Caspian Sea.

During this time, these fashions were known as barbarian, or *barbaresque*, a word equivalent to the modern epithet 'orientalism' and just as generic. Strikingly akin to the subsequent application of oriental, 'barbarian' referred to anyone of different language and custom. Apprehensions over unfamiliarity made it slide into the pejorative modern usage, usually in opposition to 'Christian'. In describing an Armenian beauty, Nerval comments that her 'clothes, less richly barbarian, recalled rather the contemporary fashions of Constantinople', an unspecified, but by implication a more couth, Christianized form of Eastern dress.[3] While barbarism now refers to uncivilized coarseness, in the realms of dress it was first applied to the defiance of austerity in favour of the novel and the new. The women of the Franks were fond of all manner of barbaresque influence and wore sleeves with a still more exaggerated taper than their male counterparts. They wore long gowns made of silk or diaphanously fine cotton from Mosul ('muslin'), embroidered with gold, as well as Indian cottons and scarves and sashes made of Chinese silk. Cyprus, Syria and Asia Minor were all sources of fustians, fine woollens and silks.

Cotton fibre had been first used in ancient Peruvian textiles and in India, spreading to Europe during the period of trade and conquest of the Roman Empire, although production remained in the East. In the in eleventh and twelfth centuries, Mediterranean trade cotton was used as an all-purpose material: not only for fabric but also for wadding and candlewicks. And although it is true that by the late-twelfth century Sicilian mills had come to dominate Western production of all manner of textiles by weaving textiles approximating the quality that the crusaders had earlier come to expect, perhaps the first textile to be manufactured in the West was *isphanis*, a cloth from Almeria.

Almeria, the city and province of south-east Spain, gets its name from the Andalusian Arabic *Al-Mariyya*, meaning 'the mirror'. Referring to the reflective sea of this part of the Mediterranean, it also conveys the interchangeable nature of what constituted Eastern and Western dress at this time. In southern

Europe, reaching into the southern Germanic principalities, Eastern dress was all but normative. Only the poorest were deprived of textiles originating from the East. By the time the Christians had begun to gain the upper hand in the early-thirteenth century, architecture, dress and decorative arts reflected profound Moorish influence. After the Christians defeated the Moors in 1212 at Las Navas de Tolosa, no effort was made to adopt different customs other than those relating to religion. The Moorish style remained constant until well into the fifteenth century, when it was deemed the height of lavishness in dress. When Granada fell in 1492, Ferdinand and Isabella accepted its surrender clad in full Moorish dress. (Henceforth a Christian city, Muslims were allowed to practice their faith unmolested.) Silk in Spain continued to be produced in handsome qualities from the mills originally established by the Moors and evolved to be the outward sign of grandeur, distinction and prosperity.

It was relatively early when oriental motifs were subjected to Western imitation and slight alteration, again blurring the line between what was oriental and what was not. Production in Italy had helped to disseminate the popular floral curvilinear, 'arabesque' designs on both church and courtly dress by widening the repertoire of their oriental originals. Wavy tendrils and floral clusters became larger and bolder and were accompanied by thistles and fruits like pomegranates and berries, presaging the liberties taken with chintz wallpaper in the eighteenth century and beyond. Velvets and silks were embroidered and embossed with such designs in a way that showed that an open licence had been taken with the oriental idiom.

Justinian's uneasiness over the economic consequences of the Western thirst for Eastern goods, particularly for fabrics, was echoed by countless others well into the Middle Ages, despite European cities having developed their own means of weaving clothing of comparable quality. Comparable but not equal—as early as the thirteenth century the Orient continued to exercise a spell over the West as the font of worldly goods of highest quality and sensuous magnificence. When it came to ceremonial garb for princes and those in high ecclesiastical office, oriental fabrics were de rigueur. Such fabrics were not limited to hats, capes, chasubles and surplices but were also used for ceremonial heraldic standards and for mitres and altar cloths. Although most examples of orientalist textiles have disappeared or deteriorated, examples of embroidery showing a Chinese-influenced fret pattern exist from the 1300s, and a painting of St Ursula by the Cologne Master shows her in a dress decorated with phoenixes in the Chinese style.[4]

'Chinese style' is a curious generalization which, like all assumed notional terms, ought not to be taken for granted, especially when surveyed from the vantage point of the difference between cultural reality and cultural influence. Both are subjective, but 'cultural reality' in the present sense refers to indigenous and endogenous perceptions of a given culture as opposed to how that culture is used as a feature, or specimen. In the latter case the culture is taken up in material signs in a near talismanic way, in which extracted signs— Chinese dragons, multilimbed Indian gods, turbaned men—are saturated with significance so as to embody a particular condition.

It was relatively early when oriental motifs were subjected to Western imitation and slight alteration, again blurring the line between what was oriental and what was not. Production in Italy had helped to disseminate the popular floral curvilinear, 'arabesque' designs on both church and courtly dress by widening the repertoire of their oriental originals. Wavy tendrils and floral clusters became larger and bolder and were accompanied by thistles and fruits like pomegranates and berries, presaging the liberties taken with chintz wallpaper in the eighteenth century and beyond. Velvets and silks were embroidered and embossed with such designs in a way that showed that an open licence had been taken with the oriental idiom.

As Antonia Finnane observes about Chinese clothing, European observers of Chinese clothing from the sixteenth to as late as the nineteenth century are relatively free of an exacting interest in the shape and cut of the garments themselves, that is to say the specifics of Chinese clothing. The emphasis was on overall differences and 'more specifically the repository of ways they had of describing what they saw'.[5] Before the modern period of eighteenth century, European and Chinese dress were similar, since clothing was largely draped, but by the time of William Alexander's illustrative publication of *The Costume of China* in 1805, the differences were pronounced. The Manchurian period in China that began in the middle of the seventeenth century made numerous distinctions of class and status, which included a dress code for the underclass, such as the servants. Why European observers were reluctant to examine Chinese clothing as something unto itself has much to do with the self-conscious nature of the observer who was ultimately tied in some way to a travelogue. As so many cultural commentators before and after Said have been apt to show, such accounts are invariably an arbitrary arrangement of peculiarities and generalities to be synthesized into a compelling narrative that would ultimately find a wide and profitable readership back home. The relics they brought back with them were typically the most evocative objects, most suggestive of what was most extraordinary—early forms of its mass-marketed cultural debasement, the souvenir, where extraordinary courts a fine line with banal and in which clothing plays a large and significant part. Indeed, the souvenirs of today are a graphic way of thinking of orientalist fashion in its most extreme sense. After all, locals seldom wear their own souvenirs.

While certain loose and inaccurate assumptions of the Orient took hold in Europeans' imagination of these fashions, this orientalism was very different from the orientalism that evolved in the seventeenth and eighteenth centuries. It was an orientalism in which the financial interests of the Western empires and the fictitious resonances of the Orient prevailed in equal measure. What is consistent, however, is the extent to which the Orient inspired envy and exuded an air of hedonism, comparable to the emotions that a city like Paris inspires to the contemporary mind.

VENICE

Since at least the ninth century, Italy prospered as a secondary producer of silk textiles, thanks to Arab, Greek and Jewish artisans, and was central to the economies of its northern cities, which communicated constantly through trade and war with the Holy Roman Empire, which was the buffer zone between East and West. While cities such as Bologna, Lucca and Milan became known for the cheaper *sendal*, a light silk cloth, Venice was not only the major port but by the fifteenth century became both Persia and China's greatest rival in silk production. In the eleventh century, Venice evolved to become a central nexus between East and West through its policy of putting its naval fleet at the disposal of the highest bidder. It thereby became a market city and an expanding point of trade. It was the best place to obtain sundry luxury goods such as spices and gems, and above all, silks and other valuable textiles. Such commerce helped to establish it as among the richest and most powerful cities in the world. The Venetians were willing travellers, and by the fifteenth century their grasp of the Eastern world was unmatched by any other region in Europe, best reflected in not only textiles but also carpets—and represented by the Bellini family, sired by Jacopo, the first great Western orientalist painter. Venice was an exciting and motley hub of commercial activity, where representatives of the various Italian states rubbed shoulders with just about every state in Europe, especially the traders: Flanders, France and England.

Venice got its silks from the Caspian region of Asia Minor such as Ghilan and Azerbaijan, which were sold in Constantinople. After Constantinople fell to the Turks in 1453, the markets shifted to the Damascus, Aleppo, Tripoli and Beirut, until they finally converged on Aleppo, Syria's second largest city, until the end of the seventeenth century. When Turkey came to occupy large tracts of Eastern Europe, this interval of over two and half centuries was marred by repeated territorial conflicts. The battle of Lepanto in 1571 slowed the Turkish advance before they were finally defeated in 1686. Earlier, with its defeat in 1538 at the Battle of Preveza, Venice had been forced to hand over naval dominance to Turkey. With its naval power on the wane, Venice's survival as a trade hub depended to a large part on the level of its finished goods: soap, paper cut gems, blown glass and, of course, woven silk, whose quality by the sixteenth century had well exceeded that of its Ottoman neighbour. In his article on Venetian–Ottoman diplomacy and trade during this period, Julian Raby notes that although Venice may have been unsuccessful in scoring a monopoly of the Ottoman market, Venetian artisans were kept enormously busy satisfying their demands. Designs were alternately European or Ottoman, with drawings often sent to accompany orders. A salient example of this cross-fertilization are the velvet kaftans in the Topkapi Palace, which, although long considered a paragon of Turkish weaving are, with the exception of three, wrought by Italian hands.[6] In fifteenth-century Turkey and Persia, Venetian velvet was an exceptionally coveted commodity.

While there is no surviving evidence of Venetian imitations of oriental carpets, carpets imported mainly from Anatolia had a large influence on Venitian textile designs. To cast one's eyes over paintings by such as Carpaccio, Crivelli and Mansueti is to see the extent to which carpets were central to Venetian life, draped over balconies, placed over tables, adorning floors. Venice was also the supplier to the rest of Europe, servicing who was perhaps the first European carpet collector, cardinal Wolsey, first minister to Henry VIII (records of his personal effects contain over 400 entries of carpets of 'Turkey making').[7] Elizabeth I appears to have had a lesser concern for such exotica until it was revived by James I, as attested to in several portraits of him.

Collecting precious textiles continued to be desultory and dwindled off by the beginning of the seventeenth century until a mutual interest was struck between Siam (now Thailand) and France, who hosted their visit in 1686. In fact, Siam placed orders from the carpet factories from the Savonnerie, which, as Louis XIII had ordained, would make rugs 'in the Turkish style'. By this time there was a relatively long but uneven history of Europeans replicating Islamic carpets, which can be traced as far back as the twelfth century, when the Arab geographer al-Idrisi reported that woollen carpets were being made in Chinchilla and Murcia in Spain and exported widely. Moreover, in John Sweetman's words, the

> tapis Sarrasinois was known in the France of Louis IX and in 1277 there were trade privileges for it in Paris. In the fourteenth century woven Islamic hangings were prized in Arras. Silks too were by then a precious part of church treasuries: a cope from Mamluk Egypt inscribed in Arabic with the words 'the learned Sultan' was in St Mary's church, Danzig, early in the same century.[8]

Typically, Venetian merchants obtained their raw silk through bartering the bolts of silk and wool that they had woven, including ribbed cloth, in the manner of the English kersey. The bulk of the silk either came overland from Bursa, Turkey's former capital, or later from Syria. By sea it came across the Caspian from Mazandran, Shirvan, Karabagh and mostly Gilan, in north Persia. By the early-seventeenth century this trade route became ubiquitous, supplying around 2,200 bales, or the equivalent of almost a quarter of a million kilogrammes.[9] By the end of the century, owing to the pressures exerted by the Nine Years' War, silk was exported more through Russia. As Edmund Herzig finds, in his essay on the Iranian silk industry during this period, by the eighteenth century, Persia (Iran) had far superseded China as the primary supplier of silk to Europe, making silk the mainstay of its export economy. The overall erratic patterns of trade by the end of the eighteenth century owed themselves to the unreliability of quality and supply; the Levant company was supplied by Armenian intermediaries infamous for diluting high-grade batches. It was not until the nineteenth century, with the introduction of mechanized reeling, that Iran regained some of its footing as an international supplier.[10] In the intervening period, Venice's own production was centred on reliable routes of supply, which resulted in more limited production that gave primacy to Venetian craftsmanship.

Thus, at the close of sixteenth century, when competition from Italian and French cities such as Genoa and Lyon began to mount, Venice concentrated on the quality of its production over the cheaper, lighter and less expensively dyed counterparts. In Syria in the late-fifteenth century, Venetian silk was among the most costly and most prized. The water- and pedal-powered looms across a steadily industrializing Europe resulted in the export of cloth of middling grade to the Middle East in a volume with which a small state like Venice could scarcely compete. Nonetheless, until the seventeenth century it remained the main port where one could obtain quality textiles from all over the known world.

What the history of the Venetian economy during this period tells us is just how closely enmeshed the Eastern and Western markets were. Venice not only obtained much of its silk from the East but reinterpreted Eastern designs for themselves which they sold back to their Eastern suppliers, a back-and-forth movement of trade and reconfiguration that would persist to various degrees until the couture of today. The Venetian velvets and dyes inspired Anatolian carpet weavers, while in Venice, since the fourteenth century, Ottoman silks were used in furnishing fabrics and sacred vestments, although seldom for secular clothing. It has been argued that the supreme popularity of Venetian luxury fabrics in the first half of the sixteenth century led to the growth of the Ottoman's reinventing of their own specialist textile industry, eventuating in what are deemed among the highest achievements of Ottoman decorative art of the period.[11] At this time the Grand Vizier Rüstem Pasha sought to reinvigorate Ottoman industry with a similar kind of protectionist policy that, as we shall shortly see, was instrumented by Louis XIV's resourceful chief minister, Colbert. Colbert wanted to address the ever-mounting dependence of the Ottoman economy on the Venetian market and to stimulate internal growth by exporting to local neighbours like Russia. He did not wholly get his wish, largely because of Venice's capacity to adapt to market need. Although the Ottomans modified their textiles in response to the Venetian designs, these changes cannot be called innovations as such; the Ottomans' preference for thick damasks remained consistent for several centuries, a symptom of what Carlo Poni suggests was the 'unchangeability of Oriental fashions and ways of dressing'.[12]

Other evidence contradicts this view however. As Raby shows, the costume albums which were a common medium for circulating fashions in Europe until the nineteenth century were, in their early incarnations in the in the sixteenth century, popular amongst both Ottomans and the Venetians. Many of the editions produced for Europeans were the work of Ottoman artists, with notable exceptions such as the celebrated work in 1590 by Cesare Vecellio, *Habiti antichi et moderni di tutto il mondo*, which nonetheless had a an entire chapter devoted to Turkish dress. By contrast, the Ottoman interest in European dress was peripheral. Raby explains that while the Europeans were already designating their special 'other', in the sixteenth century the Ottoman Empire was so vast as to look into many directions for points of reference. It was a time of prosperity in which the Ottoman Empire was receptive to myriad influences that might bolster its own interests.[13] The cliché of an intractably closed East is best reserved for a conquered Ottoman Empire. In turn, the East used anachronism as a virtue in counterpoint to Western progress, which was painted in the same colours as wanton opportunism and decadence.

TEXTILES IN WESTERN EUROPE

While the lighter and more expediently produced Dutch and French fabrics made only a limited mark on Eastern tastes, their production expanded dramatically and by the mid-sixteenth century began to dominate all but high-end production. The string of Ottoman conquests and its assertion of power until the beginning of the seventeenth century, as well as the domestic embargoes and ambivalences of trade over centuries, made domestic autonomy in textile production and other luxury goods more exigent for Europeans. By the mid-1500s Lyon was recognized as one of the world's leading textile producers, albeit on a level of quality and consistency unequal to Venice. By this time the market had become more diverse and consumers more literate in the variety of textiles available, creating a more fragmented economy in which a broader range of producers and consumers could operate. Lyon certainly had a major hand in this. The kind of threat it posed to the more artisanal Venetian silk weaving is commensurate to the difference today in both perception and truth between garments produced in Italy and those in China. The analogy is not at all throwaway, as *fabricants* of Lyon were summarily ruthless in bringing down prices by mixing first-choice silk with silks of lower grades to enlarge profits and the number of prospective buyers. Such practices had been forbidden, but the opprobrium was soon drowned out by volume and demand.[14]

The swathe of land from Flanders to Lyon belonging to the Dukes of Burgundy—a region not only contested militarily but attracting merchants and workers from all over Europe—was one of the most prosperous regions of secondary and tertiary fabric production by the fifteenth and sixteenth centuries. In the middle of the sixteenth century, as a producer of silk and fustian, Lyon employed over twelve thousand workers. Other cities in the region, such as Orléans, Tours, Nimes, Dourdan and Montpelier, also enjoyed growth and an influx of wealth—so much so that a series of new ordinances in 1540 and 1572 forbade the export of raw textiles and, conversely, the import of other stuffs like broadcloths, linens and taffetas. Turkish and Syrian markets suffered from these measures, as did Italy. In the early-seventeenth century the French wealth from its American colonies allowed it to pay in precious metals for silks from Aleppo, which almost brought Venice, reliant more on barter than currency, to its knees.

Furnished by both Eastern and local markets, the loom became one of the symbols of French economic power. Textile production would have grown into an institution rather than an association had not Louis XIV in 1685 revoked the Edict of Nantes, sending thousands of skilled labourers, manufacturers and traders, the bulk of whom were Calvinists, into persecution and exile. Burgundy was crushingly debilitated as a result. In Beaune, for instance, the exodus of a sizeable number of its 2,000 employees occupied in making broadcloth shut down the industry almost overnight. For clothing and textiles, this bleeding of skilled labour would represent a massive shift in power for the textile industry in Europe and the Ottoman Empire. It also had the inevitable side effect of making France temporarily more popular with its Ottoman and Chinese trade partners, on whom they suddenly became more reliant, albeit to the detriment of the already-ailing treasury.

COTTON AND CHINTZ

Cotton textiles are something of a national industry in India, which, like China, can be dated back to around 3000 BC. By the sixteenth century it was the industry on which India depended, connecting it not only to Africa and the Middle East but also to Indonesia and Japan. It was a market economy that brought the products of small hinterland villages to busy distributions centres such as Amsterdam and London via trade epicentres such as Ahmedabad, Surat, Lahore and Agra. Before the establishment of the East India Companies at the beginning of the seventeenth century, trade was a complex series of markets from which it is impossible to separate the Portuguese, Spanish, French and English from those within Asia itself.

An historical turning point occurred in England in 1592 when an English privateer vessel captured the Portuguese *Madre de Dio* which was carrying a large cargo of Indian cotton, a plunder that met with a jubilant English home reception. Indian cotton is also thought to have entered France through Portugal, this time less coercively, and sold in the Foire Saint-Germain from 1630. Colbert set up France's answer to the Dutch and English East India Companies, namely the *Compagnie des Indes* in 1664. Although of far more mixed fortunes than its counterparts, cotton was more than just a conversation piece. The diversity of its incarnations and uses called for a lengthening litany of words named descriptively after their salient qualities or where they were from: *toile peinte, indiennes, chites, surates,* and *patnas.* In 1683 the demand for cotton was enough to warrant India making products expressly for its European markets.[15]

For many ports, such as in Java and Malaysia, Indian cotton represented the primary currency for obtaining spices, foodstuffs and other local specialties. By the time bolts of cotton had arrived at their destinations in Turkey and Europe they had passed hands several times, especially when travelling overland. Yet this was a practice that involved risk and incurred cost, incremental with each middleman, making naval trade more attractive. With the discovery of the cape route, the Portuguese became the first Europeans to trade with Asia, yielding healthy profits owing to low costs and high demand. Sea trade courted its own risks, since pirating was a clandestine industry unto itself. Overland trade never dwindled; in the mid-seventeenth century it was still India's principal export conduit.

While the East would always be the source of curiosities, cotton was the basis of its trade. 'Cottons were central to the world: they formed long-distance commercial relationships across the Indian Ocean'. Giorgio Riello and Tirthankar Roy make the startling claim that 'Cotton textiles were perhaps the most global among the various manufactured and non-manufactured commodities entering long-distance trade in the period between 1500 and 1800'.[16] And as K. N. Chaudhuri observes, textile commerce along the various trade routes ought not only to be seen along economic lines, but also represented a veritable 'transmission of culture' whose enormity of scale is incalculable.[17] Europeans were justifiably intrigued by the variety of cottons and what they had to offer, especially with respect to the intricate designs they could hold. Indian cottons were always in demand. By the 1600s England had become alert to the fact that cottons were the material of choice in the African slave trade.[18] The amount of cottons at every level of quality changing hands over vast distances was phenomenal and impossible to gauge. One thing is certain: cotton was the sine qua non of commerce in the early-modern world, carving out lucrative trade routes and centres, facilitating the circulation of information and countless other objects and substances, particularly spices, which were the most lucrative commodities in proportion to mass. While countries such as Portugal traded actively in textiles throughout India and South East Asia, it was the way that the English harnessed the Indian textile trade to its economy that would have untold historical consequences.

The devastation of the French fleet at Gibraltar in 1704 left the country permanently crippled and, perhaps more than the destruction of the Spanish Armada in 1588, is a significant turning point for the British imperial domination of the seas, both military and mercantile. While still in bitter competition with Portugal, Spain, Holland, Sweden, Denmark and France, the British East India Companies that evolved out of the sixteenth century were to become a specific financial bulwark for the growth of its Imperial Empire. England would prove merciless in its dealings with its colonies, especially when its own technology eclipsed its colonial suppliers. Indian and English weaving industries would continue to go from crisis to crisis until, in the space of fifty years, from around 1760 to 1810, the balance of power in textile production had shifted, alarmingly for India, toward Britain.

It was a shift that had to be strategically put in motion by the industrial powers of Europe, lest they become restricted by the vicissitudes of outside markets, which they had already observed in the supply of silk. But with cotton, the volume and stakes were considerably higher. Indian chintzes had entered myriad forms of European life: wall hangings, curtains, bedding and of course clothing. It was simply too much a perceived necessity of life for it to be spirited away with an edict. In France Indian cottons were so plentiful and popular that that on 26 October 1686 the controller-general of finance, Lepeletier, took measures to prohibit further Indian fabrics from entering the country. This freeze also extended to the French printers themselves, the tertiary stage of the industry, who were ordered to destroy all their printing blocks. A little more than a year later all printed and painted cottons, irrespective of origin, were banned. These laws were enforced by yet another in 1692. Yet for all the severity of these new laws, such fabrics kept entering the country: the *Compagnie des Indes* kept unloading cargo, and local artisans kept printing. Unfortunately these restrictions were promulgated at the same time as the revocation of the Edict of Nantes, which, as already mentioned, gave good reason for skilled labourers to flee the country. A beneficiary of the exodus was England, which had begun printing its own cotton by the 1670s and notably in 1690 in Richmond, thanks to an exiled Frenchman called Cabannes. Despite inhibiting this fertile tertiary industry, demand within France for decorative cottons continued unabated. A citable instance is when, in the eighteenth century, Mme de Pompadour decorated the Chateau Bellevue with the best *indiennes* to be found.[19]

England, which had lapped up much of France's skilled labour in the textile industry, was not without its own complications, however. The fortunes of English manufacturing were somewhat reversed by the mounting influx of goods from the East India Company, which in 1685 precipitated the near collapse of the wool weaving industry. As we have seen, English artisans instructed Indian craftsmen in oriental designs that suited European expectations of what the Orient was, or should be. The craze for the lighter, more diaphanous, freer muslins and cottons continued to spread, entering into all facets of everyday life. As Joyce Appleby in her book on the economy of England during this period shows, the free trade in bullion after 1663 allowed the East India Company to expand, so that by 1680 the annual export figure reached half a million pounds. 'What had begun as the inconspicuous use of cotton for suit lining grew rapidly into a pervasive display of printed draperies, bedspreads, tapestries, shirts and dresses.'[20] In short, every quarter of society became affected. Speaking at the end of the seventeenth century, John Pollexfen affirmed that this thirst for the 'Fabricks of India' cut all boundaries, from 'the greatest Gallants to the meanest Cook-Maids'.[21] So entrenched had the rage for foreign fibres become that clothiers blamed the influx of Bengal silks for bringing the English silk industry to heel. The wool industry was also critically debilitated by this trend: England's rising interest in cotton led to dwindling imports of German linen, which in turn left Germany in a weaker position to import English wool.[22] The more venerable textiles did not stand a chance. The Indian cottons were cheaper, looked better, by and large felt better, and, to boot, were infused with exotic novelty.

It is an important point for postcolonial theorists that the beginning of travel discourse about India (itself soldered from a number of kingdoms as a result of colonization)—notably that of the early-seventeenth century adventurers Thomas Roe and Thomas Coryaote, whose accounts are frequently cited in such studies—enframed the travellers' adventures as discoveries which would soon evolve into civilizing missions, Kipling's 'white man's burden'. Simply on the face of it, the national psychological consequences of the idea that the West, in this case, Britain, 'discovered' India, lands the centre of consciousness squarely in the discoverer's camp. The seer–seen dichotomy allows the East to be open to the need for Western conception, for it to be the object of thought. As Jyotsna Singh succinctly puts it, 'English endeavours to open trade routes for commercial profit were recorded as narratives of wonder and discovery in which "India/Indies" emerges through the prism of the exotic and barbaric'.[23] As we will see in the next chapter, these terms will shift slightly in the eighteenth century once England's foot was firmly planted within the Indian states.

The English period of Indian colonization is a tangled mesh of exchanges that are all too easily oversimplified in terms of imperialist dictatorship. Not only did Britain and other European powers vie to supersede their oriental counterparts in textiles and design, but the period from 1600 onwards was the beginning of a confusing oscillation of influences, especially in the way that orientalism was remade within Europe for Europeans, followed by the redigestion of these refashionings by the Orient, either out of competition or through a hankering for what they perceived was superior prosperity. This prosperity, more precisely named industrialization, had allowed for the Orient to be produced, replicated and distributed in styles, fabrics and items (fans for example) at a rate with which the Orient itself could not easily compete. As Joseph Inikori indicates, between approximately 1750 and 1820, India was still an able competitor with England in exporting cotton to West Africa. But by the 1840s, English exports outmarched India more than twentyfold.[24] Other research has shown that during the same period English exports flowed into China in amounts that local producers could not curtail, with acute effects on Chinese textiles until the early-twentieth century.[25] Against such pressure, the competitive rallying point for the Orient was quality, which became married to less measurable notions of authenticity and origin. Curiously enough, since the late-twentieth century these fortunes have reversed, with fashion producers such as Italy and France using the cachet of quality as the only way to compete against the productive might of India and China.

The tergiversations of oriental styles were already becoming felt in mid-seventeenth-century England where Indian chintz had to be modified to suit popular taste. Although this is a somewhat trivial upheaval in the annals of textiles, it does isolate not only the displacement of authenticity within orientalist fashion but also the basic divisions within Indian textile production that eventually calcified into stereotypes. In 1643 the directors of the East India Company returned to their Indian suppliers with the wish that the patterns be placed on a white ground rather than a coloured one. White cotton had always been the default for European cotton. It could not fade and denoted status for those fortunate enough to keep it clean. While white chadors and their equivalents can be found all over the non-Western world, neither Middle Eastern nor Asian clothing was organized along the lines of a coat and a (white) undershirt that was vestigially visible around the collar and the sleeves. Other than those cases being dictated by religion—turmeric (more auspiciously called after its rarer chromatic counterpart, saffron) tinted robes, for example—India had no such default, and its craftsmen were freer to experiment with colour. To this day, the West holds to the perception of the Orient as a place where the colours are as vibrant as the passions are unbridled.

It took some time to convince the Indian dyers and printers that patterns on a white ground were more vivid. To many an Indian mind this was a denigration of a vibrant tradition that impelled them to relinquish a craft that had taken centuries to cultivate, their mordants and resists used for fixing dyes

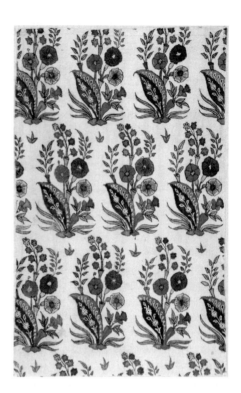

Figure 2   Seventeenth-century Indian textile, © V&A Images; Victoria and Albert Museum, London.

being far more advanced than those used in Europe. It transpired that the English also preferred their own patterns. These consisted of not only Tudor roses but also florals in an entirely arbitrary, invented 'China fashion'. But of course, the Indian textile craftsmen, accustomed to their own visual vocabulary, inflected this already highly eccentric style with their own. Heaping irony upon irony, this Indian adaptation of Chinese style became popular with the Chinese, who by the eighteenth century began producing fabrics with the hybridized Tree of Life of Indian provenance. English embroiderers responded to this Chinese/Indian style with particular relish. Charles II's household was filled with counterpanes and curtains replete with Oriental silks, dense with fine stitching, French knots and Peking knots. In Dawn Jacobson's words,

> Jacobean embroiderers took the Indian Tree of Life pattern—where a single asymmetrical tree rises from a hummocky ground and twists its way up the fabric—and made it their own, working their design in crewel wools in strong blues, greens and browns in imitation of the printed cotton brought from the Masulipatnam by the East India Company.[26]

Hence the phrase 'Indian chintz' I used earlier is not really a tautology, and it can refer both to chintz from India and chintz in the Indian style. These are conundrums arising from a history with more than one double helix. 'There can have been few more bizarre incidents in the whole of taste' comments Hugh Honour.[27] But perhaps not: The same imbrication of styles are to be seen in the tapestries woven for Elihu Yale (whence the great university) while serving as Governor of Madras (1687–92), which are noted to be in the 'Indian manner'. Yet a Dutch weaver, Van der Bank, made them and the visual details have nothing Islamic about them. Rather the trabeated buildings, fishermen and quaint blossoming trees are far more Chinese in character.[28] And as we shall see, such unrepentant confusions and liberalities taken with culture and style were but a harbinger for what was to occur in the English and Scottish textile industry in the nineteenth century and became a regular occurrence from the beginning of the twentieth century onward.

CHARLES II AND THE ORIGINS OF THE VEST

The notable 'invention' in menswear in the 1600s came from Louis XIV's cousin, Charles II, who adopted—officiated—the 'Persian vest', which had been introduced to England by visitors such as Sir Robert Sherley, who had been British ambassador to the court of Shah Abbas. In the words of John Evelyn writing in 1666, it was 'usually associated with eastern garments, and therefore presumably improper attire for a Christian gentlemen'. According to Evelyn, it was 'the first time his Majesty put himself solemnly into the Eastern fashion of vest, changing doublet, stiff collar, bands and cloak, into a comely dress after the Persian mode, with girdles or straps, and shoestrings and garters into buckles . . . resolving never to alter it, and to leave the French mode'.[29] Supplanting French fashion dominance was something Charles had long wished for, but with a struggling treasury, his ambitions proved vain. (Charles had also toyed with the banyan, the forerunner to the dressing gown, to be discussed in the following chapter.)

'Invention' here, of course, means a trend activated through a sanction resembling a regal fiat. Charles did not so much walk in with the garment as proclaim its admission into courtly life, as Samuel Pepys transcribes in his journal on 8 October 1666: 'The King hath yesterday in Council declared his resolution of setting a new fashion for clothes . . . It will be the vest, I know not well how; but it is to teach the nobility thrift, and will do good.'[30] A week later Charles paraded it to the court. Pepys reports that it was 'a long cassoke close to the body, of black cloth, and pinked with white silk under it . . . it is a very fine and handsome garment'.[31] A year later, Chamberlayne's *Angliae Notitia* observes Charles' gesture of departure from 'the French Mode' in favour of clothing 'according to the Oriental Nations'.[32] But as Esmond de Beer argues, although the vest may have been different from anything worn at the time, the Persian association only comes from Evelyn, who himself had garnered such knowledge from his travels in Bologna and Venice.[33] In 1662 Evelyn also notes evidence of 'Vests of several Colours, & with buskins after the Eastern manner' amongst the retinue of the Russian ambassador, and something similar in 1664 with a private exhibition of Chinese and Japanese garments.[34] Two years later, Evelyn comments on the lush embroideries that had arrived to London from China and the 'glorious vests wrought and embroidered on cloth of gold, but with such lively colours that for splendour and vividness we have nothing in Europe that approaches it . . . flowers, trees, beasts, birds, wrought in a kind of sleeve silk, very natural'.[35]

Well might the notation of naturalness and the East been rife by the second half of the seventeenth century, but the vest itself had already been enjoying popularity, having been adopted by the many English travellers to the East. The artisan Thomas Dallam, in his journey to Istanbul, noted this in 1599, when he joined the English ambassadorial party's parade at the Topkapi palace. Accompanying the ambassador's retinue were six merchants: 'these did ride in vestes of cloth of goulde, made after the cuntrie fation; thare went on foute 28 more in blew gounes made after the Turkie fation'.[36] Vest or no vest, more striking sallies into Eastern dress could be found in the figure of Sir Robert Sherley, a diplomatic envoy who encouraged Anglo–Persian trade in 1611–13 and 1624–7 and who was immortalized wearing flamboyant Turkish dress, including a large turban, in 1622 in a portrait by Antony van Dyck. Figure 3 is a drawing in preparation for the famous, flamboyant portrait.

Isolated precedents notwithstanding, it seems that Charles' hybrid of rural vernacular clothing and exoticism had a strategic purpose. It was a reform of sorts, as Evelyn states, in response to the perceptions of licentiousness which many believed incited God's wrath in the form of the Great Fire of 1665–6, hence Pepys' remark about teaching thrift.[37] But of course, as we now know, from this pretense at prurience grew the best excuse in men's fashion for the next two hundred years to show off sumptuous embroideries and colours, usually of the most opulently oriental kind. Tailors and needle-workers on both sides of the channel quickly emulated these new fantasies. Such motifs and the taste for 'bizarre silks', even if designed and made in Europe, still 'belonged' to the East—the presumption that they came from a place far away was doubtless part of their cachet, as it is now. After the French Revolution, when fashions reacted severely to aristocratic excesses, the vest stopped at the waist and so the waistcoat was born.

Charles' new fashion only lasted until about 1672, when reports have him returning to the French style. This reversion is attributed in part to the Treaty of Dover, which renewed English sympathies for the French and gave the English licence to follow Continental fashions more freely. During the same period,

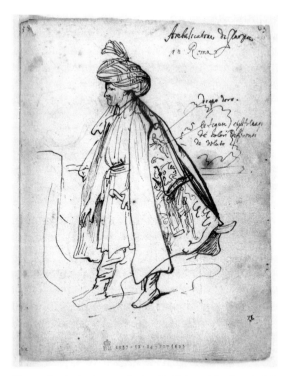

Figure 3 Anthony van Dyck, *Sir Robert Sherley*, 1622, drawing, © Trustees of the British Museum.

Parisian fashions were themselves undergoing change. Men were beginning to be fitted with a tighter-fitting knee-length coat, the *justaucorps*, which, when worn unbuttoned, would reveal the waistcoat underneath. Other evidence also suggests that vests started being worn in Paris at roughly the same time as Charles made his grand entry.[38]

Charles's efforts, however, show his acute awareness of the power that his cousin had to control people's stations through what they were allowed to wear and his ability to change what they looked like overnight. For example Louis is credited with bringing in stockings to show off his beautiful dancing legs. Boots were henceforth consigned to the muddy pursuits of hunting and war. Before they were supplanted by those made at home, stockings were first imported from China and painted with sumptuous and charming patterns and motifs. It was part of Louis's genius as a ruler that he would call on tradition in equal measure with innovations. The efforts of Charles notwithstanding, it was Louis who was the inventor of the culture of luxury in Europe and sharpened the notion of absolutism for his present age with ideas about despotism. Both ideas had strong associations with the Orient, thus unequivocally an essential component of his personal equation. As Ina McCabe observes, 'Like the Persian king or the Ottoman sultan who gave ceremonial robes (*khalat*) to worthy ambassadors and courtiers, Louis bestowed a brocade vest to male courtiers as a mark of privilege; only those bestowed the vest could be in his presence'.[39] Orientalism, redolent of absolute authority and control, was used to uphold the establishment. It is ironic to think that a century and half later, oriental references on vests and other garments would be used to signify, by degrees, opposition to it.

CHINOISERIE AND ORIENTALISM IN LOUIS XIV'S FRANCE

Chinoiserie, as we call it today, began its popular ascent in France under Louis's former mentor, Mazarin (inventories from his estate cite two pieces of serge made in Paris *en façon de Chine*),[40] and especially through the lavish use of faience tiles of blue and white Chinese flavour on which Delft in Holland had built its economy. His chief architect, Louis Le Vau, introduced it architecturally into Versailles in 1669 in the form of a small pavilion that was to serve as a retreat for the king and his mistress, Mme de Montespan. Although the Palais de Flore retained its classical idioms, Vau made sure to incorporate a sufficient amount details to make its oriental associations clear: the roof was covered in porcelain tiles and decorated with china urns and birds, rendering it reminiscent from a distance of a Nankin temple.

Historically speaking, the origins of the West's love affair with dressing up in oriental regalia are a desultory, untrackable affair. Despite having no definite beginning, what is evident is that, aside from the adoption of non-Western clothing because of habit orexchange, or just because it was better—the normal process of social acclimatization and improvement—there was more than a single set of power relations that underpinned this tendency. As we have already seen, Said and his epigones treat the adoption of orientalist modalities (to use that word, since dress itself is not much mentioned) as an expression of Western dominance, its ability to choose and manipulate signs of difference to stimulate and enforce the internal illusion it had of itself. But this is an Enlightenment idea and more tenable in the nineteenth century, during the heyday of British and French imperialism. One of the factors that allowed imperialism to flourish was the collapse of the Moorish threat, which was brought about by the late-seventeenth century. Up until then, the Ottoman Empire was held up by many princes and monarchs of Europe, most notably Louis XIV, as the paragon of absolute rule, whose tyranny was meritorious based on its perceived social stability. (Similar misprisions occur in Jean-Paul Sartre's defense of Mao three centuries later.)

With this in mind, in the seventeenth century, when the French and other Europeans dressed in 'the Turkish style', it took on a different meaning than it would a century later. As Michael Curtis argues in his book *Orientalism and Islam*, the West's view of the East prior to the eighteenth century had a different order of ambivalence than it would have in the centuries to follow, since it was equated with authority and power.[41] Montesquieu's *Lettres Persanes* were influential in bringing the image of the Orient as a place of ruthless despotism, but also of unquestioned sovereignty, something to which Louis was keenly aligned.[42] Drawing from this view, it could easily be suggested that to dress up *à l'orientale* was a way of not only ascribing to the perception of power but also defusing it, in the sense common to parody. Since the Orient was remote and obscure to most people, it was a convenient, and malleable symbol of an external threat, easy to emulate and easy to pervert.

The grasp of the Orient may still have been naïve, but this should not rule out pursuits aimed at truth and rigour. Oriental styling in which China, Turkey and Persia were abridged and anthologized came together with more rigorous pursuits of the French (and English) to get to know their non-Western neighbours. It is well known that Chinese philosophy enters into the considerations of Malebranche and Leibniz, but less well known is the extent of the infiltration of Indian, Ottoman and Chinese literature into the mainstream. Most notably, Antoine Galland's translation of the *Thousand and One Nights*, completed toward the end of Louis's reign, had an inestimable effect in sparking the contemporary imagination. No text, according to Nicholas Dew, had the same effect on its period.[43] It not only helped to underpin the nascent discipline of 'oriental studies' in what burgeoned into the discourses of anthropology and philology, but on a purely aesthetic level it provided the narrative pretext for masquerade.

Courtly masquerade probably begins with Louis's authoritarian predecessor, François I who, to unnerve his rival, the titular Holy Roman Emperor Charles V, sought an alliance with Suleiman the Magnificent. To celebrate the occasion in 1552, the Turkish ambassador paraded the Louvre in a golden gown followed by scarlet-clad attendants. That evening festivities saw the ladies of the court and Knights of Malta all donning costumes *à la turque*, accompanied by dancers dressed for the roles of the kings and queens of Mauretania. Six years later, Henri III devoted an entire royal carnival to emulate a battle between the Turks and Moors. In England, one of the first notable Oriental masques was commissioned by Queen Anne, consort of James I, in 1605. *The Masque of Blackness*, as it was called, cast the queen herself and her ladies as blackamoors, a popular disguise of the time. The event cost in the region of £3,000: members of the masque were placed in a huge shell, mimicking mother of pearl, which moved around as if buffeted by tempestuous waters. Inigo Jones designed the scenery and the costumes, in which the women were dressed as Ethiopian princesses.[44]

By the beginning of the seventeenth century, masques and carrousels had evolved into social spaces where courts could display their expansiveness and their imperial dominion, whether they really had it or not. In 1625, Louis XIII presided over a ballet of the 'Four Quarters of the World' graced with players dressed as Indians, Moors, Negroes and Chinese. Much in the way that Walter Scott, William Morris and the Pre-Raphaelite painters selectively rebirthed the Middle Ages to suit their whim, the Orient was recreated as a glittering fairytale. The participants were dressed in bright greens and blues, and bedecked with feathers and gems.

As we have already seen, Louis XIV excelled at such spectacle, which he harnessed to extraordinary effect to consolidate his power. Whereas oriental dress was once a more localized phenomenon with his predecessors, in Louis's court, dressing up as Persians, Turks, Chinese and other orientals was a favoured way of asserting control. It is of no small significance that the birth of Louis's first son was famously fêted with a horse race of three teams, the Turks, Persians and Americans. A *carrousel* for the dauphin was festooned with treasures from the Indies. At the Carrousel of 1662, the king's brother came dressed as a Shah of Persia, the Duc de Guise as a 'savage chief' and the Duc D'Enghien as a rajah. Then, in 1685, the theme for the carrousel was the conflict between the Abencerages and the Zegri.[45]

In Louis's court, where politics were firmly bound up with social perception and organization, the function of fashion to distinguish between classes reached a new register. Fashion, together with the intricately encoded movements and mores of courtly life, become the primary means by which status and rank could be asserted. It was an important vector in his court to regulate the privileges that were carefully meted out and intricately systematized. Everyone with entry to the court was expected to acknowledge its rarity and prestige and therefore be at their best and to 'dress up' for the occasion. When it came to dressing up in oriental clothing, this was very much a conceit reserved for a highly privileged social environment. The upper classes did not publicly transact their worldly affairs dressed as a Turk or a Mandarin, rather this form of deportment was reserved only for those who could not only afford costly imports and the kinds of fabrics—high-grade silks in particular—demanded by this kind of dress, but also the leisure to do so. Oriental clothing, a highly fluid yet unambiguous signifier of fashionable excess, became a mechanism by which aristocrats could participate in courtly play while also affirming their own arbitrary privileges. Masquerade was a florid, princely extreme of courtly protocols at a time in which ideas and perceptions of people and cultures could be bent so long as Louis's status at the pinnacle was maintained.

Court fashions have received their share of scholarly attention, especially in the celebrated work of Norbert Elias who argues that the elaborate fêtes in which dressing up became increasingly de rigueur was a form of covert control. It effectively distracted the upper classes from machinations that might threaten the king's power by encouraging them to compete amongst themselves in what were essentially imaginary aesthetic concerns.[46] More recently, Ina McCabe has weighed in on this thesis by adding that extravagant court fashions of this period expanded a fiscal economy, whose wider distribution of wealth was instrumental in eroding class barriers. As she maintains, Colbert was responsible for reforming the underperforming silk industry, to the distinct benefit of the middle classes.[47] Motivated that the debts that would accrue to the state already teetering financially from having to finance several expensive wars and Louis's quixotically magnificent public works, Colbert was keen to ensure that France would not be beholden to the silk trade. Lyon eventually matched Venice as a textile hub, exporting throughout Europe, including England.

But Lyon was more the exception than the rule. With Louis's expenses hanging heavily on his shoulders, Colbert adopted a series of protectionist policies, which were incongruous with a Europe that was accelerating exponentially in population, trade and industry. This is summed up frankly by Abbé de Choisy, who wrote in *Mémoires*:

> Always magnificent in his ideas and nearly always unfortunate in their execution [Colbert] believed that he could do without the silks of the Levant, the wool of Spain and the broadcloth of Holland, the tapestries of Flanders and the horses of England and Barbary. He set up all kinds of industries that cost more than they were worth. He created an East India Company without possessing the necessary funds and not realizing that the French—impatient by nature—would never have the constancy to put money into something for the space of thirty years without gaining any profit from it.[48]

LACHINAGE AND THE VISIT OF THE SIAMESE AMBASSADORS TO FRANCE

In 1686, a consort of Siamese ambassadors arrived at Louis's court, an occasion that was to leave an indelible mark on the passage of orientalist influence. One of the many effects of this visit was the introduction of *la siamoise*, light, striped linen, to French fashion. French silk manufacturers immediately began making a version of this garment. But this proved short-lived; cotton and linen proved more satisfactory, and *siamoises* were printed with wide stripes in vivid colours.

At the ball to mark the occasion, the king himself wore a costume 'half Persian, half Chinese' (*moitié à la persienne, moitié à la chinoise*). His brother disported in a number of guises, finally ending up as a Chinese grandee (*vêtu en*

Grand Seigneur chinois). The apotheosis of such celebrations took place on 7 January 1700, commenced with Louis's ball in Marly and then in Versailles by his brother's *collation à la chinoise*. In Honour's words:

> The ball opened with a divertissement, *Le Roi de la Chine*, in which thirty musicians, all dressed in Chinese costumes, carried in the king of China on a palanquin. The dancer, Des Moulins, dressed as a pagod then executed a *pas seul* which was said to be most droll. Monsieur's *collation*, organized by Jean Bérain, was a very elaborate affair. The room in which it was given appeared to be filled with pagods; three statues stood on the buffet, three musicians and two singers *en pagode* played and sang, while no less than a dozen of the Prince's officers were similarly attired and stood by each table. At the entry of the young Duchesse de Bourgogne, in whose honour the party was given, all twenty pagods, animate and inanimate, nodded their heads in unison to greet her. The napkins and the table-cloths were of oriental stuffs, the plates were of porcelain; indeed this collation seems to have been the Chinoiserie banquet *par excellence*.[49]

The postlude to this opulence came a couple of years later, when a figure dressed as the Emperor of Cathay was presented on a palanquin supported by thirty China-style courtiers. One can only assume he was a ubiquitous autocrat of the same genus as Louis himself. As with so many previous festivities in Louis's court, the person primarily responsible for all this was Jean Bérain, an early version of couturier and modern stylist. He designed the masque costumes and theatrical settings as well as hair, jewellery, fans, literally the gamut of material attributes responsible for the seventeenth-century concept of glamour.

But as Hugh Honour states, conceits in special dress took a little longer to take hold outside of the court. Regnard and Dufresny's play *Les Chinois*, which, in fact, involves precious few Chinese, debuted in 1692. Here Harlequin appears from a Chinese cabinet 'dressed as a Chinese doctor'. (Another play by Regnard and Dancourt, staged in the mid-1690s, has Harlequin donning an 'Armenian' robe in readiness to serve coffee like the first Armenian coffee sellers since the 1670s.)

It is common for architecture, decorative arts and accouterments to fall in lockstep with one another. The gaining interest in the seventeenth century in building oriental pavilions, gazebos and pagodas as garden retreats, microcosms of Eastern journeys, was one of a series of mounting trends that would begin to take root in the following century. To keep its diplomatic interests alive, in 1705 and 1712, France established its *Compagnies de Chine*, which was an attempt to rival England's monopoly in India by stimulating trade. Rival it didn't, but it continued to stimulate the vogue for things Chinese within textiles and other decorative arts. And with an eye on their competition in Dresden and Delft, Nevers and Rouen produced white and blue faience to swelling demand, while elsewhere in court, furnishings and screens 'in the Chinese manner' were the rage, visible in alcoves and private quarters. As Joan DeJean suggests, one of the ways Chinoiserie was popularized outside the court was through the antique sellers, where Chinese furniture and decorative items began to be seen among the usual furnishings, paintings of questionable merit, bric-a-brac, bibelots and bronzes. The juxtaposition only heightened their foreignness, which was certainly attractive in an age where to distinguish oneself from the crowd was a growing virtue. Their rapid popularity, coupled with the almost universal ignorance of meaning, style or provenance, made these items easy fare for copiers.[50] French designers quickly picked up on what was soon to develop into a ubiquitous visual lexicon: generic Chinese figures, effulgent floral arrangements, distorted animals, birds with wavy, feathery tendrils and gauntly angular trees. Other sources were Japanese lacquers and, as suggested earlier, Indian printed cottons. It is worth remembering that this was not an era in which anything resembling cultural propriety held sway, this was simply a matter of economics and survival, no different from the way in which South East Asia thinks nothing of ripping off Western prestige brands today. The term that grew from this adaptation was *lachinage*—literally 'Chinese-ing' or 'Chinese-ifying' (*la Chine-age*). By the end of the seventeenth century, the market was full of such objects, originals mixing with fakes, to the extent that experts are still apt to be confused. *Turquerie* was almost as pervasive and just as vague, encapsulating themes from fashion to drama that were, by process of elimination, neither Western nor Chinese.

The popularity of fans rose at a similar rate to lacquers among the ranks of the nobility, going from curiosity to necessity. They came via the Portuguese and subsequently the Dutch and English East India traders, although by the end of the seventeenth century English artisans had begun to turn their hand to making them as well. Despite documents that suggest that fan-makers were active in the mid-late-sixteenth century, during the time of Henry IV, they were not common until the eighteenth century (to be discussed in more detail in the following chapter). Both men and women made use of fans, as they did of paper parasols, the forerunner of that accessory essential for the English gent, the umbrella. Not as salutary and far less fiscally practical was the trend for wearing large diamonds in the hair and garments. It was a practice, exceptional in the East, made the rule by Louis and his court—yet another measure of weeding out the middling from the truly privileged. Fluttering coloured fans and glittering gems would have been a dazzling spectacle that had its optimal setting in the Galerie des Glaces, the great hall of mirrors at Versailles. Contemporary accounts attest to this breathtaking spectacle. By now, Eastern ambassadors began reporting to their grandees that Louis's court was threatening their own in the self-flattering display of sensuous brilliance and began to order mirrors from France in the thousands (4,264, to be exact, by the Siamese, in reply to their gift of over 1,500 pieces of porcelain).

After his death, Louis's pageant of ostentation would soon extend to the masses, who embraced luxury and finery for themselves, real or imitated. As his grandson Louis XV looked inward to his own domestic 'harem', his people and his court looked increasingly outward. The love–hate sartorial drama between France and England would continue to gain momentum, with oriental fabrics and styling maintaining a vital role.

—2—

1690–1815: Chinoiserie, Indiennerie, Turquerie and Egyptomania

See, mademoiselle, how that goes well with your Chinese-style hairstyle, your mantle of peacock feathers, your petticoat of celadon and gold, your cinnamon bottoms and your shoes of jade. . .

—Diderot, *Bijoux Indiscrets*[1]

. . . [Napoleon] entered in his new costume scarcely was he recognised than he was greeted with bursts of laughter. He took his place calmly: but he cut such a poor figure in his turban and oriental robe, looked so gauche in his unsuitable costume, that he very soon retired to take it off, and never since did he feel tempted to make a second appearance in this masquerade.

—Bourienne, *Mémoires*[2]

It is one of the great ironies (or conveniences) of this topic that the famous boutique of the French eighteenth-century seamstress Rose Bertin, who is widely regarded as the first couturier, was called *Le Grand Mogul*, named after the Muslim dynasty that ruled most of India from the sixteenth to nineteenth centuries. Frequented by Marie Antoinette, Bertin's patronage by the most exclusive clientele earned her the name the 'Minister of Fashion'.[3] The reference to the East was not intended to rankle or infuriate as it might in the later Romantic generations; rather, it carried assurance that the shop had a cosmopolitan, international scope that availed itself of oriental wealth and wisdom. It also implied a step beyond the pseudo-Chinese and Turkophilic amusements of Louis XV and sounded a note of triumph against the spate of sumptuary laws since the previous century that forbade access to printed Indian cottons. Even more than that, the reference to the exotic was the natural way for Bertin to suggest that she had a venturesome *esprit* that fed into her design; for even if the designs of the clothes were not overtly oriental, the fabrics and the patterns, visibly or through patterns of trade, definitely were. She would certainly have been making the most of the Eastern reference, since one of the most prestigious silk sellers in Paris was called the Grand Turk. Her boutique was lined with ravishing and tempting produce which, although for women, drew liberally from the myths of sybaritic Eastern tyrants, who spared themselves nothing.[4] Bertin is but one example of fashion developing into a marketable discourse in which that elusive but essential component of image is key. The Orient was also elusive, remote, the shifting signifier par excellence that could be invoked as a promise of something daring.

By the time of the early- to mid-eighteenth century, fashion had evolved beyond social mores and conversation to become topical: it was a conversation piece, a rite of passage, a social indicator—it was news. Tellingly, both the French (*nouvelle*) and English (service, product) for this concept reflect the characteristics that fashion must obey for its subsistence, namely newness. In eighteenth-century England and France, various currents of orientalism, incipient in the previous century, had become more explicit. Orientalism in product, form, sign and clothing became far more of a feature of everyday upper-class life. 'Kiosks' (the French *kiosque* was taken from the Turkish *kösk*, itself from the Persian *kus*, meaning 'pavilion') sprouted everywhere on European estates, and the large pouffes known as 'ottomans' were a special mark of domestic luxury.

Similarly, masquerade, which had its roots in the Renaissance, became all but obligatory for all kinds of eighteenth-century parties, to the extent that ornate disguise can be seen both literally and metaphorically to mark the era. As distinct from masquerades, the first masked ball per se was held in France in the year of Louis XIV's death, 1715. With French manners predominant, courtly life throughout Europe was increasingly governed by appearances, with masks both metaphoric and physical. Here oriental costume played a crucial and conspicuous role. No surprise that Revolutionary rhetoric would later make profligate use of slurs of deception and excess against the ancien régime. Oriental textiles had become normative. It was a fact of life. By now, the Mogul invoked by Mme Bertin had been supplanted by textile mills in England and France, severely denting the Indian economy and altering the terms of trade. Orientalism also made its presence felt in informal dress, in particular, with the dressing gown. By the time of Napoleon's invasion of Egypt at the close the eighteenth century, both the British and French empires had become accustomed to a steady diet of exoticism and were ready to embrace the heavy grandiosity of the Egyptian style that was credited with embodying the secrets of early civilization.

As we saw in the previous chapter, orientalism was introduced in the seventeenth century through patterns of trade that introduced cottons and silks in ever-rising quantity; these fabrics were more desirable than jute, flax, wool and linen because they were lighter, suppler and—because of that least measurable of economic variables, perception—they were different. Textiles and faiences, along with written and verbal reports of travels, aroused a collective curiosity in the educated and upper classes and were used as a cultural vector in various ways. As we saw, Louis XIV used the Orient as a paragon of stately authority, and in clothing, specifically, it was a concept that was used both to dazzle and differentiate. Costly jewels, expensive fabrics and rare accoutrements created a social landscape of covetousness and desire, where privilege was spoken, enacted and worn. By the end of his reign, these aesthetic regulatory principles had slackened and expanded to a greater public. There was more than one reason for this. In England, the unstoppable growth of imports from the East India Company caused a heated war between overseas and local industries, effectively swamping the market with affordable cottons and lower-grade silks, such that the vivid patterns could be seen as much as wall lining as on garments. If the economic dynamic was prone to be hostile, the systems of aesthetic exchange were far less. *Lachinage*, the tendency for 'style-ifying', continued to mould itself into an industry whose primary characteristic was an adaptive eclecticism. Receptive, malleable and protean, lachinage is a concept at odds with the stark binary of European versus the Oriental other. The Orient as assimilated and absorbed, thereby all but invisible, lived together with the Orient as a recognizable commodity.

Thus, while it is true that many of the *lachinages* and turqueries originated in the previous century, they were able to take hold in the next through a series of major transformations, where France continued to be the focus. Rising population, technological advances and the gradual advancement of individual freedoms had myriad and complex manifestations. Above all, this occurred through the widening idea of display, be it personal or in the pleasures to be taken in public life, whether in its incidental or organized spectacles. Theatres proliferated, as did museums and shopping arcades, places to ogle and gape. Entertainment became an available commodity to more than the rich. In such places, as well as in public parks and gardens, nobility and commoner shared in the closest thing to a mutual experience. As suggested at the beginning of the previous chapter, the culture of heightened visibility went hand in glove with social mobility, either to assert it or to get it. 'In a country where everyone strives for *appearance*' exclaims the late-eighteenth-century aphorist Champfort in one of his maxims, 'many people are driven to believe and in effect do believe, that it is better to be bankrupt than to be nothing.'[5]

It is at this point that fashion, as a state of mind, as a broad, elastic cultural modulator and as an industry, is instituted. It may be tempting to give too much credence to orientalism within this genesis; however, it is also true that fashion histories tend to downplay it. We have already seen the overwhelming changes rendered through the introduction from India, Persia and China of superior and more manageable fabrics, not to mention the sensuous and colourful designs that were printed or painted upon them. In the eighteenth century, oriental fashions were available to more than the rich. In theatre and opera, the Turkish and Chinese tastes, which had a tendency to comingle, were formidable presences. Oriental dress was the touchstone for the very ambiguous act of formal dressing up, an activity in which self-enhancement and disguise are gloriously confused. For the spectator dressed for the occasion and the actor dressed for the occasion are, in light of the specialized drama of the public spectacle, divided more in degree than in kind.

London by the end of the eighteenth century was the most populous city in the world, and also arguably the most inhospitable. Distraction was to be afforded to more than the swelling ranks of mercantile elite. As Erin Mackie emphasizes, publications like *The Tatler* and *The Spectator* were shapers of public taste amongst the new social formations afforded by trade and heated industrialization. She explains that

> fashion in England was usually identified with imported goods and styles. The eighteenth-century beau monde sustained itself on Chinese tea and porcelain, first Levantine then Caribbean coffee, North American tobacco, and West Indian sugar (and therefore on Afro-American slaves), East Indian calicoes, French and Italian silks, French manners and French tailoring. . . . Embargoes levied on French silks and Indian calicoes in the early eighteenth century, far from checking, indeed enhanced their desirability by heightening their exclusivity and expense.[6]

Such diverse imports are to be seen against a wide and increasingly complex landscape of commercial enticement, of the dawn of the era of the culture of shopping. Curiosity was legion. Merchants and artisans were embracing orientalism of whatever flavour—Chinese, African, Turkish or Persian. It was a marketing gift. Unbeholden to any scientific standard, the manipulability of exoticism was openly exploited to service all kinds of whims. This would change to some extent in the next century, when ethnographic study became more than a gentlemanly occupation and when orientalism was even more a feature of everyday existence so as to warrant more rigorous benchmarks.

TEXTILES

England's growing presence due to its increasing commercial interests, compounded by some decisive military victories, most memorably Robert Clive's over the Bengalese leader Siraj-ud-Daula, ensured that its presence in the Indian states were secure. The leaders installed or supported by the English were to the exploitative benefit of Company officials. It was more, however, from the latent aggression of commercial administration that the English in the eighteenth century assumed governance of India. In the same breath, a new melancholy set in for a lost, unadulterated past tradition, the golden age of the eclipsed Moghul Empire. In other words, once India ceased to be a discovery, England and its European neighbours needed to rearticulate a new beyond, hence the West's deliciously vexed relationship with the Orient as something both possessed and eluded. And it was this nostalgia in the eighteenth century of such real and fictive displacement that was one of the factors that stoked the desire for masquerade.

Apart from a small proportion of luxuries, the goods pouring from India and other East Asian ports were for the large part of common utility. As Beverly Lemire is quick to point out, already in the latter half of the seventeenth century there was indeed nothing remarkable about the clothing trade, so entrenched was it in English life, civil and military. English imperial expansion serviced and called for a large military and navy who were clothed by calico and chintz shirts, neckerchiefs and the like made available in the tens of thousands by the East India Company. In the navy, cotton did not distinguish between ranks. Officers used what the common sailor used, although perhaps of a higher grade. For example, in accounts of the domestic life of one of the heroes of Trafalgar, Captain Fremantle and his wife reveal the degree to which mainstream 'oriental' fabrics had ceased to be stand-alone curiosities and had permeated the life of salubrious middle-class British life. The Fremantle's drawing room contained some elegant cane chairs; chintz cushions and upholstery matched the curtains, which were of a grand Moroccan style; Turkish rugs lay on the floor. The four servants' quarters were decorated in gay gingham.[7] From the middle of the eighteenth century it is hard to overstate the prominence of the navy in British life and, by extension, the products and the stories that the navy regularly brought home, so that the oriental had two parallel roles; it was both a part of life and a welcome distraction.

It is worth remembering that clothing in the premodern period was not ready to wear; generic garments were reserved for convicts and slaves. But by the end of the seventeenth century, England's industrial and commercial machine had advanced in production and efficiency. The denizens of the workhouses and patrician charity schools of dubious repute were likewise clothed by prefabricated clothing, much of it emanating from Eastern ports.[8] Cotton was still considered inferior to wool and linen products, but its availability meant it was a constant threat to these industries as to those of fustian, flax and linen emanating from major industrializing cities such as Lancashire. Writing in the *Weekly Review* in 1708, Daniel Defoe remarked ruefully that East India cottons had become so profuse as to overstep class boundaries: 'chintz and painted calicoes', once reserved for carpets and quilts, had graduated to 'clothe children and ordinary people' and then on to cloth 'ladies'. Nonplussed and a trifle indignant, Defoe saw the patterns on clothing as emulating 'Indian carpets', which but a few years before their chambermaids would have thought too ordinary for them: the chintz was advanced from lying on their floors to their backs, from the foot cloth to the petticoat'. The Queen herself was content to 'appear in China and Japan, I mean China silks and calico'. Defoe figures the spread of such fashions as a kind of disease: 'It crept into our homes, our closets and bedchambers, curtains, cushions, chairs and at last beds themselves, were nothing but calicoes or Indian stuffs'. In effect, Indian trade had invaded all walks of life.[9] As Christopher Breward argues, Defoe's observations were more than reactionary; they responded to a growing taste for what was new and exotic, above and beyond considerations of quality or price. And Defoe's comment about the migration of carpet designs from floor to back was more than just flippant. There had always been some correspondence between carpet and textile design, but this gathered apace in the eighteenth century. The main cause of this had been the exponential growth of the English and Dutch East India Companies, to the detriment of the Ottoman silk weavers, causing carpet production to rise as compensation. Along with the East as a prime producer, Venice ceased to operate as the Europe's prime *porta orientalis*, although carpets were one of the means by which nostalgia for the past and a fascination with the Islamic Orient were kept very much alive.[10]

Another reason for the popularity of the fine Indian floral cottons was their resemblance to the finer French artisanal silks from Lyon and Grenoble, which were naturally associated with the upper classes. Like these fashions, the calicoes could be folded and pleated in much the same way as silk, but they were not only cheaper, they were also far easier to clean. As Elizabeth Wilson explains, the restrictions on French fashions made such cottons imported by the East India Company more popular. In turn this glut had a negative effect on the English wool and silk industry. The prevention of cotton imports in 1720 caused more cotton to be spun, woven and printed within England and was one of the primary causes of launching the industrial revolution. It was also what accelerated the need for inventions, such as steam-powered looms, which began to become the norm by the middle of the eighteenth century.[11]

After the wool textile mill crises of 1685, England was forced to adopt a cautionary policy that balanced its own cotton trade with the production of more traditional textiles. But by the beginning of the eighteenth century, competition from India was severe enough to warrant a protectionist policy in 1721, outlawing all coloured, woven and printed fabrics from entering the country. However, this measure did not prevent English prints on plain Indian calicoes from being exported. As a result, India concentrated its primary production on weaving. Until it began to enforce more supervisory control, England had vociferous, at times belligerent, input into its day-to-day running, but to limited effect. The weavers were extremely mobile, able to decamp and reestablish themselves in a short period.[12]

Eventually, by the end of the eighteenth century, the English transformed these ad hoc enclaves by undermining their independence, making them wage earners and by controlling the supply of raw cotton. Once the restrictions on English coloured goods had been lifted with the so-called Manchester Act of 1736, providing for a linen warp to be incorporated into a cotton weft, a greater variety reentered the market in direct proportion to competition. With Arkwright's invention in 1774, all cotton fabrics were made possible in England. Such improvements in spinning engendered a broader range of quality that became commensurate to the high calibre of English printing, which often used four to six plates. As a result, consumers did not necessarily see cotton as only servicing the market's lower end. Instead, with technological gains, cotton was beginning to be seen less as the meagre substitute for silk and to have its own substantive identity.[13] Cotton printing had grown into an intricate language that took all kinds of stylistic liberties: highly decorative and vividly episodic motifs mixing neoclassical idioms with both remote and recognizable chinoiserie effects. Although this textile dates from just after the eighteenth century, it has been chosen because it is a forceful example of the wild eclecticism at play in chinoiserie, in which Chinamen and exotic flora coexist with Apollo on his chariot, as if it had always been that way.

In France in 1746, Köchlin and Dollfus introduced 'Indian' cottons to Mulhouse and to Alsace. While England continued to dominate the trade,

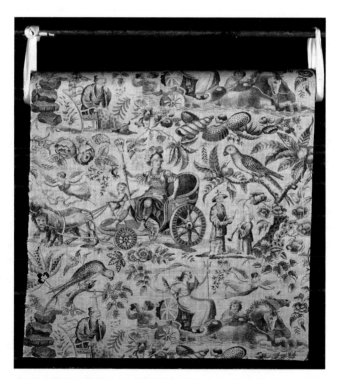

Figure 4 Furnishing fabric, 1816–20, Joseph Lockett (printer), George Palfreyman (retailer) Manchester; roller-printed cotton, © V&A Images; Victoria and Albert Museum, London.

manufacture and supply of cotton to Europe, France—specifically, Lyon—had become the undisputed leader of silk production. Without rival in its training schools for craftsmen and designers, it attracted some known artists such as Jean Revel and Philippe de Lasalle. They may be peripheral to the history of art, but their work boldly indicates the extraordinary debt of rococo textile design to Indian, Persian and Chinese influence which, we now accept, were themselves a result of a high level of translation over the last two centuries. Natalie Rothstein, in her essay on eighteenth-century silks, remarks that the prohibitions on silk supply in France and England, rather than curb the taste for the exotic—she prefers to use the twentieth-century term *bizarre*—only caused it to become more of an attraction for designers to conjure up images of what was withheld. With bogus iconography came false attribution: a silk of 1707 features a false Gujarati mark within the weave.[14] But by 1786, the Lyon silk industry had begun to suffer from the high demand for cotton gauzes and muslins, whose diaphanousness rivalled silk and which were far cheaper. The slump lasted until well into the following century.

BANYANS AND FANS

Hans Christian Andersen's story 'The Flying Trunk' tells of a poor merchant's son who, dressed in all he has—a dressing gown and slippers—is magically delivered to the Turkish land only to feel completely at home, since that was all, as the story goes, the Turks wore. Banyans and fans can be discussed together because both are associated with lounging and comfort. And both are our contemporaries: if all of us have not used a fan we have at some point certainly donned a dressing gown. It is worth beginning with this pair because they both exemplify the model in orientalist fashion that, as this book progresses, will be evident as a salient idea, namely, an obscured or altered origin. Having only an impact on the dress amongst the higher echelons of the seventeenth century, they became a recognizable feature of life in the following century. In his *Tableau de Paris,* Louis-Sébastien Mercier quips, 'Why do we not laugh at oriental clothing which doesn't change, yet our tailors constantly cut and recut cloth in different ways? It's because oriental clothing is made for the human form.'[15] Mercier may be perpetuating the tried belief of the immutability of oriental dress and custom—the West evolves and the tribal other remains static—but it is true that by the eighteenth century people throughout Europe turned to the Orient for clothing that was sympathetic to the body. It did not take long for the association of informal, liberating clothing to extrapolate itself into that of liberal thought, living in paradoxical balance with the contradictory notions of oriental despotism. By the end of the seventeenth century, men of manners and education were proud to be depicted in informal robes that showed off their prowess as intrepid thinkers and adventurous spirits. Samuel Pepys, for example, as a stamp of his progressive intellectual aspirations, had his portrait painted in a banyan, or 'Indian gown', as he called it, even if it had only been borrowed (some accounts say hired) specifically for that purpose (Fig. 5).

By the middle of the eighteenth century, orientalist costume and dress was, among other things, an outward sign of an expanded and freewheeling consciousness. It coalesced into one single item, the banyan, or *banian*, the paragon of male informal dress resulting in the *robe de chambre*, English morning dress, and the smoking jacket. By the middle of the eighteenth century it was an important hallmark of intellectual manhood. One need only think of Rousseau's 'Armenian' robe and fur hat, and his contemporary *philosophe* Diderot and his eccentric discourse of 1769, 'Regrets for my old dressing gown, or, a warning to those who have more taste than fortune'. ('In its shelter I feared neither the clumsiness of a valet, nor my own, neither the explosion of fire nor the spilling of water. I was the absolute master of my old robe. I have become the slave of the new one.')[16] For Rousseau, fashion was one of his longstanding aversions. His Oriental-inspired robes and caftans were a way of removing himself from the flows of fashion that were gaining

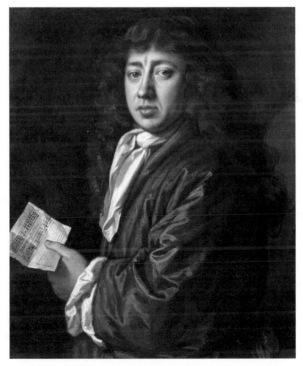

Figure 5 John Hayls, *Samuel Pepys*, 1666, oil on canvas, ©
National Portrait Gallery, London.

momentum in his time.[17] Hence again, there is the assumption that the Orient is somehow outside of time.

Although less enduring than the banyan, turbans had been used since at least the fifteenth century to denote worldliness and prosperity. This was evident in van Dyck's portrait of Sherley, but there are also countless examples, most notably, Rembrandt was in the habit of painting himself in slouched hats and turbans. By the eighteenth century, oriental costume had all but become the orthodox dress for the mildly unorthodox but erudite man, the sign linking in exotic fealty an expanding community of artists, poets, scholars, scientists, travellers and traders. And perhaps beneath their newfangled robe they may have worn a pair of nankeen breeches, whose name was from the thick, off-white cotton grown around Nanking in China.

Something of a highpoint of this tendency finds itself in the portrait of Linnaeus in Chinese clothing. It is often alternatively described as Saami (Lapp) costume, which suggests a fascinating hybrid. To whatever degree we might argue of what is predominant or accurate, what is most striking is the need for enlightened men to resort to exoticism and 'primitivism' (the ancient and indigenous races within Europe were as much part of this designation) to separate themselves from both aristocrat and bourgeois. From the late-seventeenth century onward, countless portraits exist of such men in more and less authentic exotically themed clothing, specially donned for the occasion in what might be called the official academic dress of exotic freemasons. It was therefore in support of a frame of mind that was different from the dressing up in court life. This encounter between the two classes was prophetically dramatized in Molière's *Bourgeois Gentilhomme* in 1670, whose protagonist, Jourdain, is mocked by Louis XIV's courtiers for wearing a banyan of printed calico, presumed for the nobility. By this time, oriental clothing was not just a status symbol; it had begun to take on a more formal function of sidestepping the tight standards of courtly dress. It was able to do this precisely because foreign codes were vague and potentially malleable codes and thus not subject to the same court mores and observances. So in the more informal atmosphere of the Chateau de Marly, women were instructed to wear the Ottoman *deshabillé*, or morning dress.[18]

Seen from the perspective of Enlightenment ideals of progressive thought and free exchange of ideas, it is maybe unsurprising that the origins of the banyan are to be seen alongside the birth of the coffee house in London and Paris. Coffee, the signature drink of Paris, was first publicly consumed in the Foire Saint-Germain in 1672 at the stand of an Armenian by the name of Harouthioun, clad in a flowing robe *en Arménien*. His example would become the rule with the drink-sellers, or *limonadiers,* hence. Whether in stalls or in the grander cafés, it became customary to be served in an elegant, copious robe, vibrant with printed or hand-painted designs. Armenia was the symbolic origin,

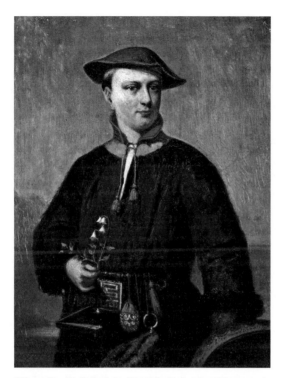

Figure 6 Attributed to Hendrik Hollander, *Linnaeus in Saami costume*, c. 1853, oil on panel. This work is probably one of several versions made by Hollander. A larger version was given to Natura Artis Magistra (Royal Amsterdam Zoo) in Amsterdam in 1852. By permission of the Linnean Society of London.

much as, say, 'Swiss formula' is tacked onto cosmetics or muesli. Top-layer garments much like overcoats had long been worn in Moghul India, Persia and the Ottoman Empire.[19] This generic surcoat is one component in the banyan's convoluted genealogy; the other is private dress worn by the shogunate of Japan.

Apart from its anecdotal rootedness in an Armenian beverage-seller, another source of the banyan is the Japanese *yukata*, an unlined, cotton, kimono-like garment that doubled as both a dressing gown and as summer clothing. These were simpler versions of the more imposing, traditional robes worn by the shoguns. In her spirited analysis of the banyan, Beverly Lemire tells of certain seventeenth-century Dutch traders of the United East India Company who, as a sign of esteem, were presented by the shogun with a special lacquered tray supporting a meticulously folded garment. When worn back in Europe, the silk gown with its patterns 'had an honorific association, as well as being constructed of distinct and sumptuous fabrics'.[20] As something that conferred status upon the wearer, it did not take long for its popularity to spread. It was quickly reproduced using fabrics from India. Moreover, as authentic as it sounds, the English name banyan is itself 'an intriguing cross-cultural eliding of terms' first recorded in 1518 in Duarte Barbosa's voyage to the subcontinent. It was a word for Indian merchants subsequently applied by the English for a fashionable home gown with particular overtones of social mobility. Meanwhile, in France the robe was designated Armenian in accordance with the intermediaries of Eurasian trade; in Holland it was alternatively called a Japanese robe, or cambay, after the Western port. As Lemire states, the meanings of the garment

> varied from country to country: denoting a commercial elite in India (in the English sense), the Japanese origins of the robe or a great Indian port (in the case of the Dutch), or the dynamic Armenian trading community (in the case of the French) . . . Banyans were replete with an amalgam of meanings, defining urbane, successful and erudite masculinity.[21]

This rather complex sartorial interplay was topped off with the 'Siamese hats' in vogue after the 1686 visit. John Singleton Copley's 1767 portrait of Nicholas Boylston shows the sitter in a soft, pink hat and sleek, green silk banyan ornamented with audaciously large flowers. While the hat might look silly to us now, Boylston almost purrs with urbane confidence. Like the banyan, these soft bell-like hats assumed their own life after a while, evolving into similar interior lounge wear, including into nightcaps, the tassel a familiar but little remarked remnant of faded Ottoman glory. It also now easy to see the East–West origin of today's pyjamas, which frequently meld the flowing, unobtrusive features of Chinese and Eastern garments with that of the suit, which makes itself known in the v-line collar when accompanied by a buttoned front (Fig. 7).

The fate of fans from the late-seventeenth century onward was not dissimilar. By the mid 1700s, fans and fan sticks numbered among the regular imports from China, including spices, sugar, tea and silk. Historically traced to ancient Egypt, the fans most familiar to Europe, the folding fans, hailed from Japan and were introduced to sixteenth-century Europe by the Portuguese through its Chinese trade connections. By the mid-eighteenth century, fans were made in varying oriental styles and in different degrees of chinoiserie hotchpotches produced in France, England, China and India.

At this time the volume of imports from China was disconcerting English and French fan-makers. In France alone in 1770, over 6,000 people worked in the fan industry, and the first 60 masters in Paris in 1673 had by 1753 swelled to 150. As in Louis XIV's time, fans continued as components to some highly auspicious events.[22] All over Europe, fans were made for specific use in christenings, mourning, weddings or birthdays. Art history has given

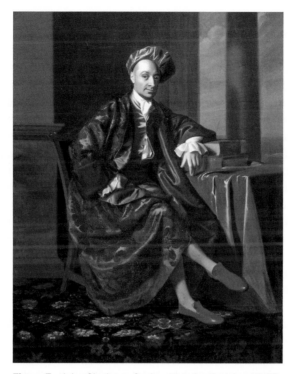

Figure 7   John Singleton Copley, *Nicholas Boylston (1716–1771)*, 1773, oil on canvas; Harvard Art Museums/Fogg Museum, Harvard University Portrait Collection, Painted at the request of the Harvard Corporation, 1773 Photo: Imaging Department, © President and Fellows of Harvard College.

fans rather short shrift, despite them being the primary means by which men and women of station could literally wear, or at least carry, a work of art. This said, by the middle of the eighteenth century they were commonplace accessories. The East India Company Letter Book of 1699 records the import of 20,000 fans from Canton and Amoy. In the following year it comments on such plentiful stock that 'they will not turn to account', and that only those of the finest lacquering and ivory would find purchasers. About fifty years later, English fan makers chose to make their complaints official, begging parliament to restrict imports at the risk of jeopardizing the livelihoods of 'Hundreds of Poor artificers . . . imployed in Painting, varnishing and Japanning'. As a ploy for survival they presented the Princess Dowager of Wales with a 'Fan superior to Indian fans'.[23]

As Indian textile printers adopted their own Chinese-style inventions that passed for authentic, fans had a similarly uneven evolution. Fans probably began in ancient Egypt but only caught on in Europe in the late-fifteenth century. By 1673, fan-making France had entrenched itself sufficiently to warrant guild status. Portuguese traders disseminated folding fans, which originated in Japan, throughout China. There are technically two types of fan: folding or flat. The latter were the more genuinely oriental but the least favoured in Europe. The folding fans manufactured in China throughout the eighteenth century never caught on amongst the Chinese themselves. A closer look at the history of German porcelain at this time reveals a curious analogy: Chinese producers were painting religious and classical designs in deference to the European taste.[24] Indeed, the Chinese productions gleaned from European sources could as easily be dubbed 'Europerie', as A. Hyatt Mayor presciently suggests.[25] This period was an iconographic climate of undaunted recreation, the visual equivalent of literary pastiche, or of what had become conventional in music: variations on someone else's theme. The items from exotic lands prized by the fashion-conscious elite were far from authentic but were subject to quite pronounced modification. While the eighteenth century is filled with the flavour of the *honnet homme*, authenticity only became a by-word in art, design and fashion with the revolutionary classicism by the end of the century. Before this time, objects and fashions were radically altered and made to fit into an expanding idea of abundance.[26]

Needless to say, chinoiserie fans were typically those that favoured stylistic, often lavish, amalgamation. Best known as the *brisé* fan, they were made of individual sticks joined with thread or ribbon, incorporating a range of materials including cloisonné enamel, lacquer, ivory, kingfisher feathers and filigree

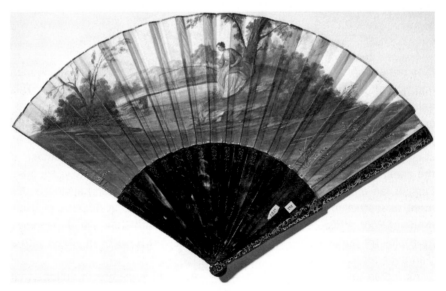

Figure 8   Fan; Naples, Italy, 18th century; watercolour, tortoiseshell, gold and skin, © V & A Images; Victoria and Albert Museum, London.

of gold and silver. These and later designs in the following century, like the cockade and asymmetric fan, remained for China exclusively something for export. The other type, the pleated fan, was made from pivoting sticks and ribs mounted with material—paper, cloth or kid leather—and outer guards. This Neapolitan fan is particularly curious for the way it articulates a rather crisp transposition of visual idioms. To have women fishing is unconventional to eighteenth-century easel paintings; here she has simply taken the place of the jolly piscatorial Chinaman.

Precious few of the earliest examples of the Chinese exports from the sixteenth and seventeenth centuries survive. Consistently made for a Western market, they were made of ivory and pierced to give the sense of filigree lacework. The painted designs they carried were hybridized Chinese–Western, sharing many characteristics of the porcelain produced at the time, again purpose-made for the Western market, especially the varieties of *famille verte* and Chinese Imari. Ivory continued to be a material of choice until the end of the eighteenth century, although by this time cheaper, less sought after materials such as silk began to dominate production. The period from 1790–1820 saw lacquer fans take over, and together with the traditional repertoire of figurative vignettes of chinoiserie landscapes we see freer, more abstract patterns from plant tendrils, vines and flowers, frequently punctuated by the owner's monogram.

The Stradivarius of fans was the 'vernis-Martin' variety of the mid-eighteenth century, duly named after the enamel-like finish and the workshops of les Frères Martin in the area near the Bastille, the Faubourg Saint-Antoine. Fans of this make were recognizable through their copal–rosin base, emulating the famed varnish of Japan and China. Around 1748, the Martin brothers were honoured with the title of 'manufacture royale', which not only denoted state legitimacy: they were expected to syndicate their enterprise and disseminate their standards and findings. The fans known under this appellation were a set of sticks of ivory or mother of pearl, imbricated and fastened by means of a rivet at the base and a ribbon at the circumference. They were sought after because of their resilient sheen and their resistance to cracking. Their form of decoration melded touches of neoclassicism with chinoiserie figures, ornament *à la perse* and other decorative units drawn from ceramics in which the East–West distinction is all but lost.[27] The highest quality exceptions remains unaffected by the market, but the sheer bulk of Chinese production asserted its pressure, especially since it was superior in imitating the French, who themselves had imitated and adapted from the Chinese—yet another case of knotted genesis due to taste and patterns of adaptation and trade.

Chinoiserie painted designs were not as predominant in the early stages of the French fan industry, when in the late-seventeenth century it was deemed proper to have paintings with sufficient pomp, like the Fest of Belsheazzar from the Old Testament. By the end of the eighteenth century the tightening order of restrictions on salon painting carried over into fan painting, whose subjects had recognizable family groupings: birds, flowers, landscapes, genre subjects, and of course, historical and religious themes. (Painters sometimes circumvented proscriptions by placing scenes within decorative putti to give them a prim, theatrical look akin to genre painting.) In Germany, Holland and Italy, fan painters were not as controlled, while in England there was a fever-ish war with their Chinese competitors; each were copying the other. It is now difficult to tell English and Chinese *brisé* fans of this period apart, as it is to draw a line between chinoiserie and what is authentically Chinese. As Chinese painters imitated Western images, the imitation of Western painters of Chinese imagery eventuated in yet another hybrid. Thus the competition of the local and imported fan industries caused chinoiserie design to a fusion of two separate styles. Cultural authenticity, as it will emerge over and again in this book, is a crafted, vetted and malleable concept that is continually adapting to outside contingency.

During the reign of Louis XVI, fan designs became more austerely clas-sical characterized by a more linear furnishing style that departed from the sinuous and feminine Louis XV style. References from bucolic antiquity vied

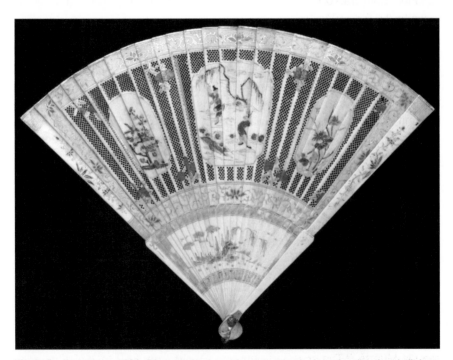

Figure 9   Fan; China, 1720–30; artist/maker unknown; carved, pierced, painted and gilt ivory sticks, © V&A Images; Victoria and Albert Museum, London.

more prominently with looser, more lyrical chinoiserie designs. Chinoiserie became diluted within hedonistic pastoral fantasies, coeval with scenes from aristocratic life, sometimes alluding to contemporary events. In the ensuing Revolutionary and Directory Periods, all signs of the previous regime were neurotically eschewed, chinoiserie central among them. Observing a stricter neoclassicist aesthetic, fans became more austere in colour and design, tended more often to monochrome and were decorated with *paillettes*, or spangles.

CHINOISERIE DESIGN AND ART

Ornamental design books were the best way of circumventing the reliance on expensive imports. Anonymous designers to prominent painters would participate in compiling image and pattern books, which would become the new mainstay of the industrial age, determining anything from architecture to textile design until well into the twentieth century. As well as ensuring a steady, responsive audience for artists, these anthologies were also the best mediums for travellers to market findings from their adventures overseas. One of the earliest known examples is from Mathias Beitler from 1616. Johan Nieuhoff's *Illustrated Embassy of the East India Company of the United Provinces to the Grand Tartar Cham Emperor of China*, published in Amsterdam in 1668 and London in 1669, was a veritable bible for ornamentalists across Europe. In England, John Stalker and George Parker's *Treatise on Japanning and Varnishing* (1688) is perhaps the first source book on chinoiserie and was therefore sought after. It was not confined to oriental finishing, for it was full of buildings of unusual proportions, remarkable birds and oriental figures with the unmistakable mix of Persian and Chinese. In its wake, hundreds of upper-middle-class girls were painting oriental designs as part of their educational regimen, and with that appeared dozens of charlatan teachers learned in the ways of a style that was, itself, largely made up. While others were produced in Holland and Germany, this and Peter Schenk of Amsterdam's *Picturae Sinicae* (1702) would continue its influence until the early-eighteenth century. The more these were produced, the more they were copied, spawning yet more variations.

Individual artists profited handsomely from this industry. Fan designs, along with textile and interior painting, were lucrative bread-and-butter assignments for even some of the best artists of the time, including Oudry, Watteau, his followers Lancret and Pater, and Huet. In the early part of the eighteenth century, it was Watteau who set the mood for chinoiserie imagery with his *Figures chinoises and tartares*, a thirty-part suite for the *cabinet du roi* at the Château la Muette.[28] The chateau was destroyed and the paintings along with it, but her designs survive through engraving produced by Boucher, Jeaurat and

Auber. Boucher, who never renounced the spell of chinoiserie throughout his long career, produced his *Suite de Figures Chinoises* (1735), one surmises, in Watteau's honour. His most famous example of chinoiserie can be seen in his cartoons executed by the Beauvais tapestry works for the Salon of 1742, commissioned by Louis XV's resilient mistress, Mme de Pompadour.

Exceeding Boucher in dedication to eighteenth-century chinoiserie was Jean-Baptiste Pillement (1728–1808). The son of a painter and master of looms, apprenticed as a designer of cartoons at the Gobelins factory, Pillement's career was always destined to be oriented toward the decorative arts. He travelled extensively throughout Europe, including Austria, Poland and Italy was a highly receptive artistic barometer and an adept artistic manoeuvrer. When he arrived in London in 1754, he observed a recent boom in the involvement of artists in crafts and manufacturing. At the time, France had the monopoly on style books, motivating Pillement the year after to publish his first independent folio (implying something slenderer than book, in this case six designs), *A New Book of Chinese Ornaments*, which was followed by second folio two years later, followed by several more in years hence, placing Pillement at the forefront of the European chinoiserie tradition. Copied or used as variations on a theme, these designs had an untold effect on all manner of decorative arts: fans, fabrics, tapestries, wallpapers, faience and porcelain, enamels, silver and furniture decoration. Pillement's paintings and designs were quickly reproduced by engravers, notably by J. C. Canot, who published three sets between 1758 and 1759. Numerous other folios continued to be published until he was slowed by the French Revolution, producing approximately twenty-one for his English period and twenty-eight in France.[29]

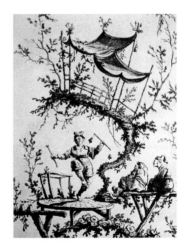

Figure 10 Jean Pillement, chinoiserie design, mid-eighteenth century.

Pillement decorated rooms in Austria, Poland, Russia, Portugal and Flanders. In 1764, he discovered a new method of printing silk with fast colours. Because of the adaptive nature of his designs, sparse evidence of this survives, presumably used for both furniture upholstery and dress fabrics. Pillement's subtlety, wit and sense of free play are hardly possible to describe without access to the pictures themselves. What they reveal is that eighteenth-century chinoiserie was a decorative armature that was the antithesis of the modern anthropological binary of cultural authenticity of the other versus the selective perception of the imperial gaze. There was no anthropological mission. Musings of cultural truth were in their infancy. Rather, the chinoiserie developed by Pillement and reflected on cloth, fans, faience and decorative patterns from Vienna to Versailles was a highly fecund device of imaginative improvisation. As the quintessence of otherness it was used as the modus operandi to signal differences in the representation of people, filigree, flora, fauna, what you will. By the first half of the eighteenth century, the clichés that had begun to take shape in the baroque period had become well and truly entrenched: long-necked birds; magnificent insects; monkeys; Chinamen with long, droopy moustaches and wide sleeves; arbitrary outcropping rock formations; spiky trees; splayed-roofed pagodas (feasibly sharing the landscape with classical ruins)—all assembled in a rambling riot of decorative excess.

These are the rule; the best artists and designers—most of whom remain anonymous—of this period chose chinoiserie as an art of exceptions. If an artist wished for slippages from convention, in what was recognizable and had corollaries in the immediate world, then it was to chinoiserie that they turned, the equivalent of today's science-fiction fantasy. Dawn Jacobson comments that Pillement's figures appear as from 'a fairyland conjured out of gossamer and stalks of grass, and the humans inhabiting it fanciful little creatures who dance and tumble around so effervescent and lively that they seem more creatures of air than earth'.[30] Similarly, but more soberly, classicism had it copious share of undisciplined interpretations. But unlike chinoiserie, it was answerable to academic scrutiny and had to be moored in some way to classical references and to the rigours of classical training. Chinoiserie's only brief was to look unlike the natural or classical world, to be lavish and intoxicating; its only limit to stretching the exotic was the threshold before it became grotesque or strange.

MASQUERADE

As it evolved from the Renaissance until the eighteenth century, the birth of modern fashion occurs together with the self-conscious sense of dressing up.

Specialized dress had always been used to denote function or station with respect to ritual and class, but the factor of self-consciousness was added with Louis XIV, who understood how manipulable such denotations are and who also understood the power of appearances to coax, convince and assert his power as well as to demarcate social activities. We saw in the previous chapter how orientalism was an important ingredient to such determinations, especially in asserting wealth amongst the wealthy. By the end of Louis's reign, in 1715, both Paris and London were large cities of growth hitherto unseen, affording far greater opportunities to the middle classes than only a half a century before.

More than today, opportunity in this period meant social advancement, either out of the mire or toward a noble title. Since society was a meritocracy built on title and wealth before knowledge and ability, it was based on appearances over utilitarian principles. In short, the birth of the concept of fashion is coterminous with a culture of perception, role-play and changing appearances. The bigger cities of Europe were places where people could literally 'dress for success'. The seeds of the public ritualization of being fashionable were sown in Louis XIV's time, but it also became the subject of satire and drama. In Molière's *Bourgeois Gentilhomme*, Jourdain is devout about finding roles that will best win him acceptance, up until the sartorial excesses (involving orientalist garb) toward the end of the play. He exclaims, 'What is real and what is acting life?', which applies to the condition of the actor but also the courtiers in the first audience.

At the end of Louis XIV's reign, Chinese, Turkish and Persian costumes were but a relative extreme of dressing that extended well beyond the once closed realm of the upper class. Instead of setting classes apart as they had formerly, during masked balls and other festivities, these fashions supplied the shell in which the signs of social differentiation could be subsumed. In other cases, as with the banyan, it could be used as a hallmark of worldly distinction and used so frequently that special costume became mere clothing. And in philosophical literature such as we find in Montesquieu, Voltaire or Diderot, the voices of political criticism, sharply monitored by the king's censors, were channeled through figures wearing oriental dress. By the eighteenth century, as we have already seen, orientalist dress had already enjoyed a healthy pedigree. There exists a book from 1587, now in Jerusalem, of watercolour drawings of Turkish and Persian figures, themselves possibly copies from the designs of Nicolas de Nicolay from twenty years before, which were subject to continued scrutiny, including from Rubens, who copied them into his 1600 Costume Book.[31]

But as Terry Castle argues in her book on masquerade in England during this period, masquerade occupied a precarious place. On one hand it embodied the eighteenth-century imagination with new possibilities, including new worlds—where Turks and rope-dancers, judges and Indian queens played side by side—but on the other it was nostalgic, already criticized at the time by the modern voice defending reason over deception and materialism over illusion, a sentiment that would climax in the revolution.[32] To these eyes especially, orientalism, references to Turkey and turquerie connoted tyranny. This became all the more pronounced with the Franco–Ottoman *rapprochement* of 1756. To quote the sardonic moralist Champfort: 'The real Turkey of Europe is France. A score of English writers use the expression, "countries of despotism such as France and Turkey." '[33] Add to this the association of eroticism with masquerade, perceived by its middle-class detractors as a recrudescence of the bacchanal, where anonymous assignations were made dressed as devils, dervishes or saturnine Turks; so much so that in 1721 in England there appeared the leaflet *Short Remarks Upon the Original and Pernicious Consequences of Masquerades* which advocated the activity as 'a Congress to an unclean End'.[34] Together with other stereotypes, the vision of the Ottoman savage was already hackneyed, dividing its audience between those who found it aphrodisiac or reprobate.

The argument that eighteenth-century masquerade verged precariously on anachronism has more than a bit of sense to it if one reviews the many orientalizing motifs within plays, masques and operas in the preceding period. The language of anachronism was also something stridently exploited in the Revolutionary era to give its own newness legitimacy. At the end of the sixteenth century, opera had been invented (*Dafne*, in 1597, by Jacopo Peri and *Orfeo*, in 1607, by Claudio Monteverdi) in Italy and theatre reinvented in England. This was to prove crucial in the manifestations of oriental style in all forms of pageant, where costume and dress are finely intertwined. Evidence of orientalist court costume can be traced back to as early as 1510, when on a Shrove Sunday banquet, the Earl of Essex and his entourage appeared before Henry VIII 'appareled after Turkey fashion, in long robes of Bawdkin, powedered with gold, hates on their heades of Crimosyn Velvet, with great rolles of gold, girded with two swords called Cimeteries'.[35]

THEATRE AND MUSIC

As the sixteenth century progressed, references to the Orient became stronger, replacing or intertwining themselves with the otherwise ubiquitous classism. Turkish history plays, some set to music, were already in vogue in Restoration England, such as Sir William Davenant's *The Siege of Rhodes* (1662), Lord Orrery's *Tragedy of Mustapha, the Son of Solyman the Magnificent* (1665), and John Dryden's *The Indian Emperor* (1668). Little credence was given to authenticity. Rather, costumes were an aggregate of signs. Roman armour made a Roman, even if he wore a periwig, and orientals were known by turbans, caftans and the like in superabundant, motley display.[36]

Turkish-style influences in music also bear a mention, as it cannot be prised away from the contrivances by masquerade; they were all part of the escapist drama, whether formalized in opera or extemporized within informal masques and fêtes. It was the superabundant atmosphere created by such expensive courtly events that elicited the nostalgia of aesthetes of the following century, who would try to recreate the multisensory ambience in their own domestic settings. It is also interesting to compare the nature of influence, especially with regard to the idea of inflection or the more universally used term in fashion studies, 'inspiration'. Like fashion, Turkish influence in music was always squarely within a Western framework, used liberally and without specificity. Composers in the seventeenth century such as Jean-Baptiste Lully and André Campra availed themselves of Turkish influence, but they did so well within their own music structures. As Mary Obelkevich puts it, 'Turkish music remained but one more color on a "palette"', that is, a kind of embellishment, an incidental 'contribution to the basic musical structure'.[37] Or in the words of Matthew Head, 'signs of difference are 'relegated' to the status of details within a pre-existing European framework: Turkish music is represented not only through decoration but *as* decoration'.[38] The decorative element is key, whereas in the nineteenth century it would also take on a more scientific dimension within the nascent field of anthropology. For hundreds of years, Turkish instruments and weaponry had been prized as both curiosities and spoils of war. They were welcome accessories to oriental dress and specifically designed Turkish chambers.

Mozart's music is perhaps the most lasting remnant of musical forays into orientalism. Much like the costumes themselves and the people who wore them, Mozart's 'Turkish' music is music in masquerade, oriental flavor over a classical armature. The salient examples of this are in his violin concerto number 5 ('the Turkish'), 1775, the *Rondo alla turca* from the 11th piano sonata (c. 1783) and not least the opera, *Abduction from the Seraglio*, first performed in 1782, around a century after the siege of Vienna, at the zenith of the Turkish craze there. In his analysis of Mozart's Turkish-styled works, Matthew Head argues that they have to be understood together with masquerade's 'festive self-Othering', and not in terms of Said's 'hidden kinship'. Like its sartorial counterpart (albeit that the period didn't always separate them), musical turquerie is festive. Broadly speaking, it is blithe and upbeat, characterized by particular instruments such as the piccolo, bass drum and cymbals, lending a 'barbarous' edge that bordered on burlesque.[39] It is also uncannily biased toward the key of A, limited not only to Mozart but also to other composers such as Gluck.[40] Head advises that it cannot be separated by the '*theatrum mundi*' of all manner of staging and surrogate awareness, in which 'the visible and audible signs of difference within and beyond Europe were both simulated fantasised in the early modern world'.[41]

INSTITUTIONALIZING TURQUERIE

Just as the Siamese delegation had had an lasting effect on the court of Louis XIV, so did the visit of an ambassadorial retinue led by Mehmed Efendi in 1720–21, stamping the court with all kinds of turquerie, enmeshing itself more freely with the *lachinage* of the former century (remembering also that chinoiserie was very much alive and a central element to the germination of the rococo; Watteau's edition, *Figures chinoises* was, for instance, published in 1731). Turquerie was already in some sense an item in court celebrations, such as the Duc de Chartres's fête at Marly in 1700, inspired after the visit of the French Minister de Ferriol to Constantinople the year before. In 1713 there appeared a suite of one hundred engravings of Turkish dress, which became the template for oriental costumes, especially for painted portraits.[42] In her account of Efendi's visit, Fatma Müge Göçek describes how the cultural détente was driven by mutual political interest bolstered by the fact that the pride of neither national had been dented by recent conflict. When thinking about the adoption of Turkish style as courtly party dress, it is also useful to spare consideration of the differences between the mores of the French and the Turks. Whereas the French were outwardly vivacious and dined in an open and relaxed way, the Turks prided themselves on their austerity and ate in private.[43]

This did not prevent the Turkish style from becoming a modish characteristic of social life, despite only the most passing credence given to the details of Turkish life. Portraiture and airy genre subjects of people in Turkish clothing proved a mainstay of mid-eighteenth-century painting. In America, John Singleton Copley painted a large series of portraits in varying degrees of turquerie. Unfortunately, there is no space here to go into in detail as they are too many to enumerate with artists such as Jean-Baptiste Vanmour, Charles Jervas, Godfrey Kneller, and Carl van Loo making a career with chinoiserie–turquerie subjects. One of the more famous among these is Carle van Loo's depiction of Madame Pompadour being served coffee by an attendant, lolling about the boudoir as a sultana (*Sultan's Wife Drinking Coffee*, 1755). Its accompanying piece is a jewel of rococo *intimisme*, featuring the sultana embroidering, attended by a rapt lady-in-waiting. Here the harem meets the daily decorous pursuits of the royal household, a harmonious but luscious one that waited subserviently upon the king/sultan (*Sultan's Wife Embroidering*, 1755).

Pompadour had had a special relationship to random Turkish refinements, since it was at a *Bal à la turque* that the king cast down his handkerchief

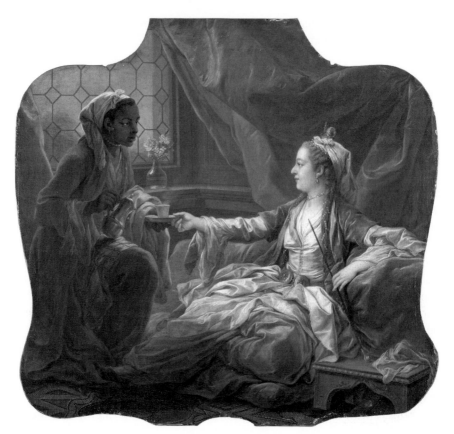

Figure 11 Carle (Charles-Andre) van Loo, *Sultan's Wife Drinking Coffee*, 1755, oil on canvas, © The State Hermitage Museum, St. Petersburg. Photo by Vladimir Terebenin, Leonard Kheifets, Yuri Molodkovets.

whereupon the court exclaimed, 'The handkerchief is thrown', knowing that it was a sign of a sultan choosing his favourite. Van Loo's success with theses and other images led to a commission of tapestries aptly named *Le Costume turc*, which ended up being taken up by his brother Amédée.[44] Madame du Barry, Louis XV's last mistress, would later assume this role, commissioning images in this style, including one of herself as a sultana-cum-concubine by Amédée van Loo and Jean-Baptiste André Gautier-Dagoty in 1771. Turkish allusions to polygamy suited Louis XV's sexual appetites, and his mistresses could effectively disguise the fact that they were not the legitimate queen. It was usurpation on a grandly metaphoric scale: Pompadour's queenly poise is to be read as being in the role of *femme savante*, the sage woman at the head of the harem, which she in effect was, having arranged the equivalent in the gaggle of teenagers she assembled for Louis's pleasure in the *Parc au*

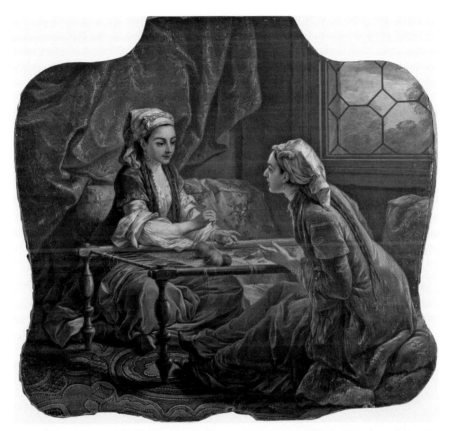

Figure 12   Carle (Charles-Andre) van Loo, *Sultan's Wife Embroidering* (pair to the painting *Sultan's Wife Drinking Coffee*), 1755, oil on canvas, © The State Hermitage Museum, St. Petersburg. Photo by Vladimir Terebenin, Leonard Kheifets, Yuri Molodkovets.

cerfs. To see her placidly embroidering is to see her as a compliant and concerned home-maker—passive–aggressive imagery if ever there were. The last years of the ancien régime saw turquerie shed itself even more into interiors and decorations. In 1777, a Turkish boudoir was completed for Marie Antoinette at Fontainbleau, and her brother-in-law, the Comte d'Artois, followed suit with a Turkish room at the Château du Temple in Paris and one in Versailles. There were places where acting and circumambient illusion could seamlessly combine.

Illusion for the sake of pleasure and play was all. In what is perhaps the most authoritative book on this theme, Aileen Ribeiro comments that

there was a certain amount of confusion over the details of Oriental dress; the term an 'eastern habit' which occurs frequently in masquerade accounts, could

cover any kind of costume that had easily recognizable features such as turbans, ermine facings to robes, and it was often extended to the dress of those
countries, like Greece, which were subject to turkey and whose costumes were
'oriental' in certain aspects. Distinguishing characteristics of the various eastern
countries were often lacking.[45]

Ribeiro details the extraordinary lengths that people would go to have themselves represented in orientalist dress.

One of the artists who stands out amongst the painters of orientalist clothing of this time is the Swiss-born Jean-Étienne Liotard, who in 1738 accompanied a delegation led by Lord Duncannon to Constantinople and stayed there
for five years. He was quick the embrace the Turkish way of life. Liotard played
a significant role in diffusing the passion for Turkish dress throughout Europe.
His affectation of wearing Turkish dress earned him the nickname 'the Turkish painter'. Known also for his fine pastels, he painted women *à la sultane*
and portraits of friends dressed up *à la turque*, such as *Monsieur Levett and
Mademoiselle Hélène Glavany in Turkish Costume* (1738–41) (Fig. 13). The
painting in many ways presages those by Ingres and Frederick Lewis. Mademoiselle Helene sits cross-legged playing the oud while Levett is enjoying an

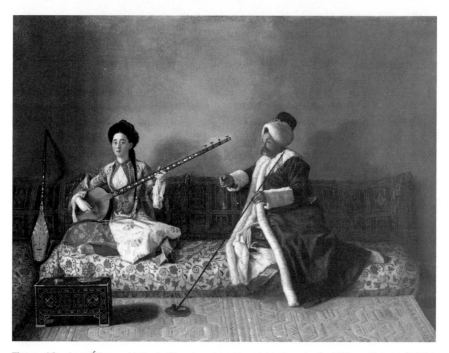

Figure 13 Jean-Étienne Liotard, *Monsieur Levett and Mademoiselle Hélène Glavany Turkish
Costume*, 1738–41, oil on canvas, © RMN (Musée du Louvre)/René-Gabriel Ojéda.

exceedingly long Turkish pipe. The detail shows the artists prowess in miniatures; the couple appear at ease with these fixtures, as if it were their own custom. In his portrait of the countess of Coventry (c. 1750), Liotard shows the sitter in an embroider overgarment known as an *entari* and a silk shalwar, or harem pants, the floor covered with a Ushak carpet. The air of both the paintings goes well beyond voyeurism or carnival toward a relaxation and sympathy for the Turkish idiom in dress and interiors. Liotard's paintings are replete with empathy and assimilation that stand in hard contrast to harsher stereotypes that persisted by European artists in his wake.

When oriental clothing was brought back from abroad, it was quickly calibrated to the mounting supply of catalogue style books, such as the *Collection of Eastern and Foreign Dresses* (1750) by John Tinney or the *Collection of the Dresses of Different Nations, Ancient and Modern* (1757) by Thomas Jeffrey. By quantity and presence alone, such contributions amounted to a self-conscious taxonomy of orientalist dress in which the emphasis always lay in typologized, distinguishing features in which foreign culture was made comprehensible through visual packaging. Terry Castle explains how the visual information was accompanied by 'pseudo-anthropological detail' to help the prospective masquerader carry out the part in a way seemly to the costume. This 'primitive ethnography', he argues, need not be understood entirely as imperial brazenness. While it may be true that in England, the tendency for dressing up in orientalist costumes coincided with its colonial empire, Castle suggests that they were also 'an act of homage—to otherness itself'. Despite being prone to stereotypes and all kinds of inaccuracies, to wear the exotic was a form of mimesis that embraced unfamiliarity.[46] By the middle of the eighteenth century it had virtually sedimented its own fairly metalanguage commenting and parodying the omnipresent institution of social appearances.[47] This is somewhere in evidence in portraits in the Turkish style painted by not just Liotard but also his contemporaries de Favray and Aved.

MARY MONTAGU AND THE SPECIAL CASE OF MASQUERADE

Before the alternative conventions of masquerade had taken root, the very special case of Mary Wortley Montagu exemplified escape through orientalist dress on an altogether different scale. Already a social and literary identity upon her departure to Turkey, Montagu accompanied her husband who had been appointed in 1717 and returned a year later. As an open-minded and confident member of the upper class who rubbed shoulders with the cognoscenti, she was alert and quizzically open-minded to what for her were extremely novel forms of dress and deportment. Her letters—written intentionally for circulation and publication—abound in comments that laud the

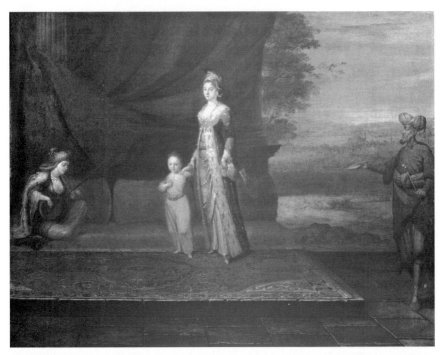

Figure 14   Attributed to Jean-Baptiste Vanmour, *Lady Mary Wortley Montagu with her son, Edward Wortley Montagu, and attendants*, c. 1717, oil on canvas, © National Portrait Gallery, London.

freedom that a veil gave her. They permitted a fluidity of movement into places normally obscured from European eyes, most covetously, the harem. With the approbation of the literary luminaries such as Alexander Pope, her letters were widely circulated.

There is a passage in her letters that is often cited, in which she describes a significant moment of wearing sumptuous Turkish dress. This is where she describes in detail her clothing as depicted in the most famous portrait of her by Jean-Baptiste Vanmour with her son, Edward Wortley Montagu, and flanked by Ottoman attendants (Fig. 14):

> The first piece of my dresses is a pair of drawers, very full, that reach to my shoes and conceal the legs more modestly than your Petticoats. They are of thin rose colour damask brocaded with silver flowers, my shoes of white kid Leather embrodier'd with Gold. Over this hangs my Smock of a fine white silk Gause edg'd with Embroidery. This smock has wide sleeves hanging halfe way down the Arm and is clos'd at the Neck with a diamond button, but the shape and colour of the bosom very well to be distingish'd through it. The Antery is a waistcoat made close to the shape, of white and Gold Damask, with very long sleeves falling back and fring'd with deep Gold fringe, and should have Diamond or pearl Buttons. My

Caftan of the same stuff with my Drawers is a robe exactly fited to my shape and reaching to my feet, with very long strait falling sleeves. Over this is the Girdle of about 4 fingers broad, which all that can afford have entirely of Diamonds or other precious stones. Those that will not be at that expence have it of exquisite Embroidery on Satin, but it must be fasten'd before with a clasp of Di'monds. The Curdée is a loose Rober they throw off or put on according to the Weather, being of a rich Brocade (mine is green and Gold) either lin'd with Ermine of Sables; the sleeves reach very little below the Shoulders. The Headdress is compos'd of a Cap call'd Talpock, which is in winter of fine velvet emroodier'd with pearls or Di'monds and in summer of a light shineing silver stuff. This is fix'd on one side of the Head, hanging a little way down with a Gold Tassel and bound on either with a circle of Di'monds (as I have seen several) or a rich emrodier'd Handkercheif. On the other side of the Head of Hair is laid flat, and here the Ladys are at Liberty to shew their fancys, some putting Flowers, others a plume of Heron's feathers, and, in short, what they please, but the most general fashion is a large Bouquet of Jewels made like natural flowers, that is, the buds of Pearl, the roses of different colour'd Rubys, the Jess'mines of Di'monds, Jonquils of Topazes, etc., so well set and enammell'd this hard to imagine any thing of that kind so beautifull. The Hair hangs at its full length behind, divided into tresses braided with pearl or riband, which is allways of great Quantity.[48]

This is in no way to be confused with conventional courtly masquerade. It was comfortable assimilation in a foreign context, not play acting amongst people who wanted to be temporarily distracted by appearing different. That Mary Montagu felt at home in the smooth, ventilated Ottoman garments is attested to in the many portraits she had made of herself in them. Together with her very real experiences of newfound womanly freedom, they were for her a tangible sign of a manageable and less restricted life for women, freed of the cumbersome, painful whalebone in corset and bustle. By using the veil in public, Montagu was able to pass unhindered and outside of the ambit of male scrutiny, penetrating into places hidden from Western eyes, like the harem. Montagu emphasizes what she refers to as the 'perpetual Masquerade' afforded women by the veil. It 'gives them entire Liberty of following their Inclinations without Danger or Discovery'.[49] Veils are fragile insulation against sexual enmity and even class discrimination. It is a restriction, as Srinivas Aravamudan observes, that nonetheless increases women's 'psychological agency'.[50]

The vividness of her account, coupled with their popularity, made Montagu one of the figures responsible for alterations in female dress. Especially in England, women had the option of more comfortable features, such as gowns of muslin or light silk gathered with a sash. Looser sleeves were made available, as opposed to the tight silk sheath around the arm, which could be gathered to the elbow when a room became hot and stuffy, which was not unusual. Another phenomenon was the fur-lined overgown placed over a simple muslin undergown, again held at the waist by ribbon or decorative rope. In either case, Turkish influence was highly moderated.[51]

There has been a fair amount of academic discussion as to where Montagu is situated according to notions of power, visibility and gender. Noting a particular entry by Montagu in the Turkish bath, where she compares the women to those painted by Italian Renaissance masters, Isobel Grundy and Cynthia Lowenstein comment that Montagu reveled in aestheticizing what she saw without delving too deeply into the less savoury aspects of women's life in Turkey. On the other hand, Elizabeth Bohls argues that Montagu's stance actually takes the place of those typically reserved for men. Her aestheticizing of the Turkish women is something different from eroticizing them, or making them libidinal scourges of the Ottoman threat.[52] Aravamudan also argues that Montagu played two types of masquerade simultaneously, one for the local population and the other relayed to her British readers. Montagu was not free of orientalist prying, but it is very much unto its own. According to Aravamudan, this very particular encounter 'revitalizes a neoclassical synthesis of Occident with Levant that is progressive and inclusionary', notwithstanding Montagu's comparison of the North African women as baboons.[53]

These debates aside, Montagu's account is still invoked as an early example of women breaking with domestic restraints and sartorial strictures. Her brief time in Turkey allowed her to experience social and somatic freedom little known to her western female contemporaries. Dressing up, especially in portraiture, would prove to have special place in England as the eighteenth century wore on. In her essay 'Women in Disguise', Gill Perry articulates how alternative modes of dress inscribed within the conventions of allegory and literature in Joshua Reynolds' portraits of women were methods of smoothing lines between public and private spaces, spaces that for women, were sharply defined. Women could 'become' natural and fecund for instance without being accused or lasciviousness.[54] Although the idioms of disguise in question were not oriental but classical and folkloric, Reynolds' portraits reveal a form of visual trope in dress that sheds considerable light on the way that fashion in the eighteenth century became as an active a tool as metaphor or transposition in poetry. It was a form of aristocratic communication through suggestion and symbols that would soon be lost.

Although this discussion has largely concentrated on England and France, the extent to which Chinese and Turkish conceits in masquerade had spread throughout other European countries should not be underestimated. Signs of Eastern influence in all forms of decoration, fashion and art are traceable across Europe to Russia, where Catherine's court were always anxious about keeping up with their Western counterparts. In Scandinavia, as in Russia, invoking the Orient was especially congenial since it represented a stark contrast in ways and climate. Extremes of taste were not necessarily the exception. In 1753, the queen of Sweden, Louisa Ulrika, was given a Chinese pavilion as a birthday present. The presentation ceremony involved a the whole court donning Chinese dress and aping what they thought were Chinese gestures, whereupon the seven-year-old prince handed over the keys dressed as a mandarin, after which occurred a Chinese ballet, itself an incongruous concept. When Marie Theresa, Marie Antoinette's mother was married to the Duke of Parma, the celebrations took the form of a Chinese fair in which teams of entertainers cavorted in a purpose-built piazza filled with special stalls and Chinese shops. Such entertainments were considered the pinnacle of fashion.[55]

Masquerade may have been the anachronism that the hedonistic elite of the eighteenth century before the revolution kept alive as a device within their own pleasurable distractions, but Montagu's dressing in Turkish clothing was the opposite. It was a device that anticipated forms of dress in which women felt autonomy rather than constraint. Orientalist dress during her stay in Turkey was a shell that gave her unprecedented manoeuvrability; and when she persisted in wearing it back in England, it remained a sign of the glimpses of independence she had while wearing it. It was thus a sign of liberation masquerading as masquerade. Paul Poiret would later write of the couturier's model that she 'had to be a woman more woman than women'.[56] In a sense, the fashion model of modernity was an atavism, plucked from a previous era. For, theatrically speaking, in the masquerade of the ancien régime, the Turk was more Turk than Turk, the Chinaman more Chinese, such is the nature of clichés pushed to state of exhaustion. Both strategies of masquerade—masquerade to conceal and masquerade as a vehicle for freer self-expression—kept to the idea that the East was a place of an ample variety of choices unavailable to the Westerner, however Montagu's example of using masquerade to liberate the self presaged the era that that was to topple old.[57] Montagu's manner of masquerade entertained some possibility, fictive or true, of new channels for subjectivity and choice. In retrospect we can see how it cast a line to women's liberation and hippies via Romantics and revolutionaries, for whom orientalist dress meant utopian disorder. A brief inspection of one of several posthumous portraits of her reveals how firmly Montagu had soldered herself into the romantic imagination. An 1844 portrait (itself a replica of an earlier image from 1836) (Fig. 15) depicts her decked out with a huge, overflowing turban, ornate trimming to her surcoat, intricate brocading and ostentatious oriental jewellery, leaving no doubt as to her sartorial allegiances. Montagu was for the nineteenth century very much a female archetype of one who had successfully and creatively embraced exoticism.

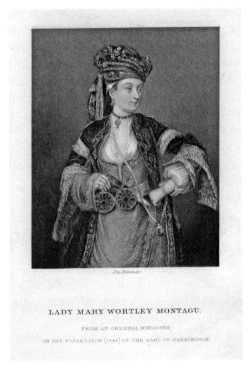

LADY MARY WORTLEY MONTAGU.

FROM AN ORIGINAL MINIATURE.

IN THE POSSESSION (1844) OF THE EARL OF HARRINGTON.

Figure 15 Joseph Brown, Unknown woman, called Lady Mary Wortley Montagu, 1844 (or after), line and stipple engraving, © National Portrait Gallery, London. Note that the NPG also have in their collection a likeness closely resembling this one, by William Greatbach, published by Richard Bentley, 1836.

LATE-EIGHTEENTH CENTURY AND THE REVOLUTION

The decade or so before the French Revolution is famous for its sartorial absurdities, from the size of the dress to the complexity of the hairstyle. Together with couturiers and coiffeurs, cosmetics in the latter half of the eighteenth century had become a competitive industry. In her excellent book on the birth of the cosmetic industry in France, Morag Martin recounts how marketers of perfumes, foundations, rouge, pomades and the like invoked the Orient to infuse their products with mystery and allure. Harem imagery abounded. One of the more famous face-whitening powders was *Serkis du sérial*, by Dissey and Piver, who went so far as to claim on their label that it was 'the favoured powder of sultans'. A disingenuous strategy this may have been, but it was also a case of a good story consorting with the truth since many of the main ingredients in cosmetics came from the Near East. 'Whether from the Ottoman Empire or further afield, exotic goods used for beauty—such as cochineal (from Goa), vermilion (from China), cinnabar, tartar, musk, rose water (from Persia), gray, amber, as well as countless spices', these were shipped in their raw form then packed or blended by French apothecaries and specialist sellers. As with silk, there were differing grades of products, and the Eastern suppliers did not shrink from attempting to circumvent the European middlemen. Whether or not the products actually came from the East, they found their way into homes with 'promises of beauty alongside cheap Oriental tales'. Martin cites Balzac's *César Birotteau*, whose eponymous hero invents a *Pâte des sultanes*. 'Eighteenth century advertisers, much like Balzac's perfumer, depended on their readers' association of their goods with literary and artistic Orientalism, bereft of any actual threat.'[58]

Together with what has already been discussed, the mass appeal of oriental allusion, however unreal and untrue, was of a piece with the appeal at the end of the eighteenth century to naturalness. One factor was Rousseau, whose contempt for the sartorial extremes of his day would have no small effect on the 'natural' fashions of the Revolutionary era. His ethos of a return to a state of nature did much to promote the use of free-flowing muslins over more cumbersome, stylized clothing.[59] The call to simple form and the devotion to all things natural was also an attribute of Enlightenment reason and its insistence on a set of core values. True enough, *nature* was one of the most frequently used words in fashion periodicals toward the end of the eighteenth century, reaching at peak during the Revolutionary and Directorial periods.[60] This was mainly with regard to the Greco–Roman style dominant in dress at the time, but especially in hairstyles, shawls and footwear, cultural references were frequently blurred, no less than the parameters of the meaning of 'nature' itself. Remarking on paintings he saw in the Salon, Mercier noted that as opposed to the powdered wigs and black coats, 'the clothing of the Hottentots is a hundred times less foreign to the brush' as it presents us with something far less jarring, meaning the contrivances of urban industrial life.[61]

Naturalness was something that Marie Antoinette ardently hoped to buy into when she had her court painter Vigée-Lebrun portray her as a shepherdess in a pleated muslin dress known as a *gaulle*, daintily holding a pink rose between forefinger and thumb. Instead of endearing herself to people with her common touch, it roused anger. The popular press proclaimed that she was dressed in a slip and had come from a harem. As McCabe observes, the irony was that although she had shed all the jewels and fineries that had burdened the public purse since Louis XIV's day, she was accused of wasting money on imports. To quell the outcry, bans were placed on imports from the Levant and England; before that she had been seen as frittering away money on expensive silks and putting stress on the industry in Lyon because of her demand for unusual colours. McCabe adds, 'as exotic imported luxuries, or their more affordable French copies, became part of more households, a philosophical debate arose about class, hierarchy and government'.[62]

Much has been made historically of the tide of vilification that Marie-Antoinette had to endure, but whatever side of the fence one stood on, the inescapable fact was that her insatiable taste for new dress designs, a highly rarified, exorbitant form of personal entertainment, contributed in no small part to a broader awareness of style and influence that germinated into an expanded vocabulary of fashion and taste. For the Queen was not alone. Her circle of ladies and then those under them were also under pressure to be a part of the tidal wave of investment in novelty. It was in this era that stylistic idioms in dress and design for the upper classes had very much meshed into an ornate allsorts, and where anyone in the know was conversant with looks *à l'italienne*, *à l'anglaise*, *à la polonaise*, together with those *à la circassienne* (an undergown with tight sleeves covered with another gown tucked up, while the faced was heavily rouge to give it a 'Circassian bloom'), *à la lévite*, *à la levantine* (an ermine-trimmed pelisse opening to an undergown and petticoat), *à la turque* and so on. It was also the case that theatre of courtly life was always in silent conversation with the theatre proper, especially with respect to fashion. There is plenty to suggest that the gown *à la lévite* derives from the Jewish priests' costumes in productions of Racine's *Athalie*. This was a relatively pared down affair involving a straight gown, with a shawl collar and back pleats, supported at the waist with a scarf, famously launched in 1778 by Marie Antoinette during her first pregnancy. (Just a year before her special boudoir in the Turkish style was completed for her at Fontainbleau.) Hairstyles and head adornments also had their fair share of oriental input from exotic flowers to centrepieces of tiger skin. In 1776, Lallemand published an *Essai sur la coiffure* from the Persian.

The thick soup of cultural reference presages modern and contemporary fashion. At this point, references to China in dress had receded and *à la turque* meant all things oriental. But it also meant that a desire to reach beyond the local or the domestic was tarred with the brush of aristocratic irresponsibility, an attitude of looking to the beyond instead of training one's ears to the mundane problems around them, of which there were many. This was so much the case that by the end of her reign, hatred for Marie Antoinette had spilled into distrust of foreignness in general—be it Austrian, Moroccan or Middle Eastern—which meant foreign foods, foreign goods, foreign clothes. An aggressive nationalism had set in that was only exacerbated when the Revolutionary wars isolated France from the rest of Europe.[63]

As is well known, the French Revolution was also a fashion revolution that marks the beginnings of modern dress: the suit, and the loose and manageable frock. When not considering the brashly ideological Phrygian cap and the incipient version of pants (*sans-coulottes*), male dress became more austere and angular. Pants, or trousers, were used as a popular strategy to differentiate from the more genteel breeches. It is true to say that they were worn by journeymen, sailors and workers, but to say exclusively is to buy into popular belief, for they were worn amongst the aristocracy who were interested in partaking in exotic languor, or 'social exoticism', to use Daniel Roche's phrase. While still confined to a minority, wearing trousers amongst the upper classes was popular among rakes and bourgeois free-wheelers.[64] It was the equivalent of high-meets-low lounge wear and associated with the myth of Eastern freedoms. Needless to say, such subtleties were jettisoned after 1789, when counterrevolutionaries set themselves apart from the shabby 'trouser-brigade' (*pantalonnades*).[65]

During the same period, women's clothing abandoned the volume and hypertrophy of the previous regime and became more streamlined and simplified, inspired after the paintings revealed from the archaeological digs of Herculaneum and Pompeii, spurred on by the rhetoric that related all things virtuous to the Roman Republic. The Turkish and Chinese tastes were jettisoned together with all outward signs of opulence as signs of the depraved and wasteful former regime. But this did not prevent the seepage of another kind of oriental influence *à la sauvage*, which was allied to the 'Otaheti' or Tahitian style, both subscribing to the Rousseauinisms that put ungirdled 'primitive' naturalness at a premium.

A welcome air of relief settled on Paris after the fall of the Jacobins in 1794. The Directory period released itself of the stately classicizing pretenses toward a culture very much as debauched as the one it replaced, except available to more people. Public tastes were eclectic and ravenous for newness. Kotzebue, a German traveller visiting Paris, commented that 'The whole world has to pay tribute to the toilette of the Parisian—one wears English cloth, Egyptian shawls, Roman sandals, Indian muslins, Roman riding boots and English waistcoats'.[66] The Greco–Roman women's fashions softened a little and took on various signs of exotic difference, finished by unusual jewelry and lavish headscarves which sometimes turned into something more assertive and turban-like, and on more formal occasions were finished with a peacock feather. The most famous turban, or turban-wearer, of the time was the writer–intellectual Germaine de Staël, daughter of Louis XVI's former finance minister, Jacques Necker. It seems that de Staël's turban was her own improvised equivalent of what the banyan had come to be for men. She was the contemporary of other protofeminists like Mary Wollstonecraft and Olympe de Gouges, for whom this orientalist touch was necessary to set herself apart from mainstream femininity. Heinrich Heine remarked of her 'enormous turban' that it was a way of presenting herself 'as the sultana of thought'.[67] Balzac would later make much of this association with the droll figure of the provincial *salonnière* Mme de Bargeton in *Illusions perdus*, whose elaborate turbans are meant to show off her literary acumen.[68]

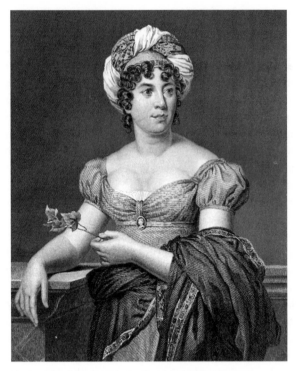

Figure 16   Germaine de Staël, early 1800s, engraving.

One only need remember back to Mme Pompadour's imitation of the sultana to find this an especially interesting remark. The ancien régime had developed its own form of matriarchy, in figures such as the formidable Mme du Deffand, whose salons had played a major part in the heady intellectual exchanges that helped to crystallize the Enlightenment. The Revolution had helped to shift the emphasis from groups far more to individuals. In the former period, the body was ensconced in all manner of finery: brocade, taffeta, silk and damask, which were decorated further with embroidery and lace. But the attraction was to the ravishing displays of fabrics and craftsmanship themselves, not, as Richard Sennett observes, 'as aids to setting off the peculiarities of his face or figure'. In the eighteenth century, bodies were more like mannequins, while in the subsequent era the body asserted its independence.[69] It did this through simplicity, concentrating on the person not the thing. One masquerade usurped another, although the modern one was—is— far harder to pick. Fashion was no longer something that intimidated with its brilliance as much as a series of more subtle devices to enframe the face— such as the cravat, or in Mme de Staël's case, the turban—to emphasize personality and point of view, or to inflect a classical ensemble (the relationship between a fashion classic originates in the appropriated classicism of this era), to accentuate one's individual discernment. Even Jane Austen wore a 'Mamluk' cap, whose feather was affixed with a crescent-shaped ornament.

An example of this is in the dress in the illustration below (Fig. 18). Made in England in 1800, it is the typical chemise-style dress that had scandalized the public when worn by Marie Antoinette and which became something of a female uniform during the revolution. It is Bengali Muslin embroidered with cotton thread. Assured and simple, this garment epitomizes what would come to be known as the 'Empire style', installed as part of the Napoleonic regime (Napoleon had just named himself First Consul in 1800), and of which the so-called Regency style of the soon to be George IV was the echo. Here the language of Ancient Rome aggressively overtook generic classicizing of the Revolution as a persuasive sign that the Napoleonic regime was the beginnings of an empire to mirror the old. Traditional discussions of these fashions commonly emphasize the Greco–Roman origins of this dress, which made women's bodies less confined and more statuesque, but less mentioned is the way in which it reinvigorated demand for Indian muslin. Steele adds that the classical antecedents of this dress cannot disregard the Creole roots that came from the sugar trade in the Caribbean that was a major source of France's eighteenth-century wealth. The bluish tinge with which many of such dresses were tinted came from the tropics, not from Greece or Rome.[70]

The lightweight, golden-coloured shawl, or pashmina, is finished with bold red paisley designs, which had started to enter into sartorial currency and which would become one of the signatures of the Anglo–Indian fashions of the nineteenth century. The pashmina (meaning 'soft hair' in Persian and Kashmiri), such as the kind seen here, became especially popular after the Egyptian campaign. During this time, Napoleon sent them to Joséphine by the

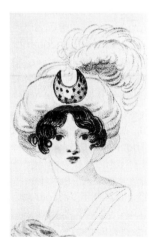

Figure 17   Jane Austen in a Mameluke turban: illustration in *The Fashions of London and Paris*, February 1804.

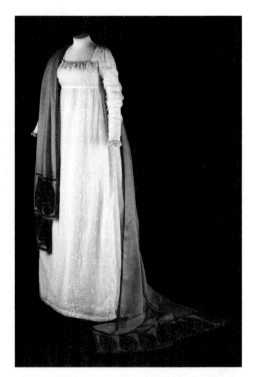

Figure 18 Muslin gown and cashmere shawl, c. 1800; Bengali cotton; Gift of Miss Frances Vickers, © V&A Images; Victoria and Albert Museum, London.

hundreds. She first responded to with studied distaste: 'They may be beautiful and expensive with the advantage of lightness, but I very much doubt that they will ever be fashionable.'[71] Yet they became her signature item. Ironically, or perhaps in uncanny synchronicity with contemporary trends, Joséphine stemmed from a white Creole family who owed their wealth to sugar trading. Her youth in Martinique saw the influence of the more natural dress of the ancien régime, with its incidental debt to her own local culture and that of the Indes. In addition to the shawls, and neat *fichus*, it was not uncommon to have one's hair simplified and more natural *à la créole*. Joséphine's biographer Ernest Knapton reports how it was during these years before the Revolution. Joséphine's aunt Fanny would have herself coiffed *à la giraffe* when visiting Buffon's museum of natural history.[72]

As the socially astute Joséphine knew only too well, accessorizing was the most important factor in female dress of her day. The white dress had become ubiquitous, and its simplicity and austerity had to remain untouched to maintain an image of flawlessness. (It is worth noting, however, that late in Napoleon's reign, cotton imports were irregular due to the British blockade, which meant that trade routes to France from the Levant were almost exclusively by land; the situation was made worse when in 1814 France was forced to consume English cottons.) Like Marie Antoinette before her, who enlisted Rose Bertin as the main gainsayer of fashion concerns, Joséphine's primary advisor on fashion, or more specifically fashionable accessories, was Louis-Hippolyte Leroy, whose firm was the leader in a quickly expanding retail market of feathers, perfumes, gloves, lace, scarves and shawls.

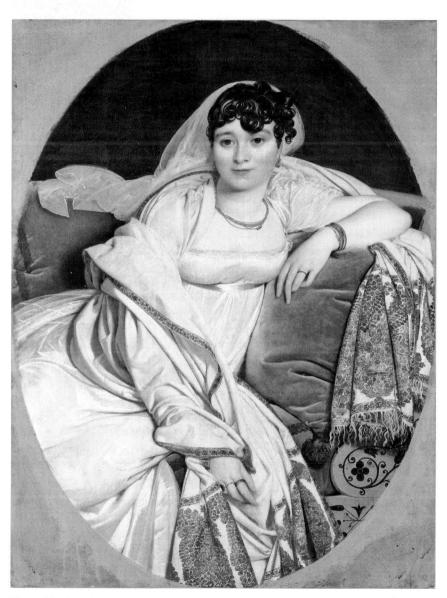

Figure 19   Jean-Auguste-Doninique Ingres, *Mme Rivière*, 1805, oil on canvas, © RMN (Musée du Louvre)/Thierry Le Mage.

As we shall see more in the next chapter, shawls became the most common fashion item for women in the first half of the nineteenth century. They came in various forms—muslin, percale, gauze, plain or heavily embroidered—but cashmere was by far the most coveted. Unlike silk, cashmere came from alpine goats, not worms, and was harder to cultivate in Europe, which meant its rarity prevailed. The painting below (Fig. 19) is the famous early (1806) portrait by Ingres of Madame Rivière, who is shown lolling in a shawl with the very popular 'pine cone' motif like the one in the previous illustration. This is first of a long love affair that Ingres would have with the cashmere shawl. Other ones, uncannily like it, feature in at least two other portraits by Ingres over the next ten years. Ingres knew of Francis Smith's *Eastern Costumes* (1769), sketched Lady Montagu's tomb, and maintained a curiosity for orientalist accessories throughout his life, from turbans to vividly striped fabrics to hookahs to shell jewellery, inserting them into his portraits of women.[73] When it was purchased by the state in 1870, the painting came to be known as '*la femme au châle*' (woman with the shawl) because, as one Ingres scholar remarks, it is 'almost the soul of the painting'.[74]

EGYPTOMANIA

Like the other styles in its extended orientalist family, Egyptian influence can be charted back to Hellenistic culture and to the Alexandrian cults of Rome. As but one of the many imports that reflected their vast and heterogeneous empire, Roman Emperors frequently welcomed Egyptian influences, whether in architecture or jewellery. The permeations of Egyptian style are yet more proof that notion of classical style is very much an ideological construction spearheaded by luminaries like Winckelmann and Schinkel in Germany and the Adam brothers in Britain, who moulded the style for themselves to reflect their Enlightenment ideals of rational harmony. This said, Egyptian style, Egyptianizing, Egyptian influence became a style with its own autonomy and a recognizable retinue of traits, Egyptomania, with Napoleon's invasion of Egypt in 1798. From a military perspective it was a tragic botch, but it was a turning point for European imperial perspectives. A dimension of the Egyptian style is its boldness and confidence in having made a significant incursion into the Middle East, not long ago a great empire.

Like all styles adopted in a packaged form from the eighteenth century onwards, it survived on the myth that it hailed from an imperviously pure source, anchored in a series of stereotypes made through the familiarity wrought by repetition. Quintessential Egyptian traits that have existed for over the last two centuries include sphinxes, Cleopatra, asps, cats, stylized bodies that were flattened and contorted, blue lapis, and architecture that was thick and authoritative. As one of the earliest great empires, Egypt was suffused with mystery, and by erecting mausolea (a particular favourite for the Egyptian style), decorating rooms and wearing Egyptian-style jewellery and clothing, the cognoscenti of the early nineteenth century could appear to be participating in the very origins of civilized life which predated Judeo–Christian codes for millennia. By plundering a culture earlier than theirs, they could keep their revolutionary credentials intact, while also safely subscribing to the heaving massing of Egyptian architecture which was sympathetic to the mentality of a large and unified Napoleonic Empire, and after, as something remote and mythic, nostalgic of his failed promise.

Technically speaking, the contemporary vernacular fashions in Egypt at the time of Napoleon's arrival had very little to do with the lofty Egyptian style. The troops would conveniently refer to the local denizens generically as Turks, to whom, in fashion and face, they were superficially the same. Women's fashions that made their way to Paris were consistently generic, such as the tunics *à la mameluck* or *à la Juive*, in vogue in 1802–3. For men, traces of the Egyptian campaign permeated every level of the military; there were countless forays in Eastern clothing, as in the comic episode of the young Napoleon, cited at the beginning of this chapter. It seems that despite this comedic contretemps, Napoleon was not entirely deterred, since he used his re-entry into Paris as an opportunity to feign a usurped inheritance to the once-proud and dazzling Mameluke cavalry, whose defeat in the Battle of the Pyramids at the beginning of the campaign (July 1798) was one of his few real victories in a string of mishaps and failures. Marie Tussaud in her memoires recounts how in his triumphal return, Napoleon was 'dressed in the costume of a Mameluke, in large white trousers, red boots, waistcoat richly embroidered, as also the jacket which was made of crimson velvet'.[75]

From the time of Napoleon's campaign until the 1830s, Egypt remained a crucible of Anglo–French imperial rivalry, both symbolically and materially. Artefacts, ideas and clothing were ways of staking one's claim to a global empire and to showing interest in faraway historical secrets. Maya Jasanoff in her account of the relationship between conquest and collecting in this period makes clear that the Middle East and especially Egypt was a place where people were able to reinvent themselves, to make good their past and to stake their claim to a different identity. When the last of the Bourbons, Charles X, ascended to the throne in 1824, although hostile to what he saw as the illegitimacy of the Napoleonic era and everything associated with it, he proved to be a consummate Egyptophile, supporting the Egyptian hall in the Louvre that was opened in 1826. British jockeying for dominance in the Nile Valley also piqued French interest in Egypt.[76] For the French, the cheapest and easiest way of asserting provisional ownership was through Egyptian decorative objects and in Egyptianizing accessories, whether the trimming on gloves, exaggerated tassels or handbags.

MILITARY COSTUME AND WEAPONRY

When the grisly details of the campaign had subsided to into a haze of exotic grandeur, Egyptian details were worn as a sign of intrepid courage. Officers, irrespective of whether they had served in the campaign or not, began to adopt Middle Eastern touches, from scarves and sashes—frequently cashmere, as a sign of status—around the waist and adopting a sabre à la mamelouk, to bedecking horses with leopard skins, symbolic trophies of ferocity tamed. In Egypt, Napoleon sought to form his own élite corps, enlisted from the vanquished Mameluke cavalry, with mixed success. From this came escadron des mamelouks de la Garde impériale, which was to remain a permanent fixture of the army in the early years of the nineteenth century. By the early 1800s, most of its number had never been to Egypt, but it was an excuse to wear oriental-inspired uniforms or adopt the relevant flourishes as in, for instance, the Marmeluke sword in David's first portrait (1816) of the parvenu officer Henri-Amédé de Turenne, who only took up service in 1805 and therefore had no first-hand knowledge of the Egyptian–Syrian campaign. Today, the Turkish scimitar, with its arced handle and blade, is used in the ceremonial uniform of the US Marine Corps.

These adaptations were of no special interest to the Eastern European nations who since well into the fifteenth century had been warding off the Ottoman threat. Most accessible to popular memory is perhaps Vlad Tepes, the historical inspiration for Bram Stoker's Dracula, who spent his youth under Ottoman service before defecting back to his home in Wallachia, now Transylvania. Vlad wore the free, brightly coloured tunic and studded belt of Turkish soldiers and, most noticeably, the cylindrical hat faced with a single plume affixed with a gem worn by pashas and senior officers (he rose to the equivalent of colonel in the Ottoman Army). Such plumes were not freely obtainable in Europe and could mean a trophy, or, in Vlad's case, knowledge of Turkish ways of warfare and torture.[77]

Areas of south-east Europe, particularly Serbia, were touched by the Ottoman influence, such as the 'Dellys', the troops from the late-sixteenth century that volunteered for the sultan's army. They were lovers of ostentatious finery, cladding their armour and horse with ornamentation and plumage as badges of their courage. For several hundred years, Eastern Europe, now Romania, Moldavia and Hungary were sites of considerable threat and turbulence, where European and Ottoman culture in many respects overlapped. This region began to be freed from the Ottoman rule with the Great Turkish wars, beginning with the siege of Vienna in 1683 and culminating in the submission of the Ottomans at the hands of Prince Eugene of Savoy and the Treaty of Karlowitz in 1699. Thus the Ottoman influence of nothing out of the ordinary and can be seen in countless historical examples, from the distinctive shape

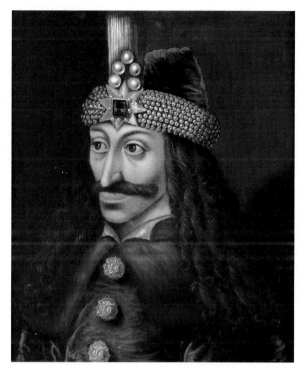

Figure 20 Anonymous, *Vlad IV/Vlad Tepes* (Vlad the Impaler), second half of the sixteenth century, © Kunsthistorisches Museum Wien, Gemäldegalerie.

of Ottoman shields to the decoratively angular shapes of armour and other military clothing. In civilian clothing, slumped loose hats and the free use of tassels were adopted traditional wear of the region, as were bright floral designs amongst women's' clothing. By way of analogy, Spain too retains signs of occupation by the North African Moors in its national identification of with the *Maja* dress from Andalusia.[78] The bright red and black needlework so jealously held as indigenous to Saxony and Transylvania owes itself in no small part to bright Turkish designs, not least from those found on carpets. (It was not until the mid-eighteenth century that European production, specifically in France and Holland, began to rival the favoured *rubia peregrina*, the madder plant from Turkey which gave their textiles their distinctive vibrancy and durability and which also accounted for their stupendous costliness.[79]) There were other accessories that lived on, such as beading, weapons and armour. The scimitar continues to be employed in much Eastern European traditional ceremonial dress.

Oriental weaponry would have a lasting fascination on the European imagination. It was a quintessential talisman of the Orient, and its combination of beauty and peril, with all the subtending sexual connotations. In one of Balzac's early novels set in 1799, *Les Chouans*, the heroine Marie contemplates killing her rival Mme de Gua:

> She had thrown into one of the boxes an elegant dagger, once upon a time carried by a sultana, with which she wanted to arm herself when venturing to the theatre of war, like one of those wags who gets hold of one of those albums for ideas for when they travel; but she was less seduced by the prospect of having to spill blood than by the joy of carrying a pretty *cangiar* adorned with small stones and toying with its blade, pure as dew.[80]

The *cangiar*, or *kandjar*, is a Turkish or Albanian cutlass with a large pommel. It would have been especially rare to have had one at this time, for these items were to spill into France only a few years later. Balzac was most likely undeterred by such details. But what this passage illustrates is the transgressive import of such objects. They became archetypes for the Romantic consciousness, springboards for all kinds of fanciful and inaccurate forays into lavish nonexistent scenes and unrealizable desires.

−3−

1815–1871: Turkophilia, Afromania and the Indes

I wish to be perspicuous and the black,
  I say, unlocking the recess, pull'd forth
A quantity of clothes fit for the back
  Of any Musselman, whate'er his worth;
And of variety there was no lack—
  And yet, though I have said there was no dearth,
He chose himself to point out what he thought
  Most proper for the Christians he had bought.

The suit he thought most suitable to each
  Was, for the elder and the stouter, first
A candiote cloak, which to the knee might reach,
  And trousers not so tight that they would burst,
But such as fit an Asiatic breech;
  A shawl, whose folds in Cashmere had been nurst,
Slippers of saffron, dagger rich and handy;
  In short, all things which form a Turkish Dandy.

—Byron, *Don Juan*, Canto V, stanzas 67 and 68

Yet neither high Egyptian nights nor the black and opulent coffee with cardamom seed nor the frequent literary discussions with the Doctors of the Law nor the venerable muslin turban nor the meals eaten with his fingers made him forget his British reticence, the delicate central solitude of the masters of the earth.

—Jorge Luis Borges, 'Translators of *The Thousand and One Nights*'[1]

Byron did more than dress his poetic dramas in oriental costume. For him the Orient was the poetic tool of escape. He was an archetypal figure even in his own day, and among the first of what would be a healthy line of artists, poets, novelists, journalists, dandies, venturesome aristocrats, travellers, elegant vagabonds and winsome eccentrics for whom orientalist clothing was a key to an outside—the first and most visible escape from convention.

Byron's poems, Hugo's *Orientales*, Nerval's travels to the Orient, the conceits of Flaubert are among the more lasting of what had become its own industry: cultural, personal and economic. For the arch-Bohemian Théophile Gautier, orientalist dress was a certain way of expressing dissatisfaction with the corseted bourgeois values of the industrial West by identifying with an external state that was less physical and more the province of imagination. It suggested the promise of a sensuous beyond, which surpassed the immediate circumstances in pleasure and possibility. While amateurs used orientalist dress as a means of skirting the borders of straight-laced society, artists enlisted it for self-promotion. They could literally wear their difference on their sleeve. To much of nineteenth-century Europe, orientalist dress was typically used as an attribute, not of assimilation to Eastern ways of life but as something more self-serving: it was one of the nineteenth-century artist's most important tools in the Romantic box of vainglorious tricks.

It is therefore telling, but no more surprising, that the painting most responsible for keeping the Byronic myths afloat is a sham in more ways than one. Byron is depicted in vermilion Albanian robes and headscarf in a smugly heroic pose that suggests that he is a habitué to such roles. Completed eleven years after Byron's death in 1824, Thomas Phillips' portrait is associated with the poet's departure for Missolonghi to join the Greeks in their war of independence against the Turks. Well known is that he never fought in the war—he died prosaically of fever; less well known is that the picture was taken from a sitting in 1813, when Byron had chosen to dress himself up from clothing he had acquired four years before, and long before he would ever have entertained fighting for Greek independence. Today the portrait is assurance that he is the fair embodiment of the orientalist escapades of alter-egos Childe Harold and Don Juan (see Figure 21).

As Richard Martin and Harold Koda state in their catalogue to the exhibition of orientalist dress at MoMA in 1994, 'Orientalism is never a narrow-gauge or scholastic enterprise in fashion. Rather, it is a fantasy, often a composite and customarily syncretised'.[2] It is a statement that can as justly be applied to Byron's poetry, and contemporaries such as Southey, as it can be to fashion. For in this period, orientalism had become immensely fluid and now a common resource, mined by all but the lowest strata of society, as opposed to just the very rich. For Coleridge and Wordsworth as for Byron, the translation in 1704–7 of the *Arabian Nights* by Antoine Galland was more than a literary event; it had a liberating influence on their spirit and their poetry.[3] As John Beer explains,

> There was more to Arabia than the *Arabian Nights* and poetry, also. The Bedouin tribes, whose independent and wandering life must have appealed deeply to a young man such as Wordsworth, knew it as home. His desire to fortify his own philosophy by discovering isolated figures who had achieved wisdom far from

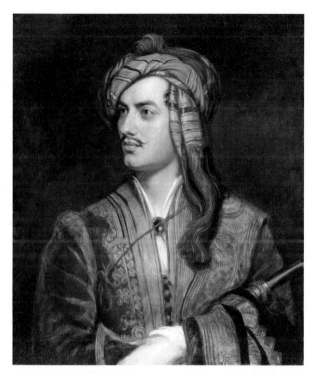

Figure 21. Thomas Phillips, *George Gordon Byron, 6th Baron Byron*, (1813) replica c. 1835, oil on canvas, © National Portrait Gallery, London.

the sources of conventional learning had been answered in the Lake District by his encounters with shepherds and wandering solitaries; but the Bedouin tradition, with its suggestions of civilisation that might combine rigorous thinking with adeptness in the skills of horsemanship was even more appealing. The knowledge that mathematics had flourished early in that part of the world gave rise to a welcome sense of a desert wisdom embodying the very contradictions he could trace in his won society, the intellectual discipline of mathematics existing side by side with a feeling for the refreshing power of romance.[4]

Orientalism had steeped into European society as more than just a place of reverie; it represented very real alternatives to contemporary ethics. This is well in evidence when one turns to Shelley's works about individual and social expressive liberty, from *the Revolt of Islam* to *Prometheus Unbound*. Here the East is used as a device for finding alternatives to what were believed to be exhausted Western principles. Several factors nourished reasons for the East being the greatest theme for the English Romantics. By 1812, through both trade and conquest, British India had become a discernible empire unto itself that was as profitable in providing a repository for imagination and desire as it was for commerce and trade. It fulfilled needs of personal expression whilst also being the idiom for a political, universalizing consciousness. It was also during this time Christian missions were directed toward India in a proselytizing mission that made it the new cultural frontier. As the symbol of alternatives par excellence, the East was a cultural metaphor, a decoy and a vector for such discussions, particular within educated circles.[5]

The progressiveness of wearing obviously non-Western clothing in the previous century had opened itself out into a much broader structure of ideas, hedging its way from the private realm to more robust external pronouncements. Nicholas Dew in his book on the orientalism of Louis XIV's court contests Hugo's lapidary statement in the preface to *Les Orientales*: 'au siècle de Louis XIV on était helleniste, maintenant on est orientaliste' [the era of Louis XIV was Hellenist; today we are orientalist].[6] As we have seen in the two previous chapters, Dew's claims to the extent of orientalisms during this period are well made, yet he may be missing the thrust of Hugo's statement, which is to highlight a mentality that is much harder to characterize according to trappings or material examples. This mentality does not have to do with the simple emulation of Eastern attributes and mores so much as embracing, or committing to, the desire to overstretch one's creative impulses. Hugo can be interpreted as suggesting that one imbibed orientalism, or wore it like an invisible skin, as it was the defining component to free and creative spirits. Similarly, Byron, particularly of the later period, favoured the theme of how an irregular life may in fact be more moral than one of orthodox piety, and of course orientalism was the objective correlative to his special heterodoxy. Orientalist fashions, seen together with all other orientalisms, from ideas to objects, not only had transgressive import but also represented the desire to overstep borders and thresholds, national and spiritual. When we come to the figure of Pierre Loti later in this chapter, we will see that the assimilation of Eastern clothing and beliefs becomes such an intricate matter that an argument, Saidian or otherwise, that aligns the liberties taken by Westerners together with the Western power to do so seems coarse and misaligned.

Bookended by the end of the age of Napoleon and the outbreak of the Franco–Prussian War of 1870, this period is a golden age of orientalism. The extraordinary discoveries afforded by Napoleon's Egyptian campaign, not least of which is the decoding of the Rosetta Stone, secured orientalism as field of serious rational inquiry. As in the example of Byron and with innumerable cases in his wake, three kinds of orientalism competed for attention. One was scientific and philological, another was commercial, and the third was an eclectic theme park of artists and artefacts, where accuracy played an inversely proportional role to distraction.

Before the century was to draw to a close, these various phenomena, from distraction to disinterest, found their home in the Society of French Orientalist

Painters, presided over by the figure of Léonce Bénédite until his death in 1925. Inspired in 1889 after the Algerian exhibition pavilion at the Universal Exposition, it was the most significant statement of French imperial expansion and art. All elements of orientalism became matters of serious study, and art was a place where the Orient in its complexity could be put up for interpretation. Thus the fancy that we associate with orientalism was also married to serious scrutiny, where fashion and decorative arts played an integral part. Bénédite, who had a sincere, albeit self-mythologizing devotion to orientalism, was a proselytizer of orientalist style in art and design. In the 1880s, before the Society was formed in earnest, Bénédite lectured at the Central Union of the Decorative Arts about chinoiserie and the indebtedness of French fashion to the Orient. As Roger Benjamin notices, Bénédite must be credited for offering up orientalism as a separate category.[7] His efforts are not to be seen in isolation however, but as the culmination of influence that, in the nineteenth century amounted to the transition from an idea that represented the peripheral and the imperfectly known, to an enmeshing of acceptable and imperfect knowledge but circumscribed and codified within everyday European (and American) life.

This is also the era when certain precepts about the 'primitive' and the oriental became conflated and solidified, which persist to the present day. As Sally Price observes, the primitives did not conform to Western bourgeois ways and were neither rigid nor conformist but obeyed nature's rules, not ones supplied by mercantile self-interest. 'Primitives are also seen, from a Western perspective, as non-conformists', were sexually free and socially uninhibited. Thus social rigidities of ritually oriented societies were conveniently overturned. Primitives were known to be communal and socially aware. 'Together', Price suggests, 'these associations are capable of casting Primitive societies into the mould of an artistic counterculture or bohemian community in the Western sense.'[8] By definition, primitives were untamed—the name Aboriginal, used to lump together the many Australian indigenous peoples, simply means primal or originary—and therefore both more exciting and truthful to man's inner nature. Since Rousseau, the idea of nature and truth were catch-cries for all sorts of alternative methods and views. Orientalism, and most conspicuously orientalist fashion and dress, stands at the epicentre of these countercultures, which converge in the notion of Bohemianism.

The emergence of Bohemianism was a rather striking extreme of a much greater transformation of dress, which is essentially the change from premodern to modern dress. As Richard Sennett describes in *The Fall of Public Man*, the late-eighteenth century witnessed a more pronounced separation between the private and public spheres, in which the latter became eroded in favour of the former, which was itself a register of individual experience. With romanticism, there was, argues Sennett, a greater emphasis on personal authenticity that eschewed overt decoration in favour of a visual rhetoric of naturalness. Sennett likens the ornate dress of the eighteenth century to something akin to a theatrical costume; the body was like a mannequin, which was geared almost entirely for a public world. By distinction, romanticism celebrated individual authenticity and truth.[9] And in the words of Entwistle, 'The idea that character is immanent in appearance became increasingly popular in the nineteenth century'. She goes on to state that romanticism 'prioritises the "natural" over the artifice and superficiality of appearance'.[10]

But this is only partly true, at least when held up to the light of the dress of the Romantic Bohemian. Pantheism, talk of inherent rights and letting children be children were very much in vogue, but naturalness, when it comes to clothing, is another matter altogether. Orientalism holds a place on both sides of this spectrum, for it was a presence within free-flowing muslins and shawls, but it was also at the service of artifice. Artifice was favoured by the new brand of Romantic artist who had to draw attention to himself to the point of spectacle to attract a clientele. Walter Benjamin's observation stands out in this regard: 'Baudelaire knew that the true situation of the man of letters was: he goes to the marketplace as a flâneur, supposedly to look at it, but in reality to find a buyer.'[11] Self-consciously free-spirited, artists saw themselves as the new spiritual aristocracy. It was they who need to look different, at once desirable and threatening. But it also behooved the artist to be truthful to his own individual 'nature'. The sartorial syntax of naturalness could take the form of invoking natural desire, which could amount to long Bohemian tresses and a brazen 'oriental' red to highly contrived hairstyles. Either way, as far as the 'civilized' West was concerned, both pure naturalness and exoticism were quantities that were foreign, and somewhere in a far-off, imaginary space they met.

The post-Revolutionary association of freedom—an abstract, malleable concept—with orientalism meant that in the first decades of the nineteenth century, overtly orientalist clothing[12] underwent a recognizable shift. Chinoiserie, which had dominated Paris and London for almost two centuries, was on the wane. Its slow demise was because it was twice tarred with the brush of the autocratic despotisms of both China and the ancien régime. Chinoiserie in decorations, textiles and accessories was a highly ornate style that was stamped with the hedonism of privileged excess. It did not lend itself to expedient improvisation. It was expensive, and its flaunted detail required skilled specialist workmanship, which had been all but wiped out in the Revolution by violence or discouragement. As Hyatt Mayor points out, the rococo and chinoiserie were opposites to the next generation ' "Gothick", whose stamped-out, serial ornaments helped to make them favourites for mass production in the early days of the industrial revolution'. Chinoiserie's intricacies made it a far more specialized artisanal affair; it was at the 'whims of small, incredibly secure coteries who thought and acted in ampler elbow-room than any society ever enjoyed before or since'.[13] Its florid details were anachronistic to the more modern taste and prone to satire.

For example, Charles Lamb, in his essay 'Old China' (1823), mocks the style's effeteness, the men with 'women's faces' and the women 'with still more womanish expressions', one of whom exerts herself with 'a dainty mincing foot' in a preposterous setting.[14] Chinoiserie would enjoy a short and desultory revival during the Second Empire of Napoleon III, particularly in their love of lacquered furniture, but overall it remained a reminder of an aristocratic age of no restraint, no industry and limited obligation. This era was treated with sentimental nostalgia by many, such as the Goncourt brothers' set of essays under the title *Art of the Eighteenth Century* (1875), which did much to foment the rococo revival evident in the curlicues of art nouveau. With the rococo must come chinoiserie. But when chinoiserie was revived at this time it was through the lens of Japonism, as opposed to how it had been in the previous centuries, the obverse.

BOHEMIANISM

As many historians of bohemia are quick to warn, there is nothing monolithic about it. Its contemporary association is Puccini's opera *La Bohème* (1896), based on the famous Henri Murger work, *Scènes de la vie bohème* (1849). Its histories also vary remarkably. Elizabeth Wilson's *Bohemians: Glamorous Outcasts*, is unusual in the way it oversteps the usual anchorage of the idea in mid-nineteenth-century Paris and London to characterize a certain cultural pathology which she sees beginning with Byron, of a type who seeks sovereignty through unconventional behaviour.[15] Bohemianism is, after all, still an idea that is loosely applied today for arty people with contempt for property and whose thirst for adventure, in the form of travel or elicit substances, is greater than their need for security. As a result, they are considered by the mainstream as outside the realms of propriety: they are deemed irresponsible and feckless, since they exist outside the boundaries of common decency. While I still ascribe to the socio-historical grounding of the idea of Bohemianism, Wilson's far broader strokes suit me as well, since they embrace the gamut of activities climaxing in 1970's hippie-dom, in which orientalist dress plays a central part, which will be the subject of a later discussion. Mary Gluck, one of the best historians of Bohemia in recent years, propounds a more restrained but similar view to Wilson's. Gluck makes the distinction between what she calls 'classic' Bohemia and what she terms 'ironic' or 'popular' Bohemia, which 'never ascribed to the myth of autonomy . . . It rejected all stable aesthetic truths or moral absolutes as incompatible with the unprecedented experiences of modernity'.[16] Her focus is less on orientalism and more on primitivism and the mediaeval revivalism, which was used as an avenue of tribal mystery or archaic escapism that trumped the utilitarian obviousness of academic art and the mercantile middle classes that it served.

What remains important for the moment is the manner in which Bohemia can be classed both as an historical phenomenon as well as a pan-historical mentality that is in opposition to what is perceived to be middle-class insularity and indifference to the bourgeois cult of security and conformity. Seen in this light, the Bohemian seeks the dissolution of the status quo first through aesthetic means that lead to a subjective liberation that supports free, uninhibited creative thought. The exotic is, needless to say, as important an item in the arsenal of stylistic and social displacement as ever. But a caveat must be put on the exotic at this point: it could either be oriental or anything that was different from common appearances which, by the 1830s, was becoming increasingly normative when it came to the state of male dress. Thus, to quote Gluck:

> Young men to be seen everywhere, sporting Venetian outfits from the sixteenth century, Polish military uniforms from Brandenburg, Hungarian hussars' mantles, and oriental robes of all kinds, which were worn as personal markers of artistic identity and distinction.[17]

The aesthetic amalgamations in chinoiserie thus became more eclectic and less focused on a single (imaginary) state. Whereas chinoiserie must be seen as a gesture of fealty in autocratic despotism and in terms of hypothetical colonization, or colonization achieved solely through aesthetic means, orientalism for the artistic avant-garde after the fall of Napoleon was more an exercise of escape than of claim.

There is much argument about the stance of Western lovers of the Orient at this time. Said, as we know, made Nerval's *Voyage en Orient* (1851), an account of his travels to Cairo and Beirut, a centrepiece for his *Orientalism*. Although Nerval was critical of European intervention, Said argues that he cannot escape the prejudices of being a privileged observer. He, like Fromentin and Flaubert, carries with him the confidence of colonization, spurred on by the French conquest of Algiers in 1830. One of the longstanding criticisms of Said's first book is that his main source is literature. While it is undeniable that the French and British, as with any other European nation, had no compunction about stereotyping its colonial and Asian counterparts within the areas of textiles and dress, as we have seen so far, the complexities of trade and cross-cultural exchange make a guilt-inspiring opposition seem obtuse. It is not my task to dissect the authors who have inspired Said's well-known critique but rather to look at many of them and their contemporaries according to what they wore. As I have already acknowledged in the introduction to this book, the act of wearing the dress of the other does assume a certain degree of sovereignty, but this consideration is not exclusive or general. I have continued to expose the different ways in which so-called oriental, non-Western styles are themselves the result of elaborate channels of construction. This was the case with the banyan: born in Japan and nurtured in India under European eyes for consumption by Europeans to show that their outlook was more than just European. When it comes to suggestions of power, the awareness of the colonial misdemeanours were mixed. For many of the artistic avant-garde, the ideological concerns voiced by Said were not high on their agenda. Neither are they to be called to task for this, since aesthetic preoccupations can themselves be political. And what is most important to remember is that orientalism in dress within the Bohemian's wardrobe was one of the ways in which he brought the establishment, that is the forces of colonization, into account. The Bohemian thereby became the other in more than one way: in the face of the ruling classes he 'became' the oriental as much as he became the more himself, that is the individual, the flâneur or dandy, the free aesthetic subject who refused to be subsumed by the codes of the industrial bourgeoisie.

The mid-nineteenth century was also a period steeped in deep self-consciousness about dress in a way that was different from the previous era, for the simple reason that appearances were prone to be more deceptive as opposed to reflective of (God's) law. Dress could therefore be a source of some anxiety, since people could be suspected of false identities: novelists from Balzac to Proust took great relish in the contretemps that sprang from situations brought on by the confounding of class, status and dress.[18] It was Balzac who coined the term *vestignomie*, the vestimentary equivalent of physiognomy, where instead of reading someone's face, one read the manner of dress. The implications of this for orientalism are immense but also complicated, since it could be used as signifying difference but also sidestepping it, for the 'primitive', while ethnographically inferior, was free of class. For the bourgeois, orientalism in silks and cashmeres spelt exotic luxury and rarity, whereas other, less expensive examples of orientalism—fezzes and vests and the like—for the Bohemian meant displacement of class structures and a scrambling of the 'vestimiognomic' code. Since the middle-nineteenth century, positivist viewpoint saw character as ultimately congenital, whereas the Bohemian took exception to this and saw it as aesthetically spiritual. The primitive–orientalist inflection within Bohemianism was both a debasement and a transcendental raising in one and the same moment of issues of class and character.

Writing toward the end of the nineteenth century, Jerome K. Jerome, in his satirical classic *Three Men in a Boat*, offers a less auspicious view of orientalist-style clothing:

George has bought some new things for this trip, and I am rather vexed about them. The blazer is loud. I should not like George to know that I thought so, but there really is no other word for it. He brought it home and showed it to us on

Thursday evening. We asked what colour he called it, and he said he didn't know. He didn't think there was a name for the colour. The man had told him that it was an Oriental design. George put it on, and asked us what we thought of it. Harry said that, as an object to hang over a flowerbed in early spring to frighten the birds away, he should respect it. . .[19]

Jerome is not writing about Bohemians, but this vignette allows a less-earnest perspective of a style that in conservative, 'respectable' circles could be received as outré and lurid.

The great Bohemian stalwart who remained devout to orientalist dress was poet and journalist Théophile Gautier, a close friend of Baudelaire, and fellow disciples to an aesthetic orient, Jules Barbey d'Aurevilly and Nerval. In an letter to Nerval, Gautier proclaimed, 'It seems to me that I've lived in the East; and when I disguise myself in the carnival with a caftan and a tarbouche I feel I am wearing real clothes again. I have always been surprised not to understand Arabic fluently. I must have forgotten it.'[20] This is far more than a fanciful remark; it is part of a lifelong preoccupation that straddled the inner orient as a wellspring of creative energy and the sartorial orient, the best manner of dressing, and thus *performing* the artist, which he saw as the artist's duty, especially in regard to asserting artistic individualism. 'It is strange' wrote Gautier some time before he went to Algeria, that

we believe we have conquered Algeria, and Algeria has conquered us. Our women already wear scarves interwoven with thread of gold, streaked with a thousand colours, which have served the harem slaves, our young men are adapting the camelhair burnous. The tarbouch has replaced the classic cashmere skull-cap, everyone is smoking a nargileh, hashish is taking the place of champagne; our Spahi officers look so Arab one would think they had captured themselves with a smala; they have adopted all the Oriental habits, so superior is primitive life to our so-called civilization.

If this goes on, France will soon be Mahometan and we shall see the white domes of mosques rounding themselves on our horizons, and minarets mingling with steeples, as in Spain at the time of the Moors. We should indeed like to live to see the day. . .[21]

When Gautier finally did travel to Algeria in 1845, he returned wrapped in a *bernous* and holding a baby lion. He was forever identified with Middle Eastern forms of dress, especially the fez or other tasselled caps. Someone who saw him just before his death in 1872 observed: 'On his head was a red knitted cap; the tassel drooping down on his curling hair gave it the appearance of a tarbouche [a cylindrical style Turkish hat] and recalled our journey to Egypt, where we had all adopted the oriental fez.'[22]

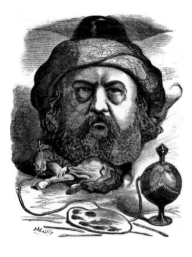

Figure 22 Hyppolite Mailly, *Théophile Gautier*, late 1800s, engraving.

This was more than mere affectation. As perhaps the most influential critic of the Second Empire, Gautier's besottedness with the Orient in dress and otherwise ensured that it maintained a steady, popular endorsement. Gautier extended his love of the Orient into many different spheres of experience— this is crucial to the understanding of the oriental and other unconventional clothing worn by Bohemians. It was far from a sartorial conceit but a way of showing one's belonging to a more distant, imaginative and demographic frontier. In his homage to his friend Baudelaire, Gautier speaks of a 'singularity that appears to elide all affectation, mixed with a certain exotic savour and like a distant perfume from countries more graced with sun'. With Baudelaire, the Orient pervaded his presence as subtly as a vague air, like some Brahmin of verse. Elsewhere he compares the way Baudelaire composes his poems to his idea of oriental clothing: 'Baudelaire mixes the sons of silk and gold with the sons of the crudest, toughest hemp, like those Oriental fabrics that are both splendid and coarse. . .'[23] Baudelaire was sent to Calcutta at the age of twenty, an experience that had an indelible effect, but in the face of his peers this was the exception. For the Bohemians and Romantics, the Orient was excessively aestheticized and was the portal for artistic work.

Such aestheticization was not lost on the moneyed bourgeois of course. One of the ironic social truths of Bohemianism in clothing and real estate is that it is subsequently enlisted by polite society. Examples, such as Gautier's red vest used as a revolutionary counterpoint to the ubiquity of black male dress, were eventually sanitized to hints of colour of a scarf, coat lining or cravat. This, and the fact that middle- and upper-class men had made a domestic tradition of dressing gowns since the seventeenth century made orientalist men's clothing associated with relaxing in the interior the norm. It is also because of the association of orientalist clothing with leisure that the term *mufti* came to be vernacular in circles such as the military for wearing civilian dress. Oddly enough, a mufti in Arab culture is an expert empowered with rulings on Muslim law—not exactly the most casual undertaking.

Although pipes had been around for centuries, cigars had begun to be smoked at the close of the Napoleonic era. Smoking cigarettes had become more acceptable after the Crimean War (1854–6), even to the extent that repairing to a chamber set aside for that purpose formed part of the after-dinner ritual. Hence the smoking or lounge jacket, which not only served to mark the end of formalities but also to protect the dinner suit from tobacco smoke. Its allegiances to the interior were built into this garment's fabric: it had quilted lapels and tassels similar to mid-nineteenth-century furniture, and was made of either silk or velvet.[24] A fez, tarbouche or floppier version thereof, also fitted with a tassel, was used to protect the hair. An interesting and not often used footnote to such affairs is to be found in King Carol I of Romania's Peles Castle. Despite its free-form antiquarian idiom, it was the most technologically modern castle of its period, filled with theme rooms in a regal microcosm version of domestic theme park. It was decorated with several sumptuous oriental theme rooms: the Alhambra room, which had its own fountain, and the Arabian smoking room. Ironically, such mid-to-late-nineteenth-century follies were of a piece with the exhibition pavilions and department stores of the same period, the era that ushers in aesthetic packaging, be it for commercial ends or for leisure. But these latter two exist only in images. To visit these places, still very well preserved, is to see the way that the so-called old-world treated leisure as a serious business, where apparel and interior were in close-knit comparison.

TRAVELLERS, ADVENTURERS AND EXILES

For the artists and poets who spent lengthy periods in North Africa and the Middle East, oriental dress was not as much a matter of posture as expedience and adaptation. Punctuated first by Vivant Denon's remarkable suites of drawings on the Egyptian campaign, throughout the nineteenth and into the twentieth century, artists sought a creative revival in North Africa and the Middle East. A memorable event in art history is Delacroix's visit to Morocco in 1832 as part of the diplomatic delegation of Charles de Mornay, which was staged as a goodwill mission to appease the Sultan Moulay Abd al-Rahman after the French annexation of Algeria. After Chassériau, the next in line for artistic orientalist honours is Eugène Fromentin, of equal repute as both a writer and painter. His *Une anné dans le Sahel* (1859) is one of the masterpieces of the period that combines memoire and critical reflection on orientalist art and fitting modes of representation. His exhortation to avoid ethnographic detail came in no small degree from his sensitivity to the discomfort of the local populations of North Africa to the prying forensic eyes of European artists, writers and scientists. Fromentin's writings were not free of its glib prejudices, however, for they abound in generalizations about Moorish sloth and are peppered with goggle-eyed eroticization. In one passage in particular, he eyes the iridescent clothing of a woman, her hands and feet made luminous by a liberal application of henna.[25] Such raptures prove localized. His presiding verdict is that the Moorish race lacks style: 'The Moors do not have any style; this applies as much to their person as with whom they mix.' Their clothes lack mass and proportion and add nothing to their air of dignity. Instead of their clothes being loose, Fromentin believes them to be too tight: 'with their coats close to their body, their pants like dresses and their belt that many wear loose, it is as hard for old men to look magisterial as it is for young men to avoid looking effeminate'. But, he allows, he is talking very much from an artist's point of view, 'with an *artistic* prejudice'.[26] From more than one perspective, there is more to this than Fromentin will allow. It does drive home that his judgments are from the hip, and subjective. The aestheticization of the other has its positive face, especially when we turn to the following passage, which reads like notes for a painting. Allowed to explore the possession of an acquaintance, his delight in the store of clothes is like Aladdin stumbling upon a treasure trove:

> It was an Arab cabinet full of the richest variety of clothing: summer coats, winter coats, small vests sprayed with gold embroidery, with enormous buttons of gold or silver; caftans of linen or silk, negligé pantaloons, casual and ceremonial, from simple Indian cotton or muslin to heavy brocade thick with silk and gold; then an assortment of *fouta* [a length of cloth like a sarong] to encircle the body, light wimples to complement a turban, headscarves and sashes, all of it called names it would be useless to now to say and of the most striking variegated colours.[27]

This is where Fromentin and his contemporaries came into their own: as aesthetic consumers, as rash fantasizers of the unexpected and dazzling. At least that is how they described it. Such accounts and the paintings that sprang from them were avidly consumed by Bohemians and by the eccentric elite at home.

Here is not the place to delve into the inestimable wealth of orientalist painting from the nineteenth century;[28] what concerns us here is that when they were not musing over the shortcomings of such clothing on the one hand or going into orgiastic raptures on the other, the artists all adopted to a greater or lesser degree the free-flowing robes of the indigenous population; if not to blend in, it was that the climate precluded anything else. Shortly upon his return to Paris on 20 July 1832 after six months' absence, Delacroix, having grown used to the comfort of North African clothing, complained that 'we in our corsets, tight shows and ridiculous casings are pitiable'.[29]

It was not only in Delacroix's nature as a trained observer to be sensitive to people's appearances; as de Mornay's accompanying artist, it was part of his job. Delacroix was sedulous in his task of observing, visually and verbally. There is one incident in particular where he records a reception that he as part of de Mornay's delegation received in Tangiers in which he records the dress in exhaustive detail. For both the delegates and the soldiers,

> white dominated all the costumes, which contrasted remarkably with their black or brown copper faces. Generally a brightly coloured caftan like scarlet, saffron or light blue went below the knee, and covered by a caftan of white percale or bazin, thus only allowing the inner fabric reveal itself from an opening from below, made possible by the irregularity of the folds that fell below the belt and the sleeves, which were large and drew back with each movement, leaving the arm free and completely bare. Over this brilliantly white kind of overcoat, which showed the interior garment, were crosswise sashes in gay colours over the chest carrying the sabre or the dagger at the side, or else a kind of sack or a highly worked leather scabbard. . .[30]

Delacroix goes on to describe the belts, leggings, shoes and turbans in similar forensic detail. The lengthiness of this description, he justifies, 'allows one to understand the kind of well-being I felt on seeing such an unexpected spectacle', adding that the consuls, embroiled in their own diplomatic interests, were surprised at his 'transports of admiration'. Their own official clothing struck a 'sad' and 'sombre' second. Indeed 'a god descended from Olympus to spend a little time on earth to choose one manner of clothing or another would have had no hesitation in preferring the dress of the majestic Moors, who next to us could be taken for kings'.[31]

The European mind might have clung firmly to the exoticism of oriental clothing, but it was at the same time something rather normal and part of the colonial's way of life. By the middle of the nineteenth century Europe's scrabbling for colonies was at fever pitch. This is when a slippery distinction emerged among what I, in the introduction, named inflection, adoption and assimilation. These categories might be dwelt on briefly in order to reflect on the different registers of orientalist fashion and dress. Bohemians were using oriental and other styling in the manner of inflection, to accent their persona, to emphasize their lack of conservatism, and as a badge of ownership to their aesthetic-mindedness. In this regard, orientalism is more a matter of fashion. By contrast, Delacroix, his contemporaries, and those in their wake adopted the clothing of the Orient as a way of avoiding the heat. It was also to varying degrees an assimilation, to ease the manoeuvre through the new society and to suggest an acceptance of local mores.

A later example of this, equally inscribed within cultural memory, is that of Arthur Rimbaud, who abandoned poetry and Bohemianism to run contraband in North Africa. Rimbaud was no stranger to taking on guises and was a consummate assimilator. One of his biographers, Graham Robb, cites the remarks of another Frenchman, Alfred Bardey, who had come to Aden to export coffee. In 1881 in Harar (Rimbaud was 26), Bardey recounts:

> Just as he was about to set off at the head of the little procession, Rimbaud wrapped a towel around his head as a turban and draped a red blanket over his usual garment. He was intending to pass himself off as a Muslim[. . .]
>
> Sharing our amusement at his fancy dress, Rimbaud agreed that the red blanket which orientalised his European costume might attract robbers. But he wanted to be seen as a rich Mohammaden merchant for the sake of company prestige.[32]

The blithe self-confidence of the colonist in this passage is to be contrasted when the shoe is on the other foot. Nerval, in his lengthy account, describes an encounter with a pasha (lord or general) who offers to dine 'à l'européenne', replacing stools with chairs, at which Nerval reflects on his displeasure at the infiltration of European customs in the Orient. When the pasha appears wearing a black coat, Nerval considers the fusion of cultures incongruous. The indigenous person assimilating such European customs avails himself of 'neutral terrain' without due benefit to himself. His imitation of the clothing, like his speaking French, is only for the sake of the French colonists. In short, in not acting 'himself', he is condemned to a grotesque mismatch that draws attention to his subaltern state: 'He resembled the kind of figure in a ballet who is half peasant, half noble; while showing a gentlemanly demeanour to the European, for the Asian he remains pure Osmanli.' But, adds Nerval, the expectations of his people have made the politic of such assimilation a necessity.[33]

The distinction between such temporary assimilation and long-term adoption is analogous to one's commitment to a culture inasmuch as one is willing to change religion. Liotard, who adopted orientalist dress well after his service in the East, took a stance to which his image as an artist could only benefit. It said that he had access to the covetedly exotic. The artist who perfected this kind of stance, of conflating sartorial necessity with exotic aggrandizement was Pierre Loti, the nom de plume of Julien Viaud, whose career straddled nineteenth and twentieth centuries, similar to that of his admirer, Marcel Proust.

Loti spent most of his career as a naval officer and therefore had direct access to a variety of France's colonized and allied countries in North Africa and the South Pacific. Loti made ample use of his experiences in Turkey, Senegal, Algiers and Vietnam to sprout novels that are largely *romans à clef*. In 1887, when he was thirty-seven, he produced *Propos d'exil*, a series of autobiographic sketches based in exotic locales. In the same year he wrote *Madame*

Chrysanthème, the inspiration for Puccini's *Madame Butterfly*. Loti was as experimental with sexual relations as he was with his assimilation and reinscription of cultures, and was as good a collector of foreign bibelots as he was of stories. His sexual deviance has attracted attention in recent years. Whether or not Loti slots into the lineage of what is now called gay literature[34] or is a writer invested in something more ambiguous, writers are in agreement that foreign settings were a way of cloaking an experience less tolerated at home. Insofar that orientalizing literature is used as a clothing for what in Europe were indiscrete desires and exchanges makes Loti something of climax to a particular form of literary masquerade that had come to emerge in literary follies such as William Beckford's Gothic novel about an Arab Caliph, *Vathek*, and then were canonized as an autonomous genre by Hugo and Byron. But more pronounced than these figures, Loti consciously muddied the division between his life and his fiction by dressing up. His is a memorable example that stands out amongst many undocumented others of the nineteenth century in which the adaptive clothing on travels in the East were brought home and used as imaginative posture, as a trophy and as certification that one had withstood uncommon ardours and seen unusual things. Numerous photographs survive of Loti in orientalist clothing, often smoking a hookah or in exaggerated Turkish settings. Here Loti has replaced his identity as the sailor hungry for cultural stimulation with clothing in the Bohemian vein in saying that he is an aristocrat of the world. His house in Rochefort contained a tiled room in imitation of a mosque.[35] In 1891, Henri (Douanier) Rousseau painted a portrait of Loti wearing a red fez and a languid stare. His East–West hybrid credentials were complete.

CASHMERE SHAWLS

If there had to be one item that summed up the nineteenth century in women's fashion in France, it was the cashmere shawl. In the previous chapter we saw some of its beginnings; by the 1830s it was something that any woman of quality had to own and went from curiosity to ubiquity. It was the fabric of excellence: what silk had been in past ages. Because shawls were more accessories than articles of clothing, they lent themselves to complement a wide range of fashions. Shawls quickly became sublimated into the European mind as something more than a piece of clothing; they articulated the beauty and profits of colonization.

European attempts to break the back of the Eastern monopoly also bear an uncanny resemblance to the difficulties encountered in the sixth century in securing its own silk supply. Spurred on by the insatiable demand in Europe for cashmere, during a trans-Himalayan trip in 1812, the veterinary surgeon and superintendent of the East Asia Company William Moorcroft secured the possession of fifty mountain goats. The haplessness of the story borders on the ludicrous: Moorcroft divided the male and female goats onto separate vessels, only to be met with news that the carrier of the females had been wrecked. French efforts proved just as inadequate, since the Pyrenees was inadequate to sustain the goats, which were only used to the Himalayan climate. Thus the regions of Ladakh and Kurdistan maintained their hold on cashmere production, forbidding the export of untreated fibre.

Unperturbed, Moorcroft pushed on with his obsession. His accounts of his visit in 1822 explain that there were around 120,000 textile workers in Kashmir, with weaving constituting the prime source of the region's industrial income. His accounts show that they were exported to all over Asia.[36] They varied in quality, according to commission and demand. Between 1825–6, Russia imported over two million roubles worth of shawls. Devout on making England a dominant cashmere producer, he sought to convince Kashmiri families to emigrate to England and commissioned a local painter to record the intricate designs, which we now have come universally to call paisley. At the end of his tenure, Moorcroft was given his own small collection of precious shawls by the Sikh ruler of Kashmir, Ranjit Sinh.

The beginnings of the Kashmiri shawl industry remain obscure. A popular account is that the shawl appeared during the Moghul conquest during the rule of Zain ul'Abdin (1420–70). But only a century later, during the reign of Emperor Akbar, after his conquest of the Kashmir valley, did the garment came into its own. Esteemed by the emperor himself, shawls were the benchmark of artisanal craftsmanship, of the power of personal patronage in India, and were objects of trade. They were also used as bribes, as reported by the English envoy to the Moghul court in 1616, who reported to have formally rejected one. In 1739, the Emperor of Constantinople accepted a huge trove of these presented on behalf of Nadir Shah, the Persian invader of India.

As we saw in chapter one, early examples of the shawl were in Bactria and Gandhara, but it is also said to have haled from Persia and Central Asia, the word coming from the Persian 'chal' or 'shaal'. It is perhaps vain to conjecture too far, given that it is such a simple, if not self-evident piece of clothing. But what we do know is that shawls were unknown in China until their advent by Europe. Like the origin of the banyan, but in reverse (origin in Japan, response production in India for European consumers), in around 1830 China began to produce shawls of silk crêpe expressly for the export market. Empress Eugénie, who was born in Spain, introduced them to the Parisian élite. While the Paris preferred the more restrained, whiter variety—which went with what is called the 'crinoline period' in fashion—the Spanish took to the polychrome variety. The Chinese silk shawls were so profuse, especially in the southern region of Andalusia, that they were adopted as European, their Chinese origins being stamped out, denied or ignored.[37]

Chinese imitations should not divert us from the fact that Kashmiri shawl weaving was itself always aimed at the overseas market. Chitralekha Zutshi argues that the fairest proof of this is the degree to which colours, designs and patterns were altered to target particular consumers. Not only were early examples of shawls used as shoulder mantles (*khillat*) but also as royal gifts on which were inscribed specific design befitting the transaction. Kashmir's capital, Srinigar, was populated with numerous agents who acted for merchants to inform them of demands of outside markets. It is even suspected that the plainer variety of the shawl came from the recommendation of an Armenian merchant from the Ottoman Empire because they were faster to make.[38]

It was in the first decades of the nineteenth century, spurred by the migrations and collisions of the Napoleonic years, that fashions became obsessed with national signage. Inspired also by the military wear, women took to wearing 'Spanish' and 'Vittoria' cloaks or 'Pyrenean' mantles. In the words of Penelope Byrde, 'other articles of dress were variously described as "Tyrolese", "Polish", "Hungarian", "Russian", "Algerian", "Turkish", "Egyptian" and "Circassian". "Chinese" parasols in the fashionable pagoda shape reflected a general and long-standing interest in oriental art. . .'[39] The shawl was the culmination of the craze for foreignness. Writing in June 1809, Rudolph Ackermann's *Repository of Arts* remarked that, 'Shawls are much worn; they are admirably adapted to the promenade, as they afford, in the throw and arrangement, such fine opportunities for the display of the wearer's taste'[40] (see Figure 23).

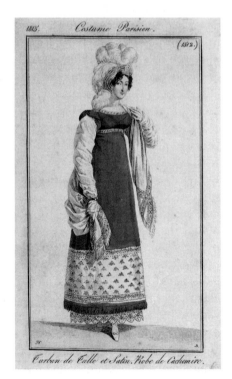

Figure 23   Women's fashion plate with turban and cashmere dress, from *Courrier des Dames*, 1815, © Getty Images.

Shawls went well beyond category of admirable apparel, however; they stretched to be a dramatic social and even political phenomenon. Zutshi goes so far as to argue that by the mid-nineteenth century, the shawl was the principal article by which Britain was able to visualize its Indian colony, and possessing one was literally to partake in Empire. On an official scale, the intense desire to discover the secrets of Kashmiri shawl manufacture can be seen as a component of the British imperial endeavour of knowledge and control.[41] 'The many Victorian narratives on shawls' she continues,

> written almost always by men and women who had never actually visited Kashmir, then, performed two interrelated didactic functions: first, they educated readers about Kashmir through Kashmiri shawls—concrete material manifestations of its beauty and exceptionality—which fulfilled the larger concern of these narratives to educate Victorian Britons about the diverse and varied geography of the British empire, and, second, they translated the specialised, scientific knowledge about Kashmiri shawl manufacture that had been transmitted to the British shawl industry by men such as Moorcroft into a more popular form, while at the same time highlighting the relationship between Kashmir, shawl production, and imperial politics.[42]

A notable example of which Zutshi speaks can be found in Thackeray's *Vanity Fair*, when Rebecca visits Amelia Sedley in Russell Square and chances upon some shawls that Amelia's brother Joseph has recently brought her from his trip to India.[43]

Kashmir shawls had a mystique rooted in the frustratingly inalienable fact that their geographic and demographic conditions were the secret to a product that could not be replicated, much like the concept of *terroir* in viticulture, where a wine's distinctive character is tied to the climate and soil of its region. But this only made the challenge greater. Kashmir and its shawls circulated in the mid-nineteenth-century British imagination with talismanic mystique. Perhaps more than any other article, the Kashmir shawl also showed how Victorian Britain used commodities to experience and reflect on its empire, its subdivisions classified according to what was produced and what could be gained (as opposed to the people deployed to produce them), with Kashmiri shawls at the apex, at least in terms of aesthetic allure.

France also managed to co-opt the shawl into its own colonial narrative. The period when the French were most with gripped by 'cashmere fever' was associated first with the Egyptian campaign and then, conveniently, with the conquest of Algeria three decades hence.[44] Walter Benjamin cites an edition of *Paris chez soi* in 1854 that describes it as an epidemic of almost pathological proportions: 'It began to spread during the Consulate, greater under the Empire, became gigantic during the restoration, reached colossal size under the July Monarchy, and has finally assumed Sphinx-like dimensions since the February Revolution of 1848'.[45] In an early phase Joséphine was bombarded with cashmere shawls from Napoleon while he was away in Egypt; an 1806 inventory lists 45 shawls. This was an exceptional number for the time in France as there was an embargo on their importation because of the blockade of trade with Britain. When Napoleon married Marie-Louise, he included seventeen shawls in her *corbeille de noces* ('wedding basket'). As Susan Hiner remarks, this was not just lip service to fashion; it had the special importance of reminding his wife that he was a conqueror of distant lands.[46] Its symbolic resonance did not just survive more than three regime changes; it escalated, for the reason that it was associated with the imperial might of what France had been and what it might be again.

It was in this regard that the French differed slightly from their British counterparts, who have their own large catalogue of narrative dalliance, but whose focus was more practical, given that they had direct access to the flow of trade. Hiner explains that in France, cashmeres were not only a domestication of the unknown but also a catalyst to erotic fantasies of adventure.[47] Silk had maybe been the source of similar obsessions in a past age, yet cashmeres embodied two specific domains of women's wear and of imperial capture. Predictably they were the dowry items par excellence, being closely associated with class, money and the ability to keep a woman. In the personal dramas, fictional and real, that subtend from such negotiations, cashmeres surfaced in all manner of literary sources. They became the subject of innumerable commentaries, news reports and stories. In 1833, a fashion publication reported how a man, after saving a drowning woman in the Seine, went back into the river for her cashmere shawl.[48] Another magazine, *Le Règne de mode*, satirized the cashmere mania with a list of questions that are all answered with the same word, 'a cashmere'.[49] It is no surprise then that cashmeres find themselves in Balzac's novels, given his fixation with money. Balzac's *Ferragus* and *La Cousine Bette* both have cashmeres as avatars of class and property. And in Flaubert's *L'Éducation semtimentale*, the shawl becomes a repository for the longing that the central protagonist Frédéric has for Mme Arnoux, whose 'brown skin' places her as Andalusian or possibly Creole.[50]

Factories in Paisley, the town near Glasgow, and Norwich, Edinburgh and Lyon began to imitate Indian shawls. Norwich led the standard, having begun in 1780s with block-printed patterns. Together with Edinburgh, it soon after took up weaving the patterns on drawlooms that included the pattern harnesses as well as the regular loom harnesses. Comparing Britain and France textile production at the middle of nineteenth century is no contest, as least with respect to quantity. In 1848, the British dwarfed French production, possessing double the automatic looms (675,000) of France (328,000), however Lyon continued to be a leader in the variety and quality. Soon after France began their production in 1804, and thanks to the invention of the 'harness' and the Jacquard loom (the latter only becoming recognized in the 1820s), weavers were able to imitate mechanically designs that were painted or embroidered by hand.[51] Fabrics were either wool or silk but not cashmere, on which India still had the monopoly. But this was not a deterrent. Lyon called the shawls generically 'cashmeres' in their exports to America,[52] which was presumably too remote from India to know the difference. Shawls were produced in all manner of materials, including damask, chenille and *barège*, and the widening of styles with improvements in dying and printing caused the magazine *Belle Assemblée* in November 1838 to comment, 'There is really quite a mania for shawls, besides those of Cashmere, which still maintain their ground, we have velvet shawls, satin, and *peluche* ones, and a great variety of fancy shawls.'[53] Much earlier, in 1810, the famous dramatist Heinrich von Kleist was already opining the abrupt changes in fashion from season to season that were sent down to Saxony from Paris and of their financial toll on those who thought they needed to follow them.[54] The ample availability of choice did not quell manufacturers' desire to find a serviceable alternative to cashmere, which by the 1830s was already commanding astronomical prices. The most notable figure to do so was Titus Salt, whose lifespan (1803–1876) roughly straddles the time of when shawls were most in vogue. In 1836 he fell upon some bales of Alpaca wool in Liverpool. He made his fortune with the alpaca spinner, thus creating 'alpaca', which became a popular alternative to both silk and cashmere. In 1980, there were as many as 20,000 registered alpacas in England.

PAISLEY

In 1686, during the first of two of their envoys to France, the Siamese Embassy brought to Louis XIV's court some examples of the vibrant *ikat* textiles. The nobility were quick to use them, calling them *toiles flammées* or *Siamoises de Rouen*. These names changed to *toiles de charentes* or cottons of Provence after the French Revolution, when there was distrust of anything foreign, to sanitize them of indigeneity. In Australia, since the 1970s the didgeridoo has been assumed to be a national instrument of the Aborigines, but it is ritually confined to northeast Arnhem Land, and its actual name is *yidaki*, didgeridoo being pidgin onomatopoeia for the sound it makes. By now this pattern or adoption to purloining has become something of a theme of this book, but the most famous example is paisley, originally known as *buta* (bud) or the 'Kashmiri cone'. But its subsequent co-option is so strong that only experts (and people from India) know the real origin; some may even be mistaken for thinking that the Scottish town took its name from the design.

Paisley, Scotland, emerged at the end of the eighteenth century as a centre for textile production, and by the 1820s it had well and truly taken over Edinburgh as the biggest producer of Indian-style affordable alternatives to the Kashmiri benchmark. Paisley was thriving not only in its production but also in its design, seeking to outdo their Indian counterparts in their own designs, expanding the visual vocabulary of the 'cone' patterns. To comply with British tastes, Scottish manufacturers modified, or 'improved' the design by introducing floral patterns into the *buta* and by making it squatter. Eventually, by force of quantity in number and variety of design, Paisley began to overtake Kashmir in public perception of what was genuine. Paisley's designs were even assumed to be coming from a long and lasting tradition.

There are a number of reasons to be ascertained about the success of this motif. One was that the design that once heralded the Moghul era lent itself to endless modifications, down to an almost fractal-like intricacy. But this could also be said of Hellenic, rococo or baroque designs as well. What really distinguished it was its asymmetry. Its fluidity and its references to the natural world could be amply drawn into neobaroque or rococo syntax, with its love of shells and plant fronds. Most relevant, though, is that it signalled an exotic wildness that was utterly at odds with the Greek revivalist styles in dress, decorative arts and architecture that only began to want by the 1840s. Because the *buta* was exotic it was different, not opposed. It is the most dominant example hitherto of orientalist inflection upon the Western design armature.

Paisley might have found its most stunning examples in clothing, but it was not confined to it. By the mid-nineteenth century it found its way onto wallpaper and decorative ironwork (exemplified in the work of Matthew Digby Wyatt). Its applications were seemingly endless. In her reflections on the stylistic colonization of Indian design, Saloni Mathur argues that hidden in the tale of stealing, reinvention and reintegration of Indian designs by the West lies a more sinister story of cultural colonization and stereotyping. The *buta* is for Mathur an emblem used by the West as the fabricated idea of India: 'The pattern bears the imprint of the colonial economy, the stamp of Victorian industrial consumption, and the reshaping of ideas about India at the point of their interpellation into Western economies of desire.'[55] It is an idea that she, as with other contemporary Indian scholars, is intent on disputing. For she believes that India as an idea remains inertly museological and debilitatingly stereotyped.

BRITISH ORIENTALIST TEXTILES AND DESIGN AFTER 1851

Prince Albert's Crystal Palace, or the Great Exhibition of 1851, marks the beginning of the ongoing taste for world's fairs and universal exhibitions. It served the double strategy of bringing the world's progress to Britain while asserting Britain's progress to the world. Its influence on the people of the day is inestimable, as was it to all manner of designers, who were able to feast on the styles of the world, a stylistic surfeit that was for the seminal architectural theorist Gottfried Semper a cause of great concern. Never before had such a variety of fabrics been seen in one place at one time, from Egypt, Turkey, Tunis and India. This panoply helped another architect, Owen Jones, to reflect on the different decorative modes and to assemble them in his *Grammar of Ornament* (1856).[56]

Three years later began the Crimean War—to which is attributed the cardigan, after Lord Cardigan—which represented a campaign of the two imperial nations to influence the territories of the Ottoman Empire, now in visible decline. This relationship with Turkey, who was now an ally against the Russians, cultivated a new wave of Turkish taste, including, not least, the Turkish and Oriental Museum on Hyde Park Corner. With the Ottoman Empire no longer a threat, it gradually began to be seen as a thing of the past and hence an object of nostalgia. This was the same time when the neo-Gothic style in architecture and design had wholly surpassed the austere Georgian and Regency styles. The Turkish style of this period was different from that of the previous century in that, in Britain in particular, it was a contradictory mixture of empirical anthropology and ornate folly. In line with the Gothic, it had a strong narrative sense, fed by writers and painters, of violence, danger and sensuality. Turkish and Alhambran settings sprang up in the museums (The Alhambra Court, the Crystal Palace, Sydenham; The Sculpture Hall, East India House Museum; Durbar Hall) and in wealthy people's homes. What was preserved was the love of the harem, sharing connotations of supine indolence and aesthetic magnificence. Given this level of availability and visibility as opposed to that of the previous century, orientalist clothing and costume carried with it a train of unspoken narratives whose contemporary corollary is that of advertising, where an object glosses a series of cultural and arbitrary references which one then wears, thereby partaking in an elaborate and loosely consensual illusion.

The world's fairs, the 'Hausmannization' of Paris that occurred between 1852 and 1870, the birth of the urban metropolis, together with the explosion of free market economy in Europe and America, ushered in the era of what Walter Benjamin called 'phantasmagoria'. Here, real and imaginary worlds intermingled without distinction, and the capitalist consumer, depending on disposition or means, was made to feel paralyzed or capable of possessing everything. The more immediately mercantile scion of the world's fairs were the department stores that began in the 1850s and 1860s (Newcastle Bainbridge in 1849; Bon Marché, 1852; Samaritaine, 1869). These began as consortiums of departments, like the separate pavilions in the Great Exhibition.

There were also large emporiums, which were places stocking rare goods. As we know from Benjamin and the many studies from the urban culture of the Impressionism to that of Victorian Britain, these were places where the main lubricant for monetary exchange was entertainment and display. Orientalist fashions and decorations played a starring role. In April 1877, *Myra's Journal of Dress and Fashion* reported that 'Messrs Halling, Pearce, and Stone have now one of the finest mantle rooms in London'. Upon entry 'one is immediately attracted by a considerable collection of choice Japanese and Chinese bronzes, porcelains, cabinets, and all the pretty trifles which, no matter how old they may be, are always new. Then come piles of Indian, Cashmere, Delhi and Chuddah shawls, mingled in admired disorder with embroidered fichus . . .'[57] Zola's *Au bonheur des dames*, which revolves around the new culture of shopping of the Third Republic, is full of descriptions of the sumptuous displays in which oriental references were never too far behind: 'silks as transparent as crystal, Nile green, Indian blue, May pink, blue Danube'.[58]

ARTHUR LAZENBY LIBERTY

The exceptional figure in this period was Arthur Lazenby Liberty. He began his career managing Farmer and Rogers's 'Oriental Warehouse' of their 'Great Shawl and Cloak Emporium' in Regent St, London. He became their competition in 1875, when he opened his own 'East India House' on the other side of the same street, later moving to Chesham House five years later with a 'North Eastern' bazaar and 'Arab Tea Room'. Liberty's success was such that by the last decades of the century he could claim all but a monopoly on supply and taste-making. A branch in Paris opened in 1880 following the 1878 universal exhibition there. It was also used to secure contacts with other continental outlets.

Liberty was one of many importers but was known for the quality of his goods, critical of the second-rate imports and approximations. When he opened his own store he filled it with the predictable stock of Imari beakers, Pekin pilgrim bottles and Buddhist altar adornments, but he soon turned to cloth-making. Weakening protective duties on French silks had saturated the market, yet all but the highest levels of production were of dubious quality. They were unsympathetic to handling, did not drape well and their colours were liable to be garish. Liberty first turned to the textiles of Japan, China and India, along with their accompanying bric-a-brac, before he convinced some mills in the East Midlands to copy these designs. Not long after, he set up his own silk printing works in south London. For these designs it is likely that he and his artisans used one of the thirteen sets of eighteen volumes of designs, each with 700 samples of cloth that had been produced by the Indian

Museum for the express purpose of making these available to British imitators. Liberty introduced Indian dyes that were unknown in Europe, and between 1888 and 1889 he visited Japan. By the beginning of the next century, Liberty's firm was an institution, recognized throughout Europe as having its own particular style.[59]

Liberty looked to the more delicate colour combinations and venerable, 'authentic' styles, particularly Persian, and encouraged British firms to improve their techniques of dyeing and printing. When Liberty eventually took control of his own printing, adapting Indian and Persian designs, they were block printed onto plain Indian silk. But the hand techniques were not ideological or sentimental as they were for William Morris or Charles Eastlake. Liberty was confident in what machines had to offer and in their ability to service a broader market. His confidence was rewarded, and soon his company was boasting the most beautiful and affordable textiles in all of Europe. His shop was aimed against the mid-Victorian taste for the mid-brow and middling quality. Liberty's talent was to see that to be an arbiter of taste one had to educate. His shop was characterized as an Eastern bazaar that transported its visitors into the dreamy confines of a bazaar in Damascus or Baghdad. Authentic items like the valuable Kashmiri shawls were put up as exhibits, no doubt, to demonstrate how the local designs vied with the benchmarks for aesthetic authority. From 1880 the firm branched out into wallpaper and furniture. Now the oriental had finally been taken out of the Orient, with chairs of Moorish-inspired designs conceived by British designers made of mahogany.[60]

Liberty had a knack for connections, personal as well as cultural. It is due to him that artists and designers were so encouraged to dabble in oriental designs at a high level of quality and for a distinguished clientele. Referring to himself as an 'East Indian Merchant' at the beginning of his career, Liberty joined many of the various oriental-associated societies, such as the Japan Society, the Asiatic Society and the Silk Association, which retained a bit of guild-like power and were usually the first ports of call when the relevant information regarding supply, taste and ideas came to port. He mixed not only with curators, artists and designers but also with prominent members of the theatre and dance.[61] The exchange of ideas and the cross-pollination of influence were no doubt made possible on such a scale because they were tied directly to consumption. Artists and designers could design for an ample market. In the main, however, the cross-pollination was between living Britons and inert oriental objects (although on one occasion in 1885 he helped bring out Indian craftsmen to Battersea Park). Yet Liberty played a significant role in removing oriental textiles, fashion and design from the realm of exceptions. Up to this day, Liberty prints have a decidedly orientalist edge but are only now discernible to the specialist; to others they are vibrant and sumptuous. In Italy they gave birth to their own style, the *stile Liberty*. By all accounts, there is a mythology around Liberty the man and his designs that is analogous the diaphanous mystique of orientalism itself.[62]

This degree of absorption into popular perception lays the foundation stone for orientalist fashion in the next century, where it occupies two main domains, adoption and absorption on one hand and inflection and inspiration on the other. As we have seen with certain items and as we shall continue to see in the next chapter with the kimono and fez, the countries in question become as complicit in the outward signs of orientalist difference even once they have become devalued and ossified into cultural cliché. And it is this easy typologizing of the orientalist sign that couture would thrive on and thrives on still.

OTHER WOMEN'S FASHIONS BEFORE COUTURE

Several developments in female dress in the mid-nineteenth century, the bustle, the bodice and bloomers, can all be linked to Eastern origins. The first's orientalist attachments are a little abstruse but are worth mentioning all the same. Rula Razek discusses the bustle in light of the term *steatopygia* used since 1822 as medical jargon for the deformity of the 'Hottentot' women of South Africa, analysed by Henri de Blainville and Georges Caver. Around this time the 'Hottentot Venus' was exhibited at carnival events with animals and grotesque aberrations of nature. When seen in light of dress, the steatopygous figure with its slim waist and enlarged buttocks was a symbol said to incite the most primordial desire.[63]

Bodices, which complemented the bustle, were a form of female waist-coat or truncated jacket that came into vogue in the 1840s and lasted about twenty years. The Crimean War helped to galvanize their exotic potential, which had already begun two years before with interest in a bolero style of jacket in 1852. A year later, the *Illustrated London News* advised that 'Turkish vests' are perfect after-dinner add-ons; they could be decorated with braiding and embellished with gold thread.[64]

The mid-1850s witnessed less-restrictive female fashions, caused by mounting evidence of the demerits of corsetry on women's health. In 1857, Auguste Debay, in *Les Modes et les parures*, compared corsets to the barbaric act of Chinese foot-binding, adding that even though it was the French who ridiculed Turkish women for their thick waists, the Turkish women were a lot better off, laughing at the pitiable Frenchwomen.[65] Waistlines marginally widened. Bodices with less boning were accompanied by shorter, wider sleeves in a 'Chinese' pagoda shape to go with expanded dresses. Outerwear, which expanded with the skirt, was also more fashionable in the mid-1850s. One example was a semifitting mantle, or quarter-length coat, the diurnal counterpart to the more striking burnous in the Arab style with a tasselled hood, for evenings. Another garment contemporaneous with the Crimean War was

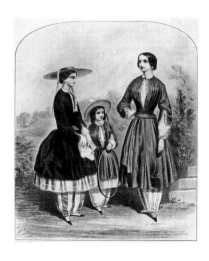

Figure 24   Amelia Bloomer, c. 1850; lithograph by Noyce, © Photo by Hulton Archive/Getty Images.

the *dolman* or *dolaman*, Turkish for surcoat, a short jacket cut to allow for the skirt's rear drapery.

A more notorious item emerged from the same period. Bloomers, named after Amelia Jenks Bloomer, had a mixed origin. Their invention has been attributed to protofeminists like Elizabeth Smith Miller of Peterboro, New York, and Fabrizia Flynn, wife of the Italian ambassador to Penrhiwceiber, in South Wales. This is mostly anecdotal apocrypha. Their origins came out of intense debate as to what garment, different from the custom of dresses, bodices and corsets, would assign women mobility but would maintain their difference from men. Bloomers transpired as ad hoc creations, for dress-reformers were not designers. They were ultimately forced to choose between Turkish pantaloons or children's pantalettes. By dint of the habitual fascination, the Turkish references ultimately took over. But as Gayle Fischer argues, the inception of such clothing was at first a practical rather than political concern. In nineteenth-century US society they were thought to be both more comfortable and hygienic than skirts.[66]

They were typically long, flowing pants that harrowed with a cuff at the ankles and were worn with a skirt. They were designed to give women greater mobility while not offending Victorian prurience, bloomers being something of a cross between pantaloons and undergarments. Anything that smacked of women's mobility was also marred by the threat of the suffragette movement, which remembered back to Mary Montagu's *Embassy Letters*, which offered a picture of greater female mobility and entitlements. In the nineteenth century, other women such as Julia Pardoe, Sophia Lane Poole, Isabel Burton, Anne Blunt and Isabella Bird Bishop travelled to Constantinople and were given a first-hand experience of a welcome reprieve in dress from what were by comparison in Europe sartorial prisons. Amelia Bloomer may not have been the first to wear them, but as the editor of the first newspaper for women, *The*

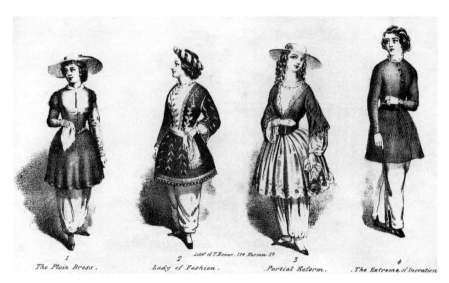

The Plain Dress. — *Lady of Fashion.* — *Partial Reform.* — *The Extreme of Inovation*

Figure 25 Examples of Bloomers: an engraving of four examples of women wearing bloomers as advocated by women's rights and temperance advocate Amelia Bloomer (1818–1894), c. 1850, © Photo by Hulton Archive/Getty Images.

Lily, she flaunted her 'Turkish trousers' as her assertion of womanly emancipation. Members of the reform movement were happy to let such references to abound, delighted by popular engravings of melting beauties, charmed by the cult of Byron and impressed by the French conquering of Algeria.[67] But as Fischer observes, women's-rights advocates were largely alone in wearing 'Turkish trowsers'. Other dress reformers such as the Mormon Oneida Perfectionist Community remained aloof from the women's movement and shunned the references to the East, references that precipitated a variety of antagonisms against its connotations of dissolute sexuality through to the heathenish celebration of Islam.[68] Fischer concludes: 'The idea of "feminine trousers" seemed a contradiction—society wondered how a female version of an exclusively male garment could possibly exist. In the case of women's rights dress reformers, the original intention of their reform was lost and re-shaped by public reaction to it.'[69]

In subsequent decades, the political and cultural overtones of trousers on women waned when they became used for women's sportswear. Physical exercise was a predictable offshoot of the more outdoor culture of urban life, and by the end of the century bloomers were the norm for cycling and beachwear. At times their activist origins resurfaced, as when Lady Archibald Campbell arrived at Marlborough House to much consternation in full trousers, wearing an 'Arabian Nights Dress' which she also wore everyday in London.[70] Subsequent highbrow manifestations came with the Viscountess Haberton, who was the founder in June 1881 of the Royal Dress Society, a group that

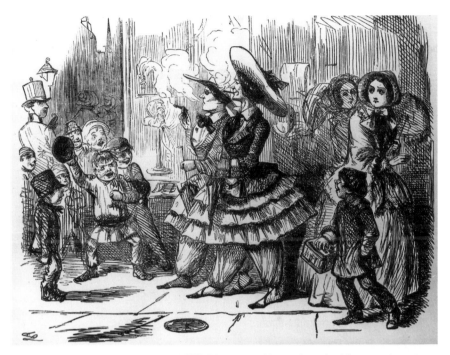

Figure 26 *Bloomerism Madness*, c. 1855, Women smoking and wearing bloomers draw stares from passers by in a cartoon entitled 'Bloomerism—An American Custom'. Drawn by Leech for *Punch*, © Photo by Hulton Archive/Getty Images.

lauded so-called healthy dress over beauty. She wore a type of trouser-skirt named the Haberton and also the more generic 'Turkish trousers'. Out of a sense of fealty and belonging, the whole of her society began to wear such garments, while others such as Ada Baillie of the National Health Society bristled at what she believed was the extremism of Bloomerism, preferring the princess gown which was still supported by the bodice, a garment that Haberton and her peers were vocal in condemning as reprobate.[71]

Paul Poiret was to make alternatives to the older style dress something of an art form, ushering in orientalism as an indispensible integer to the newly formed creative concept of haute couture. In the final decades of the nineteenth century, all styles were fair game; the exotic was far more a socially integrated concept and less based on economic or demographic rarity. Most middle-class people had a rough knowledge of the difference between Turk and Chinese styles. Orientalism was no longer the language of transgression in dress but was transformed into the rhetoric of transgression. And it is with this rhetoric that the notion of the fashion system is born, a lexicon of formal, artistic and cultural modalities which the designer, or couturier, will pick from at whim as inspiration.

–4–

1868–1944: The Japoniste Revolution, the Deorientalizing of the Orient and the Birth of Couture

What of this piercing of the sands? [Suez Canal]
   What of this union of the seas?
This grasp of unfamiliar hands,
   This blending of strange litanies?

Aves and Allah-hu's that flow
   From ulemas and monsignors—
These *feridjees* and *robes-fourreau*,
These eunuchs and ambassadors—

This *pot-pourri* of east and West,
   Pillau and *potage a la bisque;*—
Circassian belles whom WORTH has drest,
   And Parisiennes *à l'odalisque*!

—*Punch*, November 27, 1869[1]

Civilization! Read: 'the era that has lost almost all its creative power . . . in jewellery as in furniture'; and in one or the other we are compelled to exhume or import. Import what? Indian bracelets of glass filament and Chinese earrings of cut paper? No. But more often the naïve taste that underlies their making.

—Stéphane Mallarmé, *La Dernière Mode*[2]

This interval in history, from the beginning of the Meiji period of Japan and the Prussian defeat of France until the early-twentieth century, is remarkable for the way in which orientalist fashion slackened the reign of authenticity. In other words, by the turn of the century it had become a genre unto itself, whose links to race and culture existed as ideal states with sometimes the scantest basis. Indigeneity and rightful national origins had ceased to be absolutes—if they ever were—and became imaginary points of reference. Orientalism had become a means of transformation in more ways than one. In the period leading to the Enlightenment, it was a mechanism for transforming the (non-Eastern) individual and for asserting his or her independence and free will. By the end of the nineteenth century, such transformations through clothing, accoutrements and interiors had become so encoded as to be the normative mode of differentiation. Once fashion as a social and commercial institution had become enshrined within haute couture, it became both an economic modality and a social code that joined the world of material commodities with the world of qualitative abstractions (art). With fashion as an industry and as an ever-expanding complex social code, orientalist idioms were deployed to meet the expectation of the fashion industry's business of transformation from one season to the next. While science was specializing, fashion was improvising. Orientalism was, and continues to be, the generic site of difference inscribed *within* the flows of differentiation and belonging of the fashion system.

Finally, in a process older than the others, was the transformation of the orientalist garment itself within the Orient to meet Western expectations of what the Orient should be. In this auspicious genealogy of adaptation, from *brisé* fans to the *buta*, came the next great orientalist fashion institution, the kimono, the garment that encapsulated Japan as the Kashmiri shawl had the Indian Empire, abruptly eclipsing the latter as the wearable item of exotic excellence.

As artists in Europe and within the Orient tapped into their alternative 'primitive' roots, orientals from Algeria to Turkey to Japan were becoming more Westernized, 'deorientalizing' themselves in an effort to modernize to be more competitive on the world market.[3] From the end of the nineteenth century, 'tradition' becomes more orchestrated and packaged. It is something of a touristic affair, much as a quaint and entirely planned-out Chinatown exists in Singapore today to maintain the semblance of ties to an authentic past. While the West was caught up in its own orient—an immaterial, arbitrary confederate of fancies—the natives undertook a self-conscious reorientalizing to compensate for a tradition that had been subsumed by migration and modernization. With characteristic cynical mirth, Patricia Highsmith puts this well in a fictional portrayal:

> Turbaned Mahmet in his pointed, turned-up shoes and billowing old djellabah, looked more like an Arab than the Arabs. He meant himself to be a tourist attraction, photogenic (he charged a small fee to be photographed) with a gold ring in one ear and a pinched, sun-tanned visage which was almost hidden under bushy eyebrows and a totally untended beard.[4]

Highsmith's Mahmet is projecting what the audience think he should be, a personification of the Orient conducting its own orientalizing, here to attract Western interest and hopefully to make some money.

In the late nineteenth and early twentieth centuries, orientalism was a phenomenon of the second degree, a metaphenomenon. In the words of Peter Wollen, the fear that was once one of orientalism's enticements 'was now projected onto the screen'. The exotic was not exotic in the way it was before but was rather a residual and permanent component of European modern life. The exotic was a stylistic quality in vast semantic lexicon of cultures as opposed to an intrepid experience. After Japonism's assimilation into art, decorative art and fashion at the beginning of the twentieth century, the unusual, enshrined within orientalism, became expected.

JAPONISM AND THE KIMONO

The story of Japan's ascendancy in the world of art and design can be compared to what today would be called a marketing coup. By the middle of the nineteenth century, orientalism had exhausted itself in novelty, and Europe had begun to outdo the Orient in design and production. Islamic and Chinese styles had enjoyed a long historical relationship in the West. Japan opened its doors serendipitously when Europe's markets were not only hungry for new influences but their visual literacy was of a sophistication that outstripped that of previous centuries. As Thorstein Veblen famously showed, nothing drives a market more than rarity, and Japan quickly found international markets eager to get their hands on goods that had once only been talked about or spirited away in special collections.

Japan's influence on all of the arts of Europe and America was momentous. After living in isolation since the beginning of the seventeenth century, the Edo period ended in the summer of 1868 with the toppling of the Tokugawa shogunate, making way for the Meiji era. The Meiji period was less structured than the last, and the Japanese knew that the state of cultural quarantine had become exhausted and was not in the country's best interests. The reforms in domestic and foreign policy assigned a new importance to the West, whom the Japanese saw as a resource for expanding their own knowledge and power. Slightly earlier Japan had whetted the European appetite when some items were shown under the auspices of the Chinese pavilion of the Crystal Palace Exhibition in 1851—completely overshadowing their hosts. Japanese arts continued to make an impression in the London Exhibition in 1862 and then in Paris (1867, 1878, 1889), Philadelphia (1876), and Chicago (1893).[5]

During the first decades of the Meiji Reformation, Japan subjected itself to brisk modernization and reform to make itself competitive, with the ultimate aim of assuming dominance. This was to be achieved by skillfully integrating to Japan's own advantage what they saw as the best of Western mores, styles and technology. One of the first industrial areas to develop successfully was textiles where, with merciless efficiency, Japan began to supersede the rest of Asia in quality of production. Unlike the fate of Turkey, which had developed into a second-tier power and could be patronized by the West in the sense of Imperial 'othering', the Euro–Japanese or, more specifically, Franco–Japanese relations can better be described as a love affair in which each feverishly consumed the other.

Since Europe's relationship with Japan had not been allowed to evolve historically, it came to grasp Japan categorically. Japan existed as a series of chapters, or compartments: the shoguns, the Zen Buddhists, kabuki and Yoshiwara. On the other side, the Japanese fabricated their own obverse orientalism in their impressions of British male sovereignty. They were also uncritically in awe of French culture, something that Louis XIV had long before helped to foster, to be discussed later in this chapter. In the final chapter I will also explore how this image of French style was pivotal in the new wave of Japanese designers from Kenzo to Kawakubo (*Comme des Garçons*).

Japan's role in the evolution of Impressionism, Postimpressionism and Viennese Secessionism was inestimable, causing a rethinking of space and pictorial organization. It also introduced a new array of sympathetic decorative options that found their way into the paintings themselves and into design, in what evolved in the pan-European phenomenon of art nouveau. The voluptuous tendrils and floral extravaganzas had already come into being in the 1880s, but it was in 1895 that art nouveau made its official debut when the German art dealer Siegfried Bing opened the doors to his shop, the Maison de l'Art Nouveau, on the rue de Provence. Bing began his career in the 1870s importing Japanese decorative goods—woodblock prints, furniture, textiles and ceramics—from Yokohama. His new emporium, with its interiors designed by Henry van de Velde, was a haven where collection and commerce, artefact and invention were all but inseparable. Much like Liberty's in London, which at this time was enjoying the height of its success, Bing's store was part sideshow, part museum, part bazaar. Selling Japanese silks alongside prints by William Morris and lacquers together with cabinet makers, Bing encouraged French, Dutch, Belgian and Czech designers to work in the new style, which is now characterized with the belle époque, the final coruscation of old European aristocratic grandeur before its fall in 1914. Art nouveau is the modern version of latter-day chinoiserie, this time mixing eighteenth-century rococo (said to come from *rocaille*, meaning stonework) with the new Japanese decorative universe; both styles were liberal interpreters of the natural world.

Another supplier to rival Bing was the house of the Sichel brothers. Also trading out of Yokohama, it was less like Bing's gallery and more a repository clogged with Japanese goods. The volume of trade was enormous. In 1874 alone, Philippe Sichel received forty-five crates containing around 5,000 objects. In 1878, the *Gazette des Beaux-Arts* mentioned how sundry objects from enamels to embroidered satins found their way into 'a merchant's shop an immediately left for artists' studios or writers' studies'. The group of artists it lists is the pantheon of tomorrow: Manet, Tissot, Fantin-Latour, Degas,

Monet; writers include the Goncourt brothers, Philippe Burty and Zola (who in 1868 had been ennobled in paint by Manet, sitting ensconced in a Japoniste setting). The article concludes: 'The movement was established, the amateurs followed.'[6]

As we saw in the case of the shawl, some of the best ways to encounter the attitude to orientalist fashions is in literature and art. In Marcel Proust's *À la recherche du temps perdu*, there is a passage that describes the young narrator's immersion within the flamboyant, self-conscious Third Empire interior of the enigmatic Odette, Mme Swann, a former courtesan who has begun to shed signs of her former life in favour of trappings more befitting of an *haute bourgeoise*. Proust's novel is laced with subtexts and ironies, and there is often an obscured delineation between how things are and how they seem. It is a blur that easily translates into the ways in which orientalism in both fashion and dress has seeped into the West: from overt sign to something that has merged so neatly into Western culture as to become imperceptible.

> For since Mme Swann had picked up from a friend whose opinion she valued the word 'trashy'—which had opened to her new horizons because it denoted precisely those things which a few years earlier she had considered 'smart'—all those things had, one after another, followed into retirement the gilded trellis that had served as the background to her chrysanthemums, innumerable *bonbonnières* from Giroux's, and the coroneted note-paper (not to mention the coins of the gilt pasteboard littered about on the mantelpieces, which, even before she had com to know Swann, a man of taste had advised her to jettison). Moreover in the artistic disorder, the studio-like jumble of the rooms, whose walls were still painted in sombre colours which made them as different as possible from the white-enamelled drawing-rooms Mme Swann was to favour a little later, the Far East was retreating more and more before the invading forces of the eighteenth century; and the cushions which, to make me 'comfortable', Mme Swann heaped up and buffeted into position behind my back were sprinkled with Louis XV garlands and not, as of old, with Chinese dragons.[7]

This passage amenably illustrates the point that orientalism is not always an easily locatable component, nor do all its qualities or manifestations follow the same logic. If we inquire more deeply into Odette's change of face and taste, we might as well speculate that she had replaced one type of orientalism for another, since the eighteenth-century revival was caught up in Japoniste taste.

Proust supplies a more than fair setting of the interiors of the time and suggests that this act of dressing, or dressing up, was more than a theatrical conceit on the part of artists alone. Odette, whose interest and knowledge of art is as paltry as her social ambition is considerable, unwittingly conspires in the celebration of artifice that in artistic circles was known as decadence. The creation of specialist-themed interiors inspired by the pavilions of the

Great Exhibition was now no longer confined to the highest nobility. Already in 1862, the architect and designer Edward William Godwin decorated his Georgian House in Bristol with plain-coloured walls, uncharacteristic for the day, and covered them with Japanese prints, complemented by Persian carpets on the floor. He continued to do so in his other homes, which became a collector's record of his own autodidactic connoisseurship in Japanese art. In some ritualistic caricature, to harmonize with these settings, he had his successive wives and his daughter dress in kimonos.[8] He is but an early example of what would become quite normal at the turn of the century. The kimono became more than a fashion item on its own but was part of the aesthetic interior ensemble. It was more than affectation. It signalled a break with the eclectic medievalizing taste of the middle of the century.

Contemporary painters—from Alfred Stevens, James Tissot, John Singer Sargent to James McNeil Whistler—lovingly exploited Japonism's decorative repertoire of this domestic ad hoc set-designing that demanded kimono-clad women as decorative props. Figure 27, *Caprice in Purple and Gold No 2—The*

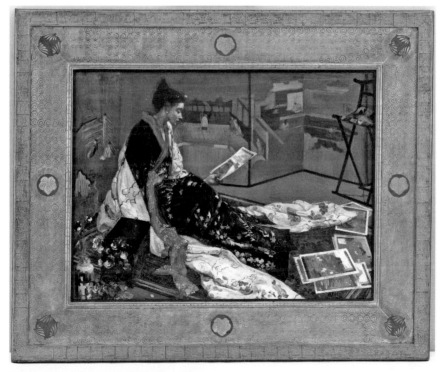

Figure 27 James McNeill Whistler, *Caprice in Purple and Gold No 2—The Golden Screen*, 1864, oil on wood, © Freer Gallery of Art, Smithsonian Institution, Washington, DC: Gift of Charles Lang Freer, F1904.75a.

Golden Screen (1864), shows Whistler at his Japoniste best: a woman clad in a sumptuous kimono, anointed in decorative silks, poring over woodblock prints, to the decorative mise en scène of the decorous goings-on narrated on a golden screen. As far as Japan was concerned, in fashion as in art, whole careers were made on interpreting on a style that the Japanese were only to happy to have interpreted. For to them, such ardour on the part of Europe spelt immeasurable possibilities of exposure, diplomacy and trade.

Early in his career, Monet painted *La Japonaise* (1876), showing his first wife, Camille, dressed in a vibrant red robe. She is standing on tatami matting, and behind her on the wall is a panoply of Japanese fans of myriad designs. The samurai appears to want to burst out from the kimono, the consternation on its white face contrasting with the come-hither expression of the woman. In the novel *Grave Imprudence*, published in 1880 by Philippe Burty, the character Brissot, leader of the Impressionists, is inspired by 'the little Japanese women . . . at the Exposition of 1876'. He paints a partially nude young woman under a red-orange robe inspired after 'costumes of *guèchas* and of *musmés*, which filled his cupboards'.[9] A slightly later memorable work is Gustav Klimt's 1916 portrait of Friederike Maria Beer, in which the subject

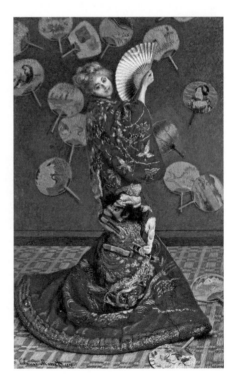

Figure 28   Claude Monet, *La Japonaise*, 1876, oil on canvas, © Museum of Fine Arts, Boston, 1951 Purchase Fund.

is wearing an ornate, flared and ermine-faced dolaman-like surcoat over an equally sumptuous undersuit with bloomer-like flared pants. The designs are of mixed origin: Japan crossed with Persian. Behind her is a scene whose energy recalls the painting by Monet. It is still uncertain from where Klimt took the design, possibly from a Korean ceramic. Klimt collected all kinds of East Asian prints, ceramics and decorative arts and fused them into his own version of Byzantine decoration. He was also a reader of Bing's short-lived monthly periodical *La Japon Artistique* (1888–91).

Toulouse-Lautrec, together with contemporaries like Whistler, Mucha, Erté and Vallaton, effectively ushered in a renaissance in printmaking after Dürer by seeing the world through a Japanese lens. The flattening and layering of planes, the simplifications of colour, decorative licence and the misalignments in space were all indebted to woodblock *okiyo-e* prints that had been a hallmark of the Edo period. Cabaret, cigarettes, bicycles and beverages were the commercial subjects. Orientalist fashions were not a high priority within these images only because the radical stylistic alterations rendered the whole world Japan-tinged. Clothing in such graphics is brought down to the same linear minima as the figures that inspired them, the artists borrowing liberally from Japanese textile designs for motifs and decorative details. Toulouse-Lautrec, who painted figures in kimonos (*Lili Grenier in a Kimono*, 1888), or in Japoniste poses or settings, also showed his devotion of all things Japanese in some photographs, many with a satirical edge. One has him languishing in all things Japanese, complete with hat, fan, doll and kimono. He stares into the distance in ironic reverie. Lautrec was no stranger to tomfoolery: another photograph affirms the irony of the first, where he sits, cross-eyed and cross-legged with two fingers raised in spiritual salute, like something out of an Abbott and Costello spoof or Emperor Ming in Flash Gordon. The most dramatic act of comedic transposition of cultures took place seven years before this photograph was taken, with Gilbert and Sullivan's hugely successful *Mikado* (1885), in which the foibles of British society were literally dressed up in Japanese dress. Its many renditions to this day attest to the fertility and malleability of the overarching Japanese aesthetic.

Toulouse-Lautrec also dressed up in other kinds of clothing and in false settings, including the Turkish style, and his fetish for other guises was as much a need to escape himself as reliving what his aristocratic forefathers the Counts of Toulouse were wont to do in previous centuries. Nonetheless, Lautrec's parlour tricks unmask the contradictions residing in the Western appropriation of the kimono. Like so many other orientalist articles in Western circulation, the word *kimono* is of modern coinage. As Anne Hollander explains, it differs from other forms of clothing like the sari and the chador, which are worn every day. Instead, the kimono is more like the Scottish kilt, which, despite also being a nineteenth-century invention, is a national identifier and

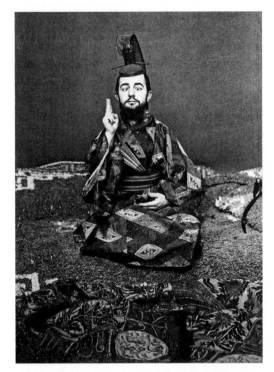

Figure 29   Maurice Guibert, *Henri Toulouse-Lautrec in Japanese Samurai Garb*, c. 1892 Vintage silver print, © Richard and Ellen Sandor Family Collection.

'invokes remote times'.[10] The kimono is a version of the garment known as *kosode*, 'small sleeve', because of the narrow openings for the hands, and they were comparatively more slender than the neutrally coloured and bulkier outer layers of courtly dress (*osode*, 'large sleeve'), which allowed for accents of colour and design to be exposed on the sleeves and around the collar. Lautrec is indeed perhaps wearing a *yukata*, the ancient informal dress that evolved into the modern day dressing gown (see Chapter 2).

The wrapped garment tied with a sash (*obi*) was truly of ancient origin, emerging first from the Chinese Sui and Tang court styles and becoming more stylized in the glorious Japanese Heian period, but that is all. Having gone through various simplifications since the Kamakura period, the *kosode* began to be worn as upper-class urban dress the seventeenth century by both civilian men and women as opposed to the more utilitarian and austere dress of the elite shoguns. It was also a solution to the impoverishment caused by the civil wars around this time. Typically, more than one *kosode* was worn in combination. Shogun dress, the *koshimaki*, meaning 'waist wrap', was dark in colour and densely embroidered with ritual and personally relevant motifs.

All such garments were heavily coded in messages relevant to age, season and occasion.

The photograph of Lautrec 'as a shogun' is therefore multiply misguided, much as a 1940s Technicolor costume drama might have sixteenth-century jousting armour in thirteenth-century open combat. His is also a relative exception to the European rule, which was for women to wear such garments. To European eyes, kimono-style dress was all but a transmutation of harem dress with its limitless erotic undertones; the geisha became the modern counterpart of the romantic harem-dweller. The gorgeously airy designs on the kimono were the newly located promise of the erstwhile Islamic *paradis terrestres*. The languid women dressed in kimonos in the paintings by European artists of the late-nineteenth century are all tinged with concubinage, the brothel never far behind. But the truth has a funny twist: in the early Edo period of seventeenth century, geisha, like actors, were all men. When the geisha assumed female form, her only function was to entertain the man. She was no carnal consort, despite what Lautrec (who lived for a time in a brothel) and his peers would make believe.

But that does not mean that this swing in orientations was all Western doing. Meiji Japan was deeply complicit in demarcating specific associations and in customizing its cultural aesthetic for Western consumption in which gender and objects were intertwined. In their march to modernization, the Meiji went to great lengths to define the role of women. Since no small part of such an effort had to do with what the West thought of them, the kimono became enlisted in rounded idea of the Japanese woman, and with a bit of Western coaxing, so did the geisha, which had gradually assumed a female face in the later Edo period. She was a schizophrenic hybrid of two rapidly coalescing constructs, that of Japanese modernity and that of newly packaged tradition. Men were expected to wear suits, and women kimonos; the new paragon of Japanese female was never without one. Women were spurred to action under the motto of 'good wife, wise mother' (*ryosai kenbo*) and encouraged to be adept in the coded practice of kimono-wearing, evidently not the Western idea of throwing on a gown and tying a girdle. Modern Japan's gendered identity was an invented one, and the kimono, the simplified single *kosode* commandeered by Meiji Reformation, was at its heart.[11]

Commerce was a principal motivation. The new woman was one of the objects at work marketing the new Japan, while the more neutrally dressed male laboured to construct it. Julia Sapin shows how department stores and world's fairs stimulated the availability of Japanese goods to Western markets. *Gofukuten*, the Japanese stores specializing in kimonos and *obi*, profited immensely from the way that foreign countries were packed into pavilions and sideshows at the various world's fairs.[12] One of the stores to benefit was Iida Gofukuten Takashimaya in Kyoto which, reminiscent of Liberty, struck up liaisons with all kinds of artists to develop designs. Sapin comments that recognition in France was as priority, and that Takashimaya's displays for the 1889 exhibition there were geared with export and approbation in mind.[13] Among other things, this meant prioritizing particular designs such as bird-and-flower painting (*kachôga*) and pictures of notable places (*meishoe*), which meant drawing from particular schools (Marayama and Shijô) where these genres were taught, thus giving cause for them to flourish.[14] She also reproduces several advertising posters, such as by Kamisaka Sekka, who went to study in the Glasgow School of Art in 1910, whose decorative elegance shows a considerable debt to belle époque posters, whose own indebtedness to Japan goes without saying.

The kimono would never retreat too far from Western fashion. It would continue to feature as itself or in a truncated form. At the beginning of the century Poiret introduced loose, free sleeves that were too much like those of the kimono than to be mistaken; in 1930, Jeanne Lanvin's 'bolero' jacket came with flared kimono-like sleeves. Chanel, too, availed herself of the brilliant florals from the silks used for kimonos, and if her line eschewed the Poiret arabesque, it did embrace the austerity within Japanese architectonics, both in the line of traditional clothing and in architecture. She also drew amply from the unisex nature of the *kosode*, in the respect that her clothing for women encroached aggressively on male dress. Moreover, Madeleine Vionnet experimented with the age-old manner of making kimonos from flat panels using only a Japanese hand-stitching, wave-seaming.[15] Since the 1980s, dressing gowns, when not made of terry towelling, have made intermittent returns to the *yukata*: long robes of decorative design gathered with an *obi*. Although something of a reinvention themselves, kimonos have also become popular wall hangings. They have become nostalgic, fictive relics of an age when things are remembered to be traditional, predictable and unchanging, belonging to a time before the advent of the age of self-consciousness and fashion—despite being born from this age.

DEORIENTALIZING JAPAN

The Meiji Reformation's quest for modernization roused the recognition, or belief, that such an enterprise could not be ventured without wearing Western clothing. It was then when the kimono was effectively born: it was used as a sign of ethnicity both to anchor national identity and to sell that identity abroad. But the near three centuries of splendid isolation had its price. Unlike China and the Middle East which had fed into European trade and back for more than a millennium, without these exchanges, Japanese ways appeared sharply discordant. This is where the power structures of orthodox orientalist discourse come into play: the overwhelming differences of Japanese mores had an attentive audience in Europe and elsewhere, while Japan at various levels had to surrender to the normative Euro–American modes of living.

As Alan Kennedy pithily describes it, 'the difference between the traditional Japanese and Western approaches to costume design is analogous to the difference between painting and sculpture'.[16] Germaine to sculpture, or the components that make up a mannequin, the West approaches dress according to an accretion of body parts, not only in tailoring but also in the evolution of styles: the bodice, made of sleeves, a back and front, accentuates the waist and the bosom, while the bustle exaggerates the behind, isolating it from the rest of the body. On the other hand, traditional Japanese clothing is conceived as a discrete whole that is based on a fabric as opposed to a garment, produced from oblong-shaped pieces of cloth sewn together with straight seams except for the buttons and lapels. 'The result is a flat, straight-edged expanse that is closer to a painter's canvas than a sculptor's armature'.[17] Nothing is wasted from the bolt of cloth. In Western terms, the tailor's 'cut' is made accountable to a particular body, whereas in Japanese terms it is relative to the garment itself. Japanese traditional dress did not fit, it hung; the tensile dynamic occurred on the vertical axis as opposed to vertical and successive horizontal axes in Western clothing. Tailoring was therefore anathema to the uninitiated Japanese sensibility.

In the 1880s, upper-class Japanese women went to uncertain lengths to respond to Paris fashions, but they imperfectly grasped the idea of fashion itself, that clothing was essentially modulated to an anonymous whim. Bustles and lapels expand and contract, feathers could be worn or not worn, hats were alternately wide-brimmed or narrow, whilst Japanese clothing, excepting the individual character of the textile, was unaccustomed to modulation. Japanese women of the time also had difficulty adjusting to the tightness of Western clothing. As if overnight, clothing was a tightened glove around the torso that had formerly had a greater freedom to breathe and move. Used only to tying the *obi* at the front, all the fasteners and rear ties were treacherously anomalous. The same incongruities applied to shoes which, in the Western sense, had not existed in Japan. Some results were ridiculously gauche. Liza Dalby, in her authoritative book on the kimono, reproduces several pictures where the East–West juncture is a less than happy one, with overcoats worn over traditional clothing or half Western and half Japanese top to bottom.

This said, as opposed to the desultory progress of women, the male adoption of Western dress was relatively swift and painless and seen as a propitious attitude for modernization. But as Toby Slade reveals, the refashioning of men was only reserved for outward appearance, while home life was still dominated by traditional forms of dress which had to do with what was appropriate to furniture and the way life was conducted.[18] Dining occurred on the floor, without chairs, for example, which can be punishing on the seams of pants. Yet the pace and impositions of modernization, and the invention of tradition to counter it, meant that sartorial modernity during the Meiji period had a political and official gloss. The bureaucratic elite, politicians and financiers adopted modern dress without demur because they knew the benefits of doing so, but other quarters were more resistant. Until the 1930s, modern dress in Japan was also predominately urban. But even such binaries between modern and traditional were slippery concepts, Slade argues.[19] The crafting of identities through responses to the outside would be a pattern of Japanese fashion and dress until the present.

One important change in Japan was in military dress, which followed a primarily French model. After 1870, when France was humiliated in Sedan and in the following year crushed by the Prussians, they fell into military disgrace. As a result, Japanese preferences switched from Gallic flamboyance to Teutonic sobriety. These two poles apparently suited two sides of the sartorial temperament: France exemplified Western excess and success, while the pared-down versions of dress were more in sympathy with the lines and in traditional Japanese dress, architecture and design. Deference to German uniform continued until just before 1905, when Japanese military dress switched to khaki, in which they defeated the Russians. This time taking from the successful use of camouflage uniforms by the British, khaki had, in Slade's words, 'an integrating force for the Japanese people, while being repugnant to all other peoples in Asia and the world'.[20] It is also curious to mention that in the 1880s with fomenting nationalism, Japanese schoolboys began to wear a uniform that resembled the Prussian ones of the day, complete with badges, buttons and differentiating symbols like stripes on the caps to differentiate one school from another.

This was an age in Japan where other nations were an adversary, a competitor, or a role model. And this was played out most obviously in clothing. Western dress was also a convenient and understandable costume for the rising bourgeoisie to adopt in their usurpation of the older ruling classes. The regular three-piece suit that became mandatory by the beginning of the twentieth century was a sign that anachronisms had been discarded in favour of prosperous bourgeois principles of reliability and hard work. But in the latter decades of the nineteenth century, Japanese tailors were still struggling to live up to the external image. Western observers ridiculed the inconsistencies of tailoring such as overly short trouser lengths and the inadequacy of the smaller Japanese male body type to carry Western style clothing.[21]

The Japanese elite were sensitive to the fact that they were potentially seen as risible parvenus on the international stage, and domestic rhetoric was rife with self-conscious diatribes about the ineffectual indolence and effeminacy of Japanese culture. One large-scale remedy for this was the Rokumeikan, or 'Deer-cry Hall'. Designed by the British architect Josiah Conder, it opened its doors on 28 November 1883, after three years' construction, paid by the foreign ministry. It was modelled on the most prestigious Parisian and London male clubs of the time but with some very official objectives, highest among them was to dispel the perception that Japan was not competitive on the world stage. Amidst clouds of cigarette smoke, whiskey, gin, German beer and hors d'oeuvres made by French cooks, the Japanese elite rubbed shoulders with foreign dignitaries, garnering their approval.[22] Slade locates four stages of the Japanese adoption of male Western dress, from 'use by eccentrics' to assimilation with the later Meiji and, finally, to the *habitus* of successive generations.[23] With institutions like the Rokumeikan, dress made its step into a wider framework of activity, namely from costume to dress; less conspicuous, more expected and into the fold of acceptable, comfortable everyday life.

Western fashion and dress had thus assumed world dominance. The suit became the unremarkable default, and everything else was other, potentially exotic. Japan's character of national mobility traded on otherness while with the other hand it played at being at one with the norm. By the 1880s, Japan was a very different place from even a decade before: women wore evening dresses to go with the men's suits; the Ministry of Education ordained that students wear uniforms in public colleges and universities, after which the private institutions followed suit, as it were. By the end of the century the silk industry had contracted in its domestic consumption, and a good three million yards of wool were being imported from England and Germany.[24] The fate of silk was also affected by diminished use in the kimono industry, where it was more the preserve of the productions at the highest end. Since Japan's reopening, the tunics and coats (*tombi*, *nijumawawasi*, *azumakoto*) worn over kimonos were made of (imported) wool. In 1881, the artisan Okajima Chiyozo introduced a technique of printing imported muslins, becoming known as *Yuzen* muslins. They were cheaper and easier to produce than their silk counterparts, and easier to clean. The first worsteds in daily used in Japan, muslins accounted for forty per cent of all textile imports. Once the technique became mechanized in 1907 in the dye-works of Inahata Katsutaro in Osaka, these statistics only increased. Another new textile used for kimonos was serge. Imported from Germany, it accompanied plainer designs and was favoured by men.[25] The kimono had therefore been readapted from and back into tradition several times over, its actual ties to the *kosode* receding with every generation.

By the 1930s the metamorphosis so strenuously begun in the 1870s was complete. Tradition became increasingly fetishized in the temples of Kyoto and in localized tea ceremonies. After Japan's belligerence and shaming de-feat in World War II, many people, intellectuals and laymen alike, in speculat-ing on a wrong turn lamented Japan's dislocation from its older traditions. Heavily influenced by Gandhi, in 1954, the left-wing critic Kamei Katsuichiro warned against the overly precipitous nature of Japan's modernization and the uneven idea of its past:

> It should certainly be a matter of the profoundest regret to the Orient that these outcries uttered in the nineteenth and twentieth centuries as Asians, in inflec-tions which varied with the particular features of the different countries of Asia, should never have achieved full expression, but should have died out without reinforcing one another. To us Japanese to die out rests with us. The cause of the tragedy lies in our vigorous, precipitous modernisation. We tried with des-perate efforts to master European civilisation, and in the act of acquiring it we lost something very precious—what I should like to call the characteristic 'love' of Asia.[26]

Fashion was not high on his mind, but as we shall see in the following chap-ter, the sources of tradition that had become codified, if not packaged out of all recognition by modernization would return with vengeance a few decades later, effectively redefining the fashions in Paris which had been first instru-mental in redefining Japan.

The Japan of the twenty-first century seems to have made its peace with the regrets that nagged Katsuichiro. It is now one of the biggest consumers of high-end ready-to-wear clothing and it excels in producing high-quality clothing (with chains such as Comme Ça Ism). By and large, urban Japanese are natty, fastidious dressers in the global Western style. However, what is noteworthy is the way in which the post-Meiji dress traditions in women's clothing, albeit in a minority, co-exist on a day-to-day level with normative clothing. More re-markable is the way that, arguably unique to any country, Japanese participate in the *spectatorship* of their own traditions. Japanese are active, proud tour-ists of their own country and, in traditional sites such as in Kyoto, will ask to be photographed next to a geisha. Cultural tourism is therefore internalized. The aesthetics of tradition are held up as cultural talismans that are distant and proximate at the same time. Tradition lives as something unchanging, essential and inviolably reliable beneath the outer carapace of day-to-day life and the exigencies of economic exchange.

Figures 30 and 31 demonstrate this very well. Figure 30 is of a woman in a kimono being photographed next to a fully made-up geisha standing beside a man who has also had his picture taken with her. Figure 31 is of a geisha posing in one of the small shrines in the historic region of Maruyama Park in Kyoto that contains the Chion-in Temple. She is not only being photographed by a professional photographer but also by a fellow geisha.

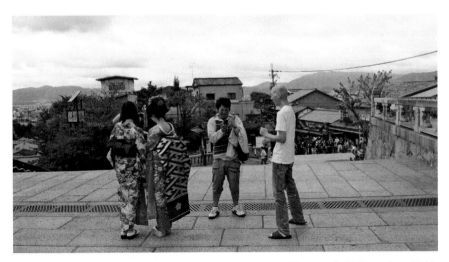

Figure 30   On the steps to the Chion-in Temple, Kyoto. Photograph 7 November, 2011. © Courtesy the author.

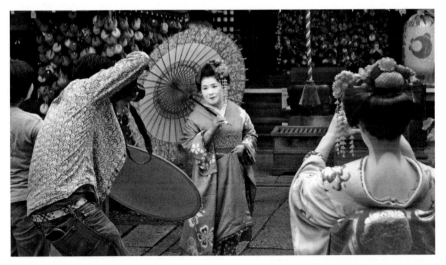

Figure 31   At a shrine in the Maruyama Park, Kyoto. Photograph 7 November, 2011. © Courtesy the author.

DEORIENTALIZING TURKEY

In Nerval's detailed account of his journey to the East, he regularly strikes out at the inadequacies of what he sees. Here his verdict on the oriental adoption of European dress is unsparing: 'For a yellow woman to dress in the European style has to be the stupidest thing in the world.'[27] He paints another merciless portrait on an occasion when he is invited to dine with a pasha:

The pasha left me for a moment, no doubt to attend to his religious matters whereupon he returned and said to me, 'We will dine in the European manner'.

And so he brought some chairs and an elevated table instead of using a stool to support a metal plate and placing cushions around it, which is what is normally done. I felt everything in the pasha's manner was to oblige me, and for all that I must confess that I dislike the way that European customs are making the Orient gradually disappear; I appealed to the pasha that he was treating me as if I were a vulgar tourist.

'You are about to see me in a black coat', he said.

My reply was justified, for a sensed that I was right. Whatever one does and however far one is able penetrate a Turk's goodwill, one must not believe that an immediate fusion between our way of life and theirs is possible. The European customs that he adopts become in certain cases a sort of neutral terrain which one gathers from rather than raising one self toward. He agrees to imitate our ways as he uses our language, but only with regard to us. He resembles one of those people who are half peasant and half aristocrat; he shows Europe his 'gentlemanly' side but in Asia is always a pure 'Osmali'.[28]

One can easily discount these observations with Saidian opprobrium as being superciliously judgmental. But what is worth savouring is that way that certain colonized nations had begun lead this double life, as we saw with Japan in the first four decades of the Meiji era.

While Japan was outwardly prospering from its newly found Westernization, Turkey had become apprehensive about itself, which it saw to be a shadow of a once great empire. While it looked melancholically inward, it also looked outward as it had never done before for remedies and improvements. Their changes of attitude make Nerval's passage seem prophetic. Like their Japanese counterparts, the end of the nineteenth century was a watershed of cultural and sartorial experimentation, an interim period when Turkish people played at being Western before Westernization became an official policy. In Japan the changes were part of a new national disposition, whereas in Turkey they were summarily enforced. The Prime Minister Kemal Atatürk recognized the importance of clothes in altering attitudes and raised such changes to the level of sumptuary law.

The changes effected by Atatürk are in truth the penultimate stages of Turkey's sartorial modernization which began somewhere earlier in the nineteenth century, around the time when Nerval was recording his travels. The period of Atatürk's stewardship as prime minister under Kemal was the definitive turning point from a military to a civil state, a change that had been occurring for over a century. These decisions, which Ussama Makdisi attributes to 'Ottoman Orientalism', embraced the West's attitudes to time and progress, whilst resisting the imperial implications that devolved from them. Turkey purposely modified and subsumed Islam to create a new idea that signified a break with the stagnant Ottoman past. 'The challenge', states Makdisi, 'before scholars of the Ottoman Empire, specifically, is to explore how Ottoman resistance to Western imperialism engendered its own interrelated forms of Orientalist representation and domination that existed simultaneously at the center and the periphery.'[29] The system of modernization that took into account its difference from the West and its need to take its cue from it exposed many different orientalist discourses that defy presumptions of static East–West binaries that persist in politics as well as clothing.

The beginnings of Turkey's Westernization became visible in 1826 under the rule of Mahmud II. A code of regulations was enacted to reform the army, which was to begin with the uniforms that were to imitate the French. This had already been attempted in 1807, at the height of Napoleonic power, but resistance to it had been so severe that it led to an insurrection that dethroned Mahmud's predecessor, Selim III. But two decades later, the fear of Turkey's military decline had begun to seep in, and the reforms were accepted. Until this time official restrictions had not been put on dress, although the Muslim accepted the need to dress in a way that separated him from the Western infidel. Bernard Lewis cites a list of informal ordinances that vaunted the virtues of the turban and exhorted men not to trim their beards. Mahmud, it seems, went a little far in some areas, such as ordering that the saddles of the cavalry be like those in Europe, weakening their manoeuverability and inciting 'disgust'.[30] The effort to reform the army had complicated psychological consequences. The progressive outward face was associated with capitulating to an enemy that for centuries had been represented as decadent and weak. These perceptions continue their currency in the present with leaders like sixth president of Iran, Mahmoud Ahmadinejad, whose refusal to wear a tie registers contempt for the formalities of Western dress.

Because headdress, particularly the turban, had for so long been a source of national identification, it was also the hardest to alter. By way of compromise, the Turkish army wore fezzes or *subaras* with their new Western-style uniforms. But the life of the *subara*, a hat of conical construction which fell to one side, was short, taken over by the fez. (The *subara* is also used in Serbian folk dress and was donned during World War I and by the Chetniks in World War II.) However, the fez was not strictly of Turkish origin, but North African. In 1828, after deliberations at the office of the Chief Mufti, it was officiated as the standard military head covering, and measures were taken to suppress any popular opposition. A year later the reform was extended to the civilian population as compulsory national dress, the robe and the turban confined to the theologians, the *ulema*. The adoption of the fez is really a metonym for the wholesale Westernizing renovation of Turkish society. With it came other directives that slippers be replaced by boots and burnous be replaced by coats. Men were henceforth expected to limit their jewellery and to keep their whiskers short. The Sultan began to receive visitors according to European protocols, and tables and chairs appeared alongside the cushions and divans.[31] This shows how Nerval's pasha was doing more than meeting his guest's approval; he was conforming to a trend that was slowly spreading across Islamic states.

The fez, then, is a symbol of Islam's early modernization and at the same time the reassertion of its autonomy from the West. For despite its sudden and enforced introduction and early misgivings that it was unsatisfactory as an Islamic head covering, a 'century later' writes Lewis, 'it became so well acclimatized that it was attacked—and defended—as the emblem of Ottoman and Islamic traditionalism and orthodoxy'.[32] The 'attack' came from Kemal and Atatürk, who outlawed its use after the World War I when Turkey's continued military failures were perceived to have chronic national ramifications calling for equally dramatic measures to resolve them.

By the second half of the nineteenth century the disparities between the crumbling Ottoman Empire and the large states of Europe were more than unpleasantly evident to the Turks who travelled abroad and to the people who heard their stories. The Ottoman Empire had relied on land trade, whereas Britain and its lesser rivals, France and Holland, had spread its reach far beyond that. The plentiful riches of Europe stoked the coals of fear of Turkish national extinction. Efforts to end the age of despotism and oust the sultan appeared in 1859 in the Kuleili Incident, an unsuccessful plot to assassinate Sultan Abdülmecid. Since Mahmud's rule, Ottoman rulers struggled to implement various constitutional reforms, tempering ancient despotism with progressive, modern liberalist values.

The reforms are generally known under the rubric of the Tanzimat ('reorganization'), spanning 1839–76. These helped to plan a market economy that ushered in a powerful working class and with it a fashion system which by definition reflects on its own capacity for change. As Reina Lewis and Nora Seni make clear, the changes in women's clothing during the period assumed a central importance to louder voices about where state and society were going.[33] Other than the fez, changes were gradual. Casting a hungry eye on Paris fashions, women of the court became arbiters of fashions that once had no presence at all. Lewis's eloquent account focuses on the changes in female visibility—both in terms of others and how they saw themselves—in this period until the early-twentieth century. She is also interested in the crosscultural fold between orientals and nonorientals and the ways in which their interaction helped shape the other: for the occidental woman the tempering of superior colonialist views about the Orient, and for the oriental woman, a change in an attitude to herself. Seeds of this had already been sown with Montagu, but Montagu always chose to draw clear lines of class and culture. Lewis insists that the restraints imposed on women, their activities, and the nature of the spaces they occupied caused female British travellers to have a very different apprehension of the Orient than the colonial male traveller. Of particular interest are the writings of Grace Ellison from the first decades of the twentieth century, whose insights in the Ottoman female experience are a seldom-cited foil to what had become clichés about Eastern men and woman alike.[34] With the debates over burqas in our present age, her writings and Lewis' study have renewed relevance.

One salient woman's voice at the end of the nineteenth century was Fatma Aliye Hanim, who published a book on Muslim society in French in 1894. An opponent of polygamy, Aliye Hanim devoted about a third of her book to woman's clothing and veiling. She discussed how the baggy trousers (*salvar*) and blouse (*gömlek*) (which had done much to cultivate the idea of the shapeless Turkish woman) had been jettisoned in favour of the *entari*, a flowing, shift-like garment which had become increasingly waisted and could accommodate a corset. According to Aliye Hanim, the *entari* was now only sympathetic to the corseted body. As Lewis points out, this had serious repercussions on all aspects of the Ottoman woman's life, from their self-perception which had broken with a womanly idea of the past, to their social interaction. The freedoms so valued by Montagu and those in her wake were severely curtailed. By the 1870s, the same sartorial partitions to be found in Japan arose in Turkey. In upper-class private gatherings, Ottoman woman could be found flaunting the latest Paris fashions, while outdoors, where they were expected to observe strict codes of modesty, they remained more or less covered. This imposition relaxed somewhat in the years before World War I. By the time of the dress reforms in the 1920s, women could be seen uncovered when escorted by a man.[35] Turkey's transformation into Western dress was thus two-sided: in private quarters women were able to express and assert themselves so long as they restricted their visibility in the public sphere.

By the end of World War I the Ottoman Empire was no more and the state of *Turkiye* was born, ushering in the new postwar regime of the redoubtable Mustafa Kemal. Sultan Abdülhamid had already abdicated in 1908, but progress until the war was far from robust. As with many of the attenuated and newly formed states after 1919, the so-called Kemalist revolution took advantage of the massive demographic and social upheavals of the time to secularize the state and to replace military organization with an efficient civil meritocracy. Understandably, coping with such a loss was difficult. Like its German counterpart, there was next to no public support in the new regime, which was blamed for the failures of its predecessor. But unlike Germany, Turkey had effectively rebranded itself, with all the connotations of the persuasive power of the visual that that metaphor implies. It is tempting to digress at length about the social upheavals that this brought on, as well as the conflicts, such as the cleansing of the Armenians in the still unacknowledged genocide that took place in April 1915. But these scattered details provide a backdrop for the rationale behind the next major wave of changes that culminated in the abolition of the fez.

In her memoir about Turkey, Barbro Karabuda describes the tensions that abounded in Atatürk's proselytizing mission to eradicate the fez, where he would travel to towns and ceremonially replace his fez with a Western hat: 'It was dreadful.'[36] She describes how to so many of the Turkish population Atatürk's actions amounted to betrayal. Since the new hats were those worn by the infidel, they were presumed, by the intransigent logic of habit and superstition, to lead to the destruction of Muhammedianism. By contrast, 'In western eyes the fez was romantic and colourful, a boon to the caricaturist and much used in the penny-dreadful type of story; but to the Turk, the fez was one of life's necessities'.[37] This national 'necessity' was ironically a fabrication that had seeped rapidly into the soil. It was adopted out of necessity as a reflex against the inexorable encroachment of the West. Finally, the informal national symbol, which was not even of Turkish origin, underwent a painful purge.

This was because the Islamic symbolism to headwear is more than just symbolic, it is physical: it is worn out of religious necessity. It was also historical, connecting Muslims across time in spiritual fealty. Moreover, it was the final article that separated the Muslim from the infidel, the mainstay against falling into the same turpitude. As Bernard Lewis expresses it, 'The rest of the Muslim's body might be Westernized, but his head remained Islamic—with the tall, red, challenging fez proclaiming at once his refusal to conform to the West and his readiness to abase his unimpeded brow before God'.[38] But to Kemal and Atatürk its unequivocal symbolism was the problem, maintaining the average Turk's contact to old-time glory and to the autocratic arbitrary rule the sultans. Wrenching the fez from the people was a traumatic measure, but the pain served the point of driving them relentlessly into the modern world. Many Turks saw it as the final capitulation to the West, the last of a string of ignominious defeats, while others saw it as a necessary break with the past, a renaissance. On 25 August 1925, Kemal officially announced that

> there is no need to seek and revive the costume of Turan. A civilized, international dress is worthy and appropriate for our nation, and we will wear it. Boots or shoes on our feet, trousers on our legs, shirt and tie, jacket and waistcoat—and, of course, to complete these, a cover with brim on our heads. I want to make this clear. This head-covering is called 'hat'.[39]

This was the first of a welter of changes, which included the Gregorian calendar and abandoning Arabic script for the Roman. Hostility was compounded by confusion: the male populace was presented with choice where before it had none. Shops were filled with all sorts of hats, high and low, wide- and narrow-brimmed. Unaccustomed to brims, they were source of yet more consternation, and many used it to remove the hat, perpetuating the stereo-type of the ham-handed oriental trespassing in Western clothing.

While Turkey underwent its changes, from the Tanzimat to the Kemalist re-forms, European men had no compunction about using the fez. Upper-middle-class men wore the floppier *subara* as part of their smoking ensemble, but it would also double as a sleeping hat. Isolated bohemians like Gautier in the mid-nineteenth century may have used it as a public signature, but it even-tually became domesticated and worn in closed gatherings. Toward the end of Thomas Mann's *Magic Mountain* there is a passage in which the straight-laced doctor, Hofrat Behrens, uses the fez to register that he has temporarily stepped out of his normal mien of clinical detachment:

> He had managed to give his appearance some carnival cheer to his clinical gown, which he also wore today in accordance as always with his duties, by donning a real Turkish fez of carmine red and with a black tassel that dangled over his ear. These two together were enough of a costume for him, sufficing to send his otherwise neutral appearance into a place of complete wantonness and wonder.[40]

Mann began writing his novel in 1912 and completed it in 1924, the year when Kemal's government was to set the wheels of the outlawing of the fez in motion. Facts such as these make this novel all the more uncannily prescient. And we can trust in the extraordinary intelligence of a writer such as Mann to suspect that the irony is more than coincidental, especially given that a leit-motif of the novel is the discord of epochal change. The phlegmatic Behrens lends himself a festive edge, an air of sublimated catharsis with a hat whose place of origin was soon to be decreed redundant.

The uncomfortable renunciation of the fez, because of its physical and historical association with society and religion of Islam, explains a great deal when applied to its female counterpart, the veil, and to the residual conflicts surrounding the burqa after 9/11 (to be elaborated on in the following chap-ter). In the veil the male's physical relationship to the fez is less metaphoric but factual. It is a material partition between the woman and the world, both a shield and a prison. Whatever may be one's attitude to the veil, it is inscribed within life and belief. It is neither interchangeable nor a matter of random choice. It is not fashion and can only be called clothing in the most empiri-cal sense. For to the most devout, it is one of the articles that endows the woman her womanhood and decrees her sacred before God, legitimating her existence much as baptism in Christianity endows one with a soul and certi-fies a religious above a merely secular life. One need only look at the verbal framing of the hijab in English: one is 'in hijab', not 'in *a* hijab', suggesting that the clothing is not a matter of one choice to the next but rather confers on the wearer a level of ritual completeness. Its meaning in Arabic has to do

with screening and separation and not with a form of dress. For Western observers, the veil had long prevailed as the sign of Eastern womanhood, the
sign that differentiated life between the sexes and social organization as a
whole. It literally connoted the harem, the wall behind which existed voluptuous womanhood.[41] For this very reason it too was targeted.

In 1935, ten years after the demise of the fez, the veil was banned. But
with mixed success—many women out of fear or observations of strict religious rules continued, and continue, to wear full traditional dress. On the
other hand, this formalization into law was taken by other women as a sign
that they were now free to dress openly, which meant the simpler and more
sporty women's fashions of the time, clothes that said that women had their
own power of movement and a mind of their own. Yet the new woman that
slowly emerged at the beginning of the twentieth century deprived the Western onlooker of the fantasies it had feasted on for the last few hundred years.
This did not prevent the West from perpetuating this fantasy for itself, helped
along by couturiers like Paul Poiret and the avant-garde artistic circles that
met around the Ballets Russes.

COUTURE, ART AND COSTUME: FROM POIRET
TO THE BALLETS RUSSES

Fashion's transformation between 1858 and 1868[42] was from unmoderated
market symptom to independent creation. Before Charles-Frederick Worth
opened his fashion house in the Rue de la Paix in 1858, fashion was defined
by its commentators, by its wealthiest exponents such as Marie Antoinette, or
boldest such as Beau Brummell, and by the private decisions made between
clients and dressmakers based on the two former influences. Worth prized
the industry away from the guilds and located it in the couturier himself, as a
matter of talent and creation. In his new role as artist–couturier, Worth mined
the history of art, especially Renaissance, Mannerist and baroque, referenc-
ing it with free abandon in his dresses—which he called his 'creations'—and
bringing what had been the purview of experts into the popular domain. His
interest in orientalism was neither avid nor overt. It was principally confined to
highly mediated styles that have already been discussed, such as the bodice-
vest, or accessories, designs and fabrics like feathers, florals and silk that by
dint of time and use had all but lost their orientalist associations. He played a
large part in ending the reign of the shawl, first by lightening them into smaller
lace then abolishing them altogether. Worth emphasized the *toute ensemble,*
demoting the role of accessories. And he made sure not to make a style or
reference too preponderant lest the idea of his unique creative genius, and
the unique item it conceived, not be preserved.[43]

Paul Poiret is the figure around which orientalist fashion in the first two decades of the twentieth century can be said to converge. He worked briefly for Worth's sons and for other established houses including Doucet, Cheruit, Rouff and Paquin and opened his own house in 1903. His early penchant for orientalism came in the form of a coat cut like a kimono while working for the house of Worth, to the dismay of the client, Russian Princess Bariatinsky, causing his swift dismissal. Together with his wife and muse Denise Boulet, Poiret designed clothing in classical and orientalist styles. In his memoir he claims that he combated against the burdensome influence of the eighteenth century with simplification and an emphasis on colour.[44] Known widely as an eccentric, Poiret was a talented showman. He took Worth's idea of couturier–creator, amplifying it into the modern idea of couturier as the unsurpassable creative celebrity. In the 1850s designers and illustrators had been dabbling in what might be named omniorientalsm—a schizophrenic eclecticism often in cross-cultural combinations that would have been unrecognizable to both country of origin[45]—but Poiret made the Orient of the Middle East a dimension of his own creative signature.

Poiret gave himself the credit for liberating woman's bodies from bustles and corsets, although this had already been in operation in the designs of Vionnet, the Callot sisters and Fortuny, who were the leading exponents of the new early-century craze of the English tea gown. As scholars such as Peter Wollen,[46] Yvonne Deslandres[47] and, preeminently, Nancy Troy[48] have shown, Poiret was remarkably adept at drawing together influences into garments that looked uniquely his own. Poiret went a step beyond Worth *père* to take his inspiration from august art history and to meld these with influences from the Far and Middle East, India and Eastern Europe, blending the classical with folk and exoticism. Poiret began to be piqued by orientalism with the exhibition of oriental art at the Pavilion de Marsan in Paris in 1906—after which he designed his famous 'Confucius' evening coat—and a large-scale show of Islamic art in Munich in 1910.

Poiret laid the platform for Chanel and Patou, who were the modern pioneers of easy lines and subtle curves. The flowing, narrow torso was topped with a scarf, or scarf-like hat, more or less turban-like, and commonly accented with jewelled or feathered aigrettes. Poiret as well as designer–illustrators who had worked with him, the Russian Erté and Georges Barbier, all had a hand in the trend that enjoyed resurgence in the 1930s and later in the 1960s, becoming what is now a standard style in the millinery repertoire.

Poiret's spring 1911 collection was an oriental feast: exotic fabrics, turbans, aigrettes, and the '*jupe-culotte*' and harem pants, which became his signatures. The *jupe-culotte*, otherwise known as *jupe-sultane* or *jupe-pantalon*, the more studied, elegant counterpart to bloomers, were sometimes pleated and gathered for maximal effect of billowing expansion and contraction. Their close resemblance to the bloomer meant they did not pass in Parisian society without a hiccup. For one, they were considered a recommendation of a form of clothing that was, with the exceptions I have already noted, informal and, from the point of view of woman's liberation and suffrage, reactionary. The sartorial line between the sexes was confounded—rhetoric of sexual inversion was rife at this time—and the woman's movement could be interpreted (although Poiret was definitely no feminist) as sanctioned in the illustrious halls of haute couture. No doubt such fears caused the inelegance of the silhouette to be decried. To others, as Valerie Steele notes, the 'harem pants' were identified as lewd because the erotic and exotic were indissolubly united. In accentuating the leg they were scandalous.[49] When translated to profits, these concerns assumed tangible importance. Conservative backers branded Poiret as eccentric and threatened to withdraw their support.[50]

One of Poiret's chief supporters was his illustrator Georges Lepape, a former student of Cormon who had also taught Toulouse-Lautrec, Van Gogh and Matisse. His penchant for thin lines lent itself to the sinuous line of Poiret's designs, which he celebrated in the booklet that came out with the collection in 1911, *Les Choses de Paul Poiret*. He shared in the couturier's Fauve-like colour, fervour for aigrettes, turbans and beaded tunic, bangles and harem slippers. The *toute ensemble* of the previous era of Worth, Redfern and Doucet appeared mannered and pompous by comparison, and Poiret meant it to be so. Now a woman was no longer presented by a homogenous package organized by the higher power of the couturier; instead she was presented with a *look* that could expand or contract at her own will. She was given a set of options to which she could add the amount and extent of accessories according to her taste and to suit the occasion. In many ways, by mediating fashion through the other of the Orient, Poiret anticipated the modern concept of 'elegant casual' which was to be put into full effect a decade later.

Up until now, oriental clothing had been used as costume (masquerade), in private (dressing gowns,) or as accessories (fezzes, turbans, jewellery and shawls), or it was absorbed and excelled at by European industry (silk, paisley). In other words, until now orientalism had either been a source of fun, absorbed, or used as tasty inflection in which the Western sartorial core remained inviolate. But Poiret's changed this. Though it may have been true that orientalism was on the rise before Poiret's 1911 collection. In 1909 Lady Ottoline Morrell noted that the wife of Neville Lytton was wearing 'gorgeous Arabian dresses'.[51] Poiret colonized this taste with the hype of personal ownership that foreshadowed the high capitalist couture that appeared after the 1980s. Formalizing the oriental other into the fold of Western dress was effectively lowering the invisible screen that occurred with masquerade and making, rhetorically speaking, the oriental equal with the European. One was no longer infecting one's dress or adopting as the intrepid Westerner ready to return later to his former, more sensible ways, one was *emulating* the oriental. But this was illusion in more ways than one. As we have already seen in this chapter, the old fear of the Eastern threat had not only descended into the innocuous, it was unfounded, since many areas of Asia and the East were busy emulating the West.

Poiret used the launch of his collection as the occasion for staging his now famous *Thousand and Two Night* party, where everyone was expected to dress in the Persian-inspired clothes of his latest collection. It was a clever ploy. His guests were literally made to wear his designs and mentally enact the ideas they evoked. As Poiret recounts, once the guests had donned their costumes, they repaired to a room where they were greeted by

> a semi-naked negro draped in Boukhara silks, armed with a torch and a yatagan [a Turkish sword], brought together and led in my direction. The first walked into a sandy chamber bedecked by blue and golden velum, fountains falling into porcelain basins. It called to mind a sun-filled patio belonging to Aladdin. Multicoloured light cast across motley vellum. The guests mounted several steps to find themselves in before a huge golden cage, gridded with twirly ironwork behind which I enclosed my favourite (Mme Poiret) surrounded by ladies in waiting singing Persian airs. Mirrors, the sorbets, aquariums, little birds, chiffons and plumage—these were the distractions of a queen of the harem and her ladies in waiting.

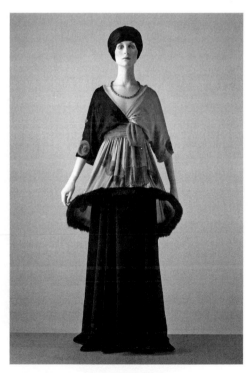

Figure 32   Paul Poiret: Sorbet, skirt and tunic evening ensemble, Paris, France, 1912, © V&A Images; Victoria and Albert Museum, London.

One then repaired to a chamber with a fountain which seemed to come from the carpet and to fall into a basin of iridescent crystal.[52]

Poiret himself was the image of the Sultan Suleiman the Magnificent, in a fur-trimmed caftan tied with a green sash, large turban and slippers adorned with jewels, holding a whip in one hand a scimitar in the other. When his wife appeared, she was wearing a 'lampshade tunic', crinoline over loose pants of light chiffon, the incipient design for what would later be the 'Minaret look'.[53] Her turban was of gold cloth wrapped with chiffon and finished with an aigrette anchored by a large turquoise.

Cast into a blinding spectacle of limitless texture and colour, Poiret's guests were sensorially stuffed to the gills with signs of pleasure. Poiret had taken Worth's premeditated choreography and transformed into a lavish theatre in which he sought to make the 'Persian' Orient his own. 'The whole party' writes Wollen, 'revolved around this pantomime of slavery ad liberation set in a phantasmagoric fabled East'.[54] As with the *jupes-culottes*, Poiret's party announced a break with past conceptions of the Orient. From an anthropological or moralistic point of view, in the seventeenth and eighteenth century for

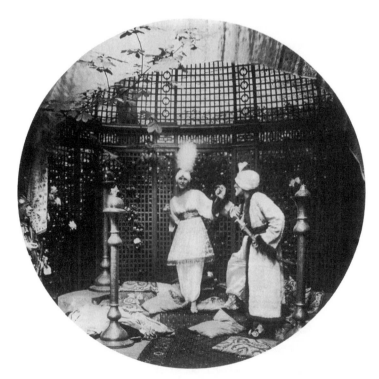

Figure 33   Paul Poiret (1879–1944) and his wife Denise at a party on June 24, 1911, photo by Henri Manuel, © Photo by Apic/Getty Images.

example, 'fabrications' of the Orient meant lies and misconceptions. 'Fabrications' however, had a different semantic ring, connoting creation and free-
association, since the euphemism 'fabricate' is to lie. With the diminution of
the Ottoman threat and its shift into Westernization, there was not much to
get wrong. After all, the Orient was participating in reshaping its own traditions. As far as art and design was concerned, and especially fashion, the Orient was a floating signifier freed of imperatives of truth or equivalence.

A parallel can be drawn here with one of the earliest and greatest works
of modern orientalist music, Rimsky-Korsakoff's *Scheherezade*, composed in
1888. Rimsky-Korsakoff stated that his composition avoided the specific to
maintain its air of mysterious wonder:

> In composing *Shekherazada* I meant these hints [the jettisoned titles such as
> 'The Sea' and 'Sinbad's Ship'] to direct but slightly the hearer's fancy on the
> path which my own fancy had travelled, and to leave more minute and particular
> conceptions to the will and mood of each. All I had desired was that the hearer,
> if he liked my piece as *symphonic music*, should carry away the impression that
> it is beyond doubt an oriental narrative of some numerous and various fairy-tale
> wonders and not merely four pieces played one after the other and composed on
> the basis of themes common to all the four movements. Why then, if that be the
> case, does my suite bear the name, precisely, of *Shekherazada*? Because this
> name and the title *The Arabian Nights* connote in everybody's mind the East and
> the fairy-tale wonders . . .

A little earlier, he stipulated that the 'aversion for the seeking of a too definite program in my composition led me subsequently (in the new edition)
to do away with even those hints of it which had lain in the headings of
each movement like: The Sea; Sinbad's Ship; the Kalender's Narrative, etc'.[55]
Rimsky-Korsakoff's own words go a long way toward helping to define the
shifting association, guiltless appropriation and generic placelessness of
transorientalism.

Similarly, Poiret created his own Orient. Poiret's clothes did not simply
evoke or invoke a place beyond itself; they participated in its continued conception. In short, they kept the idea alive and mobile. Poiret recounts how,
during his *Thousand and Two Nights* party, a gentleman was asked to fit
himself in the appropriate costume; when the he replied that his coat was
'authentic Chinese' he was informed, 'Sir, we're not in China, we're in Persia'.[56] Culturally and geographically, the 'real' Persia had long since faded
only to be remade, reclaimed in a vivacious couturier's household. It is also
noteworthy how in this instance fashion and dress intertwine with theatrical
costume (conceits that would come to a grinding halt with the outbreak of
World War I).

One source of inspiration that Poiret acknowledged was the student ball
at the École des Beaux-Arts, which in 1911 had a Babylonian theme (*bal des*

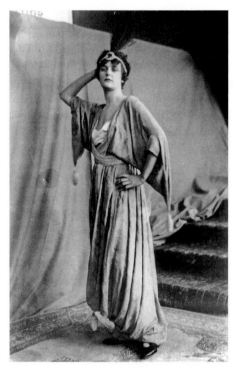

Figure 34 Model Gimbels wearing a dress by
Paul Poiret, March 1914, © Photo by APIC/Getty
Images.

Quat'z-arts).[57] For this event Poiret wore the costume that he himself had designed for the Édouard de Max for the one-act play *Nabuchodonosor*, which
had opened in January of the same year, with sets by André Dunoyer de
Segonzac. By all accounts it was a dress rehearsal for his own event, and
by his own admission, his first foray into costume design. Poiret had Nabuchodonosor in a long flowing robe and he designed for a consort of black
slaves, eunuchs and concubines. Acclaim was enthusiastic. The artist and
critic A. E. Marty enthused over Poiret's 'costumes of unimaginable sump-
tuosity and tonal beauty'. The marvellous colours were a special attraction,
remarking on the 'greens, yellows and oranges' that were counterpoised by
Max's coat 'of sombre purple'.[58] Compare this to Claude Lepape's description of the baggy trousers worn by the Negroes at Poiret's *Thousand and Two
Nights* party: 'trousers of muslin silk in Veronese green, lemon, orange and
vermilion.'[59]

It might well have been done earlier, but this is an appropriate juncture at
which to hone in on the subject of colour, and its relation to orientalism. In
many respects it appears to be a fairly weak link whose prejudices are not

worth engaging too ardently, if only because colour is by nature abstract. It is not the same as the appropriation of a motif. After all, a colour cannot be owned. But what could have been so provocative about Gautier's red vest or Poiret's chromatic cavalcades? One may start with the famous observation by Baudelaire about how male class and identity lay hidden behind the new modern uniform of the black hat and coat. This is a good place to begin but does not explain enough. An answer is essayed by David Batchelor in his book *Chromophobia*, in which he observes a marginalization of colour in Western culture. This is echoed by John Gage in his seminal *Colour and Culture*, where he suggests that to eschew colour was a sign of a more serious and less frivolous disposition.[60] Batchelor goes on to show that the blandishments of modern reason and industrial instrumentalism have encouraged the marginalization of colour to the realm of 'the feminine, the oriental, the primitive' and to the superlatively cosmetic.[61] In the most unabashed way, Poiret unconsciously played upon these notions while also bringing them into account. Whereas in the language of the suit, colour, supplied by the tie, is the accent on the monochromatic canvas of the sartorial body, in woman's wear he injected it into fashion's substance. But this would only truly take effect in the 1960s. When we look at sports and leisurewear, we can safely say that in certain line of fashion and dress, colour has happily lost its gender and exotic associations. Poiret was no doubt not alone in this, but he is an important marker in this shift in awareness. Eirik Hanssen suggests that fashion in the 1920s and 1930s in America, inspired by the Parisian examples, was a specular method of enjoyment, where colour was essential to visual impressiveness and immediacy.[62] Although the links of colour to femininity and orientalism may have eroded, it has not however marred its resuscitation in manoeuvres of contemporary transorientalism. In 2010, for example, a collection in high-key oranges, pinks and greens were immediately dubbed oriental.

The other significant influence for Poiret's 1911 collection was one that he strenuously denied: the Ballets Russes. The production of *Schéhérazade*, with its designs by Léon Bakst, had taken place the previous summer. A closer look at photographs and the original costumes reveals an uncanny resemblance. With a mind perhaps to his own self-promotion, Bakst himself remarked on how swiftly Paris fashions took up his influence. Parisians, whose knowledge of oriental taste was by now quite literate, saw something new in Bakst's designs, a particularly Russian orientalism. The production, with Rimsky-Korsakoff's mixture of folk and generic orientalist music and Fokine's choreography, as Troy argues, was a catalyst in a new orientalist revival. Now that the threat of the Ottoman Empire had vanished, they found the Ballets Russes's 'hot-house vision of the East'[63] a congenial starting point for variations on oriental themes of remote paradises and veiled sexual encounters, all of which were mirrors in masquerade of their own hedonism.

The Ballets Russes was the crucible of a very new manifestation in the love–hate affair between art, theatrical costume and fashion. It also revealed a new evolving condition of each of the three domains. Since at least the Renaissance, artists, out of interest or financial necessity, had participated in theatrical set and costume design. But with the Ballets Russes this became a far more self-conscious involvement, not least because of the myth of the (male) individual creator–genius that we know characterizes modernism. In other words, the designs announced themselves as artistic creations as opposed to the handiwork of people who elsewhere preferred to be known as artists. While Bakst was by far the most prolific and dedicated of the troupe, its director, Diaghilev, enlisted the talents of some of the greatest artists of the day, including Braque, de Chirico, Sonia Delaunay, André Derain, Goncharova, Gris, Masson, Picasso and Matisse. Bakst was always the leader in oriental conceits, but it is also surprising to note the degree of orientalist influence there was to be had in the designs up to and toward the end of the War, not least in the dazzling colour combinations.

One very specific source of references during this period was 'Negro art', *L'art nègre*, whose most enduring references remains the early Cubist works of Picasso, championed by Apollinaire, a spokesman for African 'primitivism'. The bold angularity in the costumes from Diaghilev's ballet and that of his rival, the Ballets Suédois, are attributable to this fact. Sonia Delaunay contributed to both companies. Her costume designs in these years, and later when she opened her boutique in 1925, betray a strong if at times concealed debt to African decoration. Delaunay's 'jazz' textiles were among the first such influences trickling into art deco, examples of what Rosalind Krauss has dubbed 'black deco'.[64] It was in her fabric and costume design that Sonia Delaunay carved out independence as an artist from her husband Robert and his Orphist and Futurist contemporaries. Her fabric designs took simultanist painting to extremes with geometrical patterns and vibratingly dissonant colours that were in no small way allusive of the compelling rhythms of jazz and their underpinning in the 'vitalism' of Negro dance, and, more mythically, to African voodoo. A small coterie of admirers from the avant-garde gathered around Delaunay, but approval in *L'art nègre* and its offshoots was not universal. Cocteau condemned it as 'worthless bric-à-brac'. This did not stop its cultic popularity. The avant-garde were not alone in collecting it.[65] The fashion mogul Jacques Doucet was one of its largest collectors; however, he represented a very different group who, together with Poiret and Lanvin, were more interested in the colonial grandeur of conquest in the 'primitive'. The transgression import of primitivism and the oriental had a very different face and a different audience for couture. It was centred more on leisure and distraction than on overhauling the minds of middle-class society.[66]

As is so often the case, particularly with the orientalisms of Russia and Eastern Europe, folk designs and oriental influence are impossible to sunder, as with Goncharova's exquisite creations for *The Firebird* (premier 10 June 1910) or *The Golden Cockerel* (premier 24 May 1914). It is yet another fine example of what Reina Lewis calls the 'imaginary geography of Orientalism', where Russia could be featured by western Europe as quasiprimitive exotica whereas the Russian elite had a sentimental agenda for their peasant and eastern populations. Turning folk designs and ways into cultural artefacts was a way of protecting traditions that were perceived as under threat by encroaching modernization. In this way the peasant and the folk aesthetic were preserved 'as internal primitivised others'.[67] In other words, tradition was upheld through its repeated imaginary construction. Bakst's design for Shah Zeman for the 1910 production of *Schéhérazade* easily bears this out. It is an uncanny hybrid of popular renditions of Suleiman the Magnificent and Ivan the Terrible.

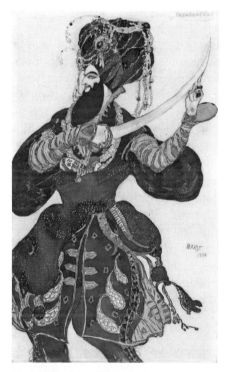

Figure 35 Léon Bakst, *Costume design for Shah Zeman*, 1910, from the Ballets Russes' production of *Schéhérazade*; gouache, pencil, watercolour, gold paint on varnish paper, © National Gallery of Australia, Canberra.

It was also at this time, from the early years of the twentieth century onward, that artists, the lions Picasso and Matisse among them, were using both oriental and primitive sources while vying for artistic supremacy. Matisse's Chinese-ifying costumes for *The Song of the Nightingale* (premier 2 February 1920) are standouts in this regard, and their luminous simplicity uncannily presage his later work. His costume for a Mandarin for example is a thick tunic of deep yellow-gold, sparingly interspersed with gilt-gold disks overlaid with lyrically spontaneous flower shapes in black.

There are two points to be made from this. The first was that artists felt free to embroil themselves in pursuits not strictly within the province of fine art, for the paradoxical reason that they wanted to keep art alive by testing its boundaries yet felt safe in the sanctity of what it was to be an artist. From a fashion perspective, it was also a symptom of modernist fashion and its separation from the kind of performance and theatre that began with Louis XIV's court and which experienced its final gasp with Charles-Frederick Worth and the Callot sisters. Fashion and dress was now seen to aid in mobility and action, not to announce the *event* of one's presence, since to the modern soul one was only the sum of one's actions.

The second conclusion to be drawn, which is relevant to the present topic, is the way in which the Orient becomes its own theatre: decultured, decentred, reappropriated—a zone parasitic on mythology and history that has lost all ties with empirical reality. Wollen, with a slightly different trajectory, is nevertheless useful here. He writes that the three figures of Poiret, Bakst and Matisse 'had more in common . . . than colour', for 'each of them created a scenography of the Orient that enabled him to redefine the image of the body, especially, but not exclusively, the female body'.[68] Wollen's notion of 'scenography', which is meant in both its specific and figurative senses, is useful here. In ways that I have already explained in this section of the chapter, the main change that we see reflected in Poiret and his contemporaries is the way that the making of the Orient reaches a tertiary phase that becomes fully realized in the fashions of the late-twentieth century and contemporary fashion. In this phase of transorientalism, the Orient as it is used and consumed in the West is but a web of signifiers whose true inheritance and ownership is difficult to trace or is wholly untraceable because it is pure invention. And while stylistic genealogies may concern us here, for the purposes of this book, they are at best of anecdotal interest to the fashion industry. Not that it hadn't been in earlier centuries, but references for orientalism were decreasingly anthropological and almost entirely backed by the narratives shaped by the West, nurtured by the Orient, and shaped into packages first in novels and operas and later in film and on television.

PAQUIN

Apart from what he would have believe, Poiret was not alone in pioneering modernist dress and freeing women from the cumbersome confection of the previous century (the larger variety which were aptly known as *cage*-crinolines). Poiret's success was to conflate the simplification and easier wearability of clothing with a kind of 'orientalist' liberation in which now-hackneyed narratives of exotic escape were knotted together with freedom of movement that were in turn tied to political freedoms. When scrutinized, this dialectic is less than plausible, but it is nonetheless easy to see the way they were brought together. Poiret's 1911 collection also concurred with the first suffragette demonstrations. The irony here is that the freedoms superficially afforded women carried less propitious undertones: women were marching in for equality in pants worn underneath their skirts. Most women could not afford the cutting edge of fashion, but the cutting edge certainly coloured the terms by which things were seen, especially given the fanfare with which Poiret introduced his line of that season. By design or comic coincidence, a history of female imprisonment, the harem, was harnessed for her freedom. Naming them *jupe-culotte* allowed them to be sanitized of such ideas while the form itself, nourished by a copious diet of literature, paintings and posters, never disavowed it. But it is also an indication of the fluidity of the orientalist concept by this time—especially in fashion and accessories—that this was allowed to occur. Anthropologically it is a solecism, but from the point of view of fashion, the ownership of traditions of some cultures became precariously shaky.

The contemporary couturier who vehemently said no to the harem pants was Poiret's rival, Jeanne Paquin. It may not have been out of the reservations that have just been raised but more to announce her difference from her competition, and simply out of personal preferences of taste. Poiret had certainly surpassed Paquin in the art of self-adulation, but his dalliances with oriental despotism were seen by others as excessive. Paquin decried the ugly line of the pants, which caused the silhouette to slump rather taper at the bottom. But her own line from the same year revealed a suspicious influence and was her most explicitly orientalist to date, using bright colours. It was a brash change, as she was accused by a critic of using 'barbaric colour effects that were not her style'.[69] Paquin was an astute businesswoman and barometer of taste. On most occasions she managed to balance between the impression of the couturier as impresario of the moment and catering to what clients want. She drew from Bakst and Paul Iribe as much as she did from other sources, mixing expediency with personal inclination.

Even though Paquin was in no way a bastion of orientalist fashions, the collision between Paris's top couturiers and their respective collections, and the debates that spawned from these, made orientalism a leitmotif in the years leading up to War. World War I was, after all, fought over imperial rivalries. By 1910 all European countries, including the old powers, France and England, were experiencing feelings of dispossession, which would ultimately lead to the dispansion of empires and the end of colonialism. When translated broadly into sociological terms, the beginning of the twentieth century witnessed a stronger self-consciousness of gender and race. Exoticism was viewed less in terms of pleasure and possession and more with nostalgia and the odour of myth. Thus, orientalism in fashion and dress became a loaded semantic device in which both the Euro–American and 'his' oriental other were increasingly complicit.

FORTUNY

The new re-revival sparked by Poiret, Paquin and Bakst has to be understood in loose terms, of course, and is better thought of as making latent orientalisms rise again to the surface, or re-enunciating already present ones. A beneficiary of this wave was Mariano Fortuny, a Spanish designer who opened his house in 1906. His chief inspiration was Venice. Fortuny would be little more than a footnote in the history of fashion were it not for his immortalization by Proust in his magnum opus *À la recherche du temps perdu*. Fortuny, whose eclecticism was well known and whose absorption of Eastern influence was as subtle and intricate as it was liberal, plays a prominent part in the novel, anecdotally and symbolically. Fortuny himself was just as proficient in painting, sculpting and architecture, and Proust had more than a voracious, subtle and detailed eye for both natural and crafted visual phenomena. Proust was responsive to how Fortuny drew inspiration from the Venetian painter Vittore Carpaccio, especially the ornate stuffs in his glorious *St Ursula* (1495) cycle. Fortuny's gowns were not especially versatile, being of the tea-gown genus, but much heavier. A mixture of Japanese and Persian elements, they were like a kimono adapted into a more flowing dressing gown ('Albertine had remained in her room, reading, in her Fortuny dressing-gown'[70]), their principal function was to show off fabric in its fleshy opulence.

Such migrations of influence are not lost on Proust. Fortuny borrowed a great deal from Carpaccio, making his influences in this regard already twice removed. Proust, whose narrator buys several gowns for his fickle lover Albertine, uses such convolutions as allegories of the misalliances of love and desire, the differing perspectives and expectations of lover and loved one. It is therefore tempting to extrapolate from Proust's vision to the many layers of influence in fashion between East and West. Seeing his lover clad in one of Fortuny's gowns, the narrator is overcome with transports of speculation about Venice, the symbol in the novel of the place of arrival, the realization of childhood dreams:

> If I had never seen Venice, I had dreamed of it incessantly since those Easter holidays which, when still a boy, I had been going to spend there, and earlier still, since the Titian prints and Giotto photographs which Swann had given me long ago at Combray. The Fortuny gown which Albertine was wearing that evening seemed to me the tempting phantom of the invisible Venice. It was covered with Arab ornamentation, like the Venetian palaces hidden like sultan's wives behind a screen of pierced stone, like the buildings in the Ambrosian Library, like the columns from which the oriental birds that symbolised alternatively life and death were repeated on the shimmering fabric, on an intense blue which, as my eyes drew nearer, turned into a malleable gold by those same transmutations which, before an advancing gondola, change into gleaming metal the azure of the Grand Canal. And the sleeves were lined with a cherry pink which is so particularly Venetian that it is called Tiepolo pink.[71]

This passage encapsulates in almost crystalline form the way that orientalist fashion is a tissue of connotation, suggestion, and invocation—and somewhere within all that are a set of facts that have been doctored, disordered by the spate of years or by the wilful reworkings of memory and desire. Proust's words sum up many of the themes of this book better than could any historical account. For Proust the gown is not just a reminder or a trigger, it delivers his imaginings of Venice, the magnificent former way-station between East and West, in a spectral form. To admirers less prone to associative embroidery than Proust, Fortuny gowns were like a worn trophy, and a conversation piece.

The other passage from Proust about Fortuny's gowns is also worth reproducing at length. Preceding the one above, it lays Fortuny gowns not only against a glittering idealized Venice but also with its painters and the designers of the Ballets Russes:

> In the matter of dress, what appealed to her most at this time was everything made by Fortuny. These Fortuny gowns, one of which I had seen Mme Guermantes wearing, were those of which Elstir, when he told us about the magnificent garments of the women of Carpaccio's and Titian's day, had prophesied the imminent return, rising from their ashes, as magnificent as of old, for everything must return in time, as it is written beneath the vaults of St Mark's, and proclaimed, as they drink from the urns of marble and jasper of the Byzantine capitals, by the birds which symbolise at once death and resurrection. As soon as women had begun to wear them, Albertine had remembered Elstir's [the painter character in the novel who also had his models, like Whistler, dress in Oriental robes] prophecy, had coveted them, and we were shortly to go and choose one. Now even if

these gowns were not those genuine antiques in which women today seem a little too got up in fancy dress and which it is preferable to keep as collector's items (I was looking for some of these also, as it happens, for Albertine), neither did they have the coldness of the artificial, the sham antique. Like the theatrical designs of Sert, Bakst and Benois, who at that moment were recreating in the Russian ballet the most cherished periods of art with the aid of works of art *impregnated with their spirit and yet original*, these Fortuny gowns, *faithfully antique but markedly original*, brought before the eye like a stage décor, and with an even greater evocative power since the décor was left to the imagination, that Venice saturated with oriental splendour where they would have been worn and of which they constituted, even more than a relic in the shrine of St Mark, evocative as they were of the sunlight and the surrounding turbans, the fragmented, mysterious and complementary colour. Everything of those days had perished, but everything was being reborn, evoked and linked together by the splendour and swarming life of the city, in the piecemeal reappearance of the still-surviving fabrics worn by the Doges' ladies. [My emphasis.][72]

These two phrases marked out in the passage are worth special attention because they too aptly characterize orientalist influence in the nineteenth century and into the twentieth: 'impregnated with their spirit and yet original'; 'faithfully antique but markedly original'. Ironically enough they also apply to the imposed, or strategic, changes that some Eastern and Asian cultures were undergoing themselves. These passages weave art, history and desire into a smooth surface, in uncannily close parallel to the way they merge in the orientalist sign.

THE INTERWAR YEARS: THE ORIENT IN EARLY FILM

As can be expected, the aftermath of World War I ushered in a period of austerity in which eccentricities were less indulged and more infrequent. This change was also reflected in the costumes for the Ballets Russes, which became more sober and classical. During the interwar years orientalist themes were a rarity in everyday wear and in private balls which, if anything, followed more historical themes. Despite its name, the 'roaring twenties' were not a shade on the grand balls of what was now hailed a bygone era. What perhaps earned the decade before the Great Depression this title was that pleasure was more openly accessible to the lower and middle classes. Rather than the ornate and mythically ancient orient, the aesthetic was more angular and industrial: dance moves were jerky and splayed and fashions were simpler, to portray an interest in a sportier lifestyle. The fashions of the 1920s conveyed a vision of the outdoors, in contrast to the spacious indoors that only the upper classes could accommodate and, by way of extension, the sequestered and privileged intimacy of the Ottoman harem.

Orientalism was all but banished in the 1920s by Chanel and Patou. Chanel famously painted herself as the counterpoint to Poiret, whom she typecast exemplifying the last breath of aristocratic excess. She invited women to participate in the versatile austerity of dress analogous to that of men. It was a revolution, writes Gilles Lipovetsky, in women's clothing that was a kind of 'tabula rasa' from the ceremonial imperatives of the past. Fashion's simplification ran parallel to the pronounced linearity of the avant-garde: Cubism and Constructivisim.[73] As a peculiar aside, in 1908 the critic Vauxcelles commented that Picasso and Braque were working 'in the Egyptian style', because of the flat, brutal angularity of their Cubist forms. France continued to consume signs of otherness and to celebrate it as the final heartbeats of its decrepit imperial past, as evidenced in the 1925 *Exposition Internationale des Arts Décoratifs*, which situated the colonies as a vital source of inspiration for the arts. Batiks and decorative silks enjoyed special attention, and the mannequins that modelled them assumed uncanny resemblances to reductive forms of avant-garde artists, particularly to Brancusi's abstracted head, *The Muse* (1912).[74] Thus, orientalism was not entirely purged or eschewed but existed in the background, in fabrics, jewellery and perfume, which I will discuss in the following chapter.

During these years the life of orientalist costume was most vibrant in the relatively new medium of film. The two actors most responsible for perpetuating orientalist archetypes in the popular sphere were Theda Bara and Rudi Valentino. Both endowed with hypnotic sex appeal, their most famous roles ensured that the equivalence between the erotic and orientalism did not flag. Because they were in a popular medium, their images and associations were engraved into public consciousness. Theda Bara—pundits like to draw attention to the anagram 'Arab Death' in her name—was one of the first cinematic sex symbols and one of the most successful actors of the silent era. She was known as 'the vamp' because she specialized in roles of femme fatale (in almost forty feature-length roles between 1915 and 1919), a role that was later taken up by Valentino's off-sider Nita Naldi. Sadly, most of her films are lost, but the film for which she is most famous was *Cleopatra* (1917), which only exists in a miniscule remnant, although numerous images remain intact. In this costly production, Bara was featured in clothing that was deemed suggestive even for her time. From Berlioz to the Pre-Raphaelites, Cleopatra had been a popular romantic theme throughout the nineteenth century, but it was Bara who made the connection in the popular consciousness between Cleopatra and the exotic nymphomaniac vixen—an oriental vamp—indelible, much as Bela Lugosi fourteen years later would ensure that Dracula was not Dracula without a tuxedo.

Equally stereotypical, and just as emblazoned onto popular perception, is Rudolph Valentino's *The Sheikh*. Maybe because it was his last film, Valentino's

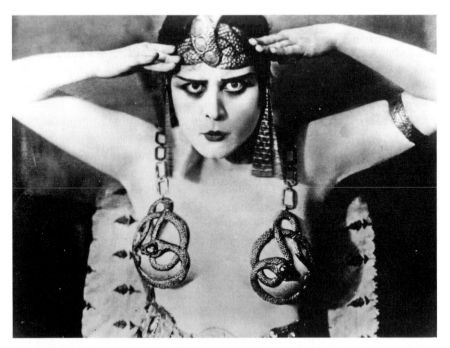

Figure 36   American actress Theda Bara (1885–1955), appearing in the title role in the 1917 film *Cleopatra*, © Photo by Popperfoto/Getty Images.

image is eternally caught up in this unapologetic orientalist travesty. It is a feast of orientalist cliché, whose sexual connotation is so hallucinatory it is worthy of an opium dream. As Miriam Hanson observes,

> exotic costumes, oriental decor, and desert landscape provoke a sensuality of vision that constantly undermines the interest in the development of the narrative. Extreme long shots show Valentino riding through a sea of sand shaped like breasts and buttocks; he prefers the skin-folds of his tent to the parental palace, and he experiences in the allegorical moonlit ruin the pitfalls of adult sexuality, the threat of castration. Though concealing dangerous abysses, the eroticized landscape becomes a playground of polymorphous desire, in which the signs of virility-sables, pistols, cigarettes remain phallic toys at best. The screen itself becomes a maternal body, inviting the component drives to revolt against their subordination. These textured surfaces do not project a realistic space that the hero, traversing it, would be obligated to subject. Rather, they construct an oneiric stage which cannot be bothered with perspective and verisimilitude.[75]

Hansen's 'oneiric stage' calls to mind Poiret's legendary party. And the comment that the settings overshadow is endemic of the way in which orientalism in fashion, costume and dress had become rudderless and unmoored from actuality.

By the end of the century, this would prove to be mixed blessing. In haute couture, orientalism would become transorientalism, a hypothetical pattern book of references and styles to be mixed, matched and reordered at a whim. This need not be criticized with the onus of postcolonial ideology, for the relative absence of ideology in fashion has made orientalism a metastasizing entity and a source of continual surprise and pleasure. But the in the domain of dress, however, the appropriation of orientalist fashion and dress by the West, so often based on narratives that have been rewritten many times over, would have sinister consequences. This would be brought to the fore in the reluctance of Europe and America to enter into empathetic dialogues about traditional Muslim garments like the burqa. Instead, it seems that for large portions of the Euro–American population, fairytale narratives of the Orient, narratives that have been creatively salutary elsewhere, prevail over pragmatic reasoning, causing the more objectionable prejudices to be played out once more.

–5–

1944–2011: Postwar Revivalism and Transorientalism

To call the toga or the mandarin's gown 'chic' is to suggest a process of change which barely existed in ancient Rome or China; the clothes of the beefeater of the samurai are eminently respectable, precisely because they are not up to date; the tarboosh was never 'all the go' for it has never gone.

—Quentin Bell[1]

I guess you could say I got carried away with Talitha's character. Not that all of what I imagined her was even true. I used her more as a fantasy to dream about.

—Phoebe Philo speaking about Talitha Getty[2]

Talitha Getty is to couture what Jimi Hendrix is to music, or Jimmy Dean is to cinema: they all died of substance abuse, only to embalm their youth in popular memory. Talitha, wife of the magnate John Paul Getty Jr., is maybe the least remembered of the three, except now in fashion circles where she remains the avatar of North African style. In an exhibition in 2008, the Bergé-Laurent foundation in Paris held an exhibition, '*Une Passion Marocaine*', of caftans and jewellery inspired by the kinds that Talitha would wear in her Pleasure Palace in Marrakesh. Dries van Noten, Robert Cavalli and Dolce and Gabanna all rose to the plate with thin and flowing dresses and pants suits, pulsing with colour and contrasts. It was an orgy of orientalism: flowers, feathers, paisley and curlicues were the order of the day, an aggressive hedonism. Yves Saint Laurent remembered the photograph taken in 1984 by (Lord) Patrick Lichfield of Talitha and Getty posing with self-conscious languor on their Marrakesh terrace: 'beautiful and damned. . . where the curtain of the past seemed to lift before an extraordinary future'.[3] Appropriately, the magazine for the latter-day eulogy of Talitha was *Harper's Bazaar*.

The photograph, and Saint Laurent's comment, can be used to formulate an insight into the kind of meanings that orientalism appears to hold for our age. Talitha represented the last age of romanticism in 1970's 'Age of Aquarius', in which men and women of Europe and America joined hands in a mass wave of Eastern revivalism prompted by Gandhi earlier in the century and given manifesto status in Robert Persig's 1974 bestseller, *Zen and the Art of*

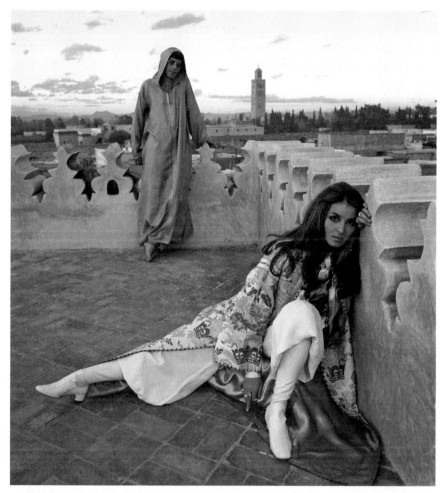

Figure 37 Patrick Litchfield, *Talitha and John Paul Getty on the Top of Their Pleasure Palace in Marrakesh*, 1969.

Motorcycle Maintenance. The decade or more after the 1968 student revolutions was an era of mass social experiment in which art and fashion played major roles. With Happenings and Earth Works, artists made a final effort to bring art out of the gallery and abolish once and for all the division between art and life. Fashion made its final foray into ecstatic wonder. The imperative was to be happy or bust. Fashion shed any inhibition with regard to colour or restraint of line. It was between the 1960s and 1980s that paisley achieved mass appeal. Finding itself everywhere, it imprinted a generation thirsty for Eastern religion and anything that preached peaceful alternatives to Cold War tension and hypocrisy. The Israeli wars with Egypt and the Arab states, the independence of India, Mao's famine, the Korean War and then the Vietnamese War—all this meant that Asia and the Middle East was ever-present to America and Europe. This was also an age of caftans, sandals and nudity. Scarves were worn in flowing abundance on heads, necks and waists and, alas, sometimes all three at once. Bra-burning and the explosion of free sex meant that the narrative of the harem was never too far away, but with feminism and gay pride its parameters had shifted.

All this would be cut short in the 1980s with AIDS, the neoconservatism of Thatcher and Reagan and the baby boomers' financial consolidation. The 1980s is now characterized as the decade of cynical retreat after the failed experiment of the protest era. It was also the era that discredited revolution as an effective transformative force within society. One way that the era now known as postmodernism can be best understood is according to this change in belief systems. It was defined as the end of what the French philosopher Jean-François Lyotard in *The Postmodern Condition* in 1979 termed the 'master narratives' such as Marxist revolution and the emancipation of the weak. That the jettisoning of faith in such change was a cause of much philosophical consternation does not concern us here. But what does is the recasting of representation from sign to 'metasign'. To the postmodernism way of thinking, originality and authenticity is moot; everything is a network, repressed or announced, of signs and representations, which are themselves derived from others and so on ad infinitum. While this had always been the case, according to postmodernism the new era conferred on these attachments and influences a particular visibility, and possibility for appearance. This liberation of representation from itself was also the cause for mourning: the end of monolithic truth meant the end of the trust in the power of art to exert major social change. It also meant that the romantic aspiration of bringing things and ideas back to their roots was forever a groundless and otiose exercise. The postmodern refrain was for many melancholically retrospective, resigned and nostalgic: 'the beautiful and the damned'.

Postmodern rejection of foundationalism had untold consequences for the idea of orientalism as it wafted into our present era. As we have repeatedly seen, orientalism in fashion is a multifaceted construction that is locatable in, but irreducible to, a slick colonialist–colonized binary of oppressor and oppressed. But orientalism survived and indeed blossomed because, as diffuse as it always was, it nourished the illusion that somewhere within it, if one looked and persevered hard enough, there was the possibility of a return to a primitive truth. This was a late Enlightenment hankering that took the shape of a particularly complex game to which the colonial, or non-Western other, was sometimes complicit. What the postmodern condition, if it can be called that, exposed, was the particularly coded character of formations of knowledge, and their 'conditions of possibility' within any given moment. According to such provisos, a truth is only the summation of a collective consensual will. In short, just as the trust in a utopian future was deemed a Marxian pipe dream; the suspension of reality and truth within orientalism was no longer sublimated; it was brought to the fore. Orientalism in fashion is worn, assumed, adopted and suggested *as something once inscribed with a dream*. In the last decades of the twentieth century, orientalism's dream-denotation is taken as a given, and its accurate cultural entitlements are relaxed. In fashion and decoration, the orientalist sign ceases to have any promissory position to an actual world whence it came and to which one might eventually escape. This condition, strategy and mindset can be called meta-orientalism, or better, transorientalism. As I have begun to define it already, transorientalism denotes a state beyond the original type but also a movement across different spheres of activity, germane to the flows and biases of globalization (the main bias is that, despite its name, it is a Euro–American concept defined largely by their terms of trade).

The position that frees orientalism from a referent is not shared by everyone. For indeed it might be argued that lurking beneath the jubilance of orientalist fashion will always be the taint of colonialism. The orientalist signifier is by nature or definition, never innocent. Sanjay Sharma and Aswani Sharma have argued passionately in this direction. For them multiculturalism is a flawed concept since it still demands an identification with whiteness that has, from the start, the power of toleration. Present-day orientalism is a 'series of imaginary mirrorings' in which the white Westerner enacts a level of otherness that eclipses the circumstances of the 'true' other.[4] To this end, multiculturalism is commodified and socially mediated in its reduction into films, foods, fads and ads. The West extracts genres and practices such as Bollywood cinema and casts it briefly into its own mainstream, captioning it, reducing a massive cultural tradition into a series of thumbnails and using it to create a new wave that in the country of origin is the norm. Asian culture is 'encountered and consumed only as an idealised, reified and exotic commodity'.[5] These are viable points in certain cases, but they miss several factors: first the enthusiastic consumption of orientalism by the (erstwhile) Orient; second the simplistic definition of 'white' and 'West' (the latter used in this book advisedly and only as a convenient foil to the equally hyperbolic 'orient'); third, the history of cross-cultural borrowing, stealing and exchange; fourth, and definitely not least, when applied to fashion and dress, the impossibility of saying where the Orient begins and where the West starts. As far as fashion and clothing are concerned, and a great deal else, its histories are often of blind beginnings, multiple origins and strategic misdirections. To make Western dominance blameworthy of voluntary internal modifications is as absurd as to make it accountable for the transition from the *kosode* to the kimono. Such an argument also discounts the ramifications of the 'Japanese

Revolution' on fashion—which I will discuss presently—that was played out a double game between old-school orientalism and its overhaul, as Japan entered the world economic stage.

We must also account for the way that Asian designers are taken with the idea of change and eclecticism, recognizing from the very first that traditions are never static. The contemporary Korean designer Hyunshin Na testifies to a process of 'transcultural style' that 'fuses' Western and non-Western elements. But this approach is not at the expense of integrity to the image of what is national or indeed indigenous. Rather, she states, the practice of 'merging' different cultures and histories can be achieved without compromising 'original meaning and content'. This is inevitable, she suggests given the nature of global trade and 'the transfer of cultural symbols' which have accelerated 'cultural interchanges'. In the discussion of her design based on the Korean traditional patchwork wrapping cloth known as the *jogakbo*, she draws attention to the way East and West historical references have been comfortably intermingled. 'My innovation comes out of the recognition of tradition, which is inescapably rooted in Korea, yet both the inspiration and execution of the work are definitely international. This internationalism freely transcends a strong Korean identity.'[6] This attitude is not by any means exclusive to all Koreans let alone Asian designers at large; however, for many designers within the 'Orient', the Orient as an imaginative construct is a repository of creative possibility, where possibility takes precedence over cultural criticism.

This is a perspective not shared by Nirmal Puwar, who discusses the palpable anger of women of Pakistani origin in Britain who witness the coming into fashion of clothes, textiles and decorations for which they were once ridiculed and reviled. A pertinent example is *mendhie*, the henna-ing in *buta*-derived curlicues on the hands, wrists and feet. Once the butt of revulsion, a sign of foreignness that might even risk physical attack when worn on white bodies, they become magically sanitized. It is as if the white Western body is the only feasible site of authentication in which the visibly ethnic is suddenly transformed into oriental chic. For Puwar, this double standard only increases the divisions that such 'acceptance' ostensibly resolves since it elicits the justifiable if irrational ire of those once reviled.[7]

Legitimate concerns such as these are all the more difficult to negotiate given the mass circulation of cultural signs in modern and contemporary society, where, with the exception of Islam, all signs are free game. In cases of cultural offense, it can also be difficult to assign an onus of guilt, given that fashion is among the most guilt-free systems there is. Transorientalism, as I explained in the previous chapter, evolved in fits and starts from Poiret onward (I have arbitrarily begun this chapter with the year of his death). It comes into full view with the birth of high-powered celebrity designers—first Yves Saint Laurent and then the likes of Versace, Gaultier and Westwood—and with the advent of the supermodel in the mid-1980s. It was both a condition of mass society and early globalization as much as it was generated by the exertions of the designers themselves. It spelled a freeing up of orientalism which was typically either responsible for registering risqué edginess or signifying a break with a previous collection, as if the designer had, in his or her head, temporarily gone off shore, gone primitive, gone oriental.

The accusations levelled at fashion since its entry into mainstream discourse since the second half of the nineteenth century, that it is effeminate, fickle and transient, are of some use to contemporary fashion practice (perhaps not fashion theory), which has made its peace both with capitalism and with the need for ideology. Fashion can be pleasantly free of ideology which—unlike art, which can be encumbered by it—gives it almost limitless potential. If one leaves aside silly comments made by the likes of Galliano (to do with Nazi sympathies), one can say that that the ethical limits within fashion can be stretched, and have. Orientalism is the ethical frontier of race and identity, which has such a long history and is so tightly bound into the evolution of fashion, clothing and dress that it in Western couture its critical dimension is lost. Echoes of racial and cultural critique abound faintly, but this frisson is exchanged for a more palatable and attractive one of sexual energy—the harem and geisha rise up yet again.

This fluidity of the orientalist sign, made more powerful by the creative flows it generates, is not lost on non-Western designers and producers. In countries as vast and varied as India, designers have asked themselves about what kinds of clothes they should be designing and with what kinds of references. Regions in Africa have focused on local traditions and industry. On the other hand, in the late 1970s, Japanese went to Paris to instigate its own new fashion revolution. And then there's the giant of China, now the world's leading clothing manufacturer. This will form the substance of this last chapter: the last hopeful light of oriental fashion in the neo-Bohemians of the protest era, the nature of orientalism in postmodern and contemporary couture and responses from the erstwhile Orient. There will also be perfume: centuries old, it is incorporated in this last chapter because it is possibly the most illustrative example of transorientalism, a free-association of values availing itself of art, history and cinema in arbitrary abandon.

HIPPIES AND COUNTERCULTURE IN THE 1960s AND 1970s

'Hippie' is still used today but is usually a pejorative for a hazy, back-to-the-earth mentality with little concern for the pragmatic values of life. Its interest in Eastern religion is drug-induced and bereft of discipline. Like all clichés, they contain a germ of truth, but the biggest strength of the countercultures that sprang from the 1960s was their defence of peace, freedom and love. It has been called a Bohemian revival, but it was both far more general in that it was a pan-Western movement, was not necessarily tied to class and was also specifically aimed at condemning the period from Eisenhower to Nixon that it saw did little to contain the threat of violence; clearly no great lesson had been learned from World War II. Understandably, hippies found their idol in Gandhi, who in the 1930s led India to independence through his policy of non-violent civil disobedience. This is not to omit others from the hippie pantheon such as Nietzsche, Thoreau and Hesse—all three of whom drank deeply from the Indian cup of religion and mysticism—or Buddha, or the sixth century Persian prophet Mazdak.

An understanding of hippies in terms of peaceful revolt (even though it was not always that way) is essential for understanding their fashions, which by the early 1970s had developed into their own substantive language that endures to this day. One of the sociological explanations of punk is that it was designed to upset its audience. That it does not any more is because it is no longer an exception but rather a recognizable subcultural genre. Ironically enough, given their differing philosophies on violence, hippies are to the late 1960s and 1970s what punks were to the late 1970s and 1980s: both did more than wear clothing, they imbibed their particular dress as a second skin to reflect an alternative way of living that frothed either rage against, or contempt of, the conventional middle classes who represented the absorption of commodity capitalism into mainstream society. In particular, hippies (and punks, to some extent) aimed their sights at the nuclear model of Protestant, male-oriented, monogamous heterosexuality advanced by packaged concepts of the postwar home made into a paradise with home appliances and pruned yards.

The first objective of the hippie was to be everything that straight-laced 1950s and 1960s were not. Today, the furore caused by the Beatles' long hair is a distant echo in any baby boomer's head, but it was only one of a raft of changes that was the beginning of the idea of *casual* we take with us today. The kind of renunciation brought about by Chanel and her generation was that of florid, overstated lines that dispensed with burdensome fashions and introduced a classic, somewhat ahistorical formality. Thus, until the 1960s, Western dress was fundamentally formal by today's standards. T-shirts and jeans may not have had anything orientalist about them, but when not going down an Apache path (the beige suede coat with tassels down each arm and across the back), almost everything else about the hippie did. Start with the ubiquitous Afghan coat, and the floral bandanna. Then there's the pyjama. These were used throughout Asia for centuries; light cotton drawn at the top with a string, usually of the same cotton. Since the nineteenth century, they were used as sleepwear, but during the hippie era they left the bedroom and resumed as street wear. Floppy meant free, and since they are conventionally without pockets, it is tempting to say that they were in accord with Proudhonist revivalism ('property is theft') and the repudiation of worldly goods. The fabrics were not all cotton. Synthetic fibres were made possible by the invention of petroleum-based products. These not only were a logical industrial by-product of the 1960s, but they began to be researched when America boycotted the import of Japanese silk during World War II.

That the hippies were as promiscuous in their voracity for Middle Eastern and Asian habits and signs as they were in their sexual habits is more than a coincidence, and lends credence one again to the eroticized orient. But aversions to their habits were not confined to the developed world. In an article written in 1972, a Canadian academic in sociology, Audrey Wipper, complains that the demeanour of the hippie who professes affinity with Africa flies in the face of the kinds of hackneyed images that Africans wished to dispel. The hippie, she contends, is the latest 'cultural invader', they are 'the spoiled children of sick, affluent societies', and their presumptions about African are grossly misplaced:

> The hippies' unkempt appearance, far from being admired except perhaps by a few rebellious youth, is looked upon with scorn. Their rejection of the very goals Africans are striving for—education, material possessions and a decent standard of living—and their adoption of certain symbols of poverty, again has overtones of westerners' mocking African poverty and aspirations. (Mr. Moi, described hippies as 'people who come to Kenya barefoot looking as if they are poor although they are not'.)[8]

She also adds voice to the African antipathy to the ' "Afro" ' which is 'merely another example of western arrogance'. African Americans, she comments, pretend an ownership over something that they know nothing about. They lay claim to an identity they know nothing about, more invented than true. She quotes the writer Kadje Konde:

> How 'natural' these nests are is a mystery to me. In the United States, where this hairdo comes from, it is called an Afro style. This implies a link with Africa, although I personally fail to see how this keeping of wild oiled bush on the skull has anything to do with dear mother Africa. From that land of drug-takers and draft-dodgers comes another shameless importation, a mast flag of a decaying ship under the guise of a hair style intended to identify American Negroes with Africans . . .[9]

An unfortunate upshot of this is that aspirational groups within Africa have felt inclined to mimic styles that originate elsewhere, styles that offer a jaundiced view of themselves. By implication, America's internal constructions of African identities, and the way such presumptions are absorbed within Africa, impede the 'real' Africa from mastery of its own cultural development. One reflex within

Africa has been to try to avoid all new Western forms of dress, with particular defensive stress lying on implications of the licentiousness of Western women.[10] Despite the indignation of such writers at misappropriations within Western countries, maybe the most egregious is the 'Mao suit' from the late 1960s, made possible by the selectively false readings by radicals like Sartre of the superiority of Maoist over Soviet communism.

It appears that despite the banter by the herbal generation about naturalness, uniqueness, respect and authenticity, the way these values were rooted in Asia and Africa—supposedly spiritually less tainted by the wayward worldly interests of the West—required some aesthetic choreographing. More than any other pattern, paisley became a talismanic badge of the 1960s and 1970s, enjoying a crazed renaissance. Paisley's ability to accrete, or build on itself, and to contain other motifs such as the floral, made it the armature for design excesses in which vivid chromatic combinations were almost always complicit. But the connection to India, via Gandhi, was crucial. Other Eastern references were far more generic and seen mostly through an Indian filter. In a spiritual sense at least, the *buta* was returned to its origins. Added to this vocabulary were designs from traditional Indian tattooing, and particularly the circular mandala henna motif that was the skeleton for an infinite array of curlicues and concentric circles.

One of the landmarks of this era was the appearance in 1967 of the Beatles' *Sgt Pepper's Lonely Hearts Club Band* album, which signalled a new stage of popular music and contained the sitar-driven track by George Harrison, 'Within You Without You'.[11] The was the beginning of what would be a lifelong friendship with Ravi Shankar and also the beginning of George and John wearing caftans and long, flowing Indian shirts, and even the dhoti, which Gandhi after the 1930s had unofficially instated as national male dress in India as active rejection of Western dress imposed by the British. Shortly after, Keith Richards and Mick Jagger took up the standard in the Indian twang in 'Give me Shelter', accessorizing their music with associated clothing: large scarves and long cotton shirts, imbuing these fashions with animal sex appeal.

The late 1960s onward was therefore not a period of invention in fashion so much as mass adoption, mass appeal and widespread reinvigoration. This is evident to in three more examples: the bikini, batik and sandals.

The earliest examples of the bikini are to be found in mosaics from the fourth century in Sicily, although two Frenchmen, Louis Réart and Jacques Heim, like to claim the invention for themselves in 1946. Réart named it after the Bikini Atoll, one of the islands in the South Pacific that was close to the nuclear testing zones used by the US in the same year that they devastated Hiroshima and Nagasaki. Réart had more than just a political tongue in his cheek when he announced that unveiling skimpy swimwear would incite a reaction of atomic proportions.[12]

With thicker oriental roots, batik, the patterning of cloth using knotting and wax prevalent in India and Southeast Asia, particularly Indonesia, became a hippie badge of honour, complementing other forms of hallucinatory designs. When from these regions, it was often on very light cloth, which felt very different and therefore more exotic than the customary thicker, more durable, American styles. In the same family of resemblances is the *festival mondial* from Senegal. It is a dramatic designs of concentric circles made from the resists achieved from stitching the cloth before entering the dye. Its dissemination in the United States was not, as one would have expected, by the black community but by the hippie generation who called it the same general names as the Nigerians, 'tie-dye'. The starburst pattern so allied to the hippie legacy is more or less a simplification of the more worked *festival mondial* design from Sudan, whose zigzag shape comes from sewing as opposed to tying.[13]

It will be remembered that traditional Japanese dress did not involve shoes; feet were bound in cloth or covered in socks and protected from the ground by a simple mechanism of a wooden base affixed to the foot by two straps meeting at the space between the big toe. Coming to view in the traders' visits to Japan and used occasionally domestically by European japonistes in the nineteenth century, they evolved into what we now know as the more disposable and informal thong, or flip-flop. Sandals were common, of course, in ancient Greece and Rome, but their reference point in the early-twentieth century was far more that of India because of the British Raj and where they continued to be worn. Their reintegration into European society began in the 1890s, most visibly with the proto-hippie Edward Carpenter.

Homosexual, socialist, anarchist, activist for free love and recycling, women's suffrage and prison reform, the memory of Edward Carpenter has waned somewhat, but he had a profound influence at the turn of the twentieth century. Buoyed by the wealth provided him by his father, Carpenter's home at Milthorpe was a communal sanctuary where guests were exposed to the incipient form of what we would now call a wholesome, or herbal, lifestyle: gardening, sewing and sandal-making. Carpenter was an adept at the latter, selling his handiwork and that of those he proselytized, in either the 'Cashmere' or eponymous 'Milthorpe' pattern.[14] In the 1960s, which Carpenter radically anticipated, sandals were more than a cool and cheap alternative to closed shoes; they were a symbol of nudity, naturalness and freedom that, at a pinch, recalled the material modesty of Brahmins.

The fashions of the '60s and '70s period still elicit a mixed reception, often involving parody, from Mike Myers' Austin Powers trilogy (1997–2002) to the Coen brothers' masterpiece *The Big Lebowski* (1998). Both of these films are telling examples of the way that hippie fashions are a recognizable feature of a way of life, analogous one might say to certain Muslim clothing; one presupposes another. The remnants of hippie clothing live on, less flamboyantly, through notions of a practical and informal lifestyle in inexpensive, versatile comfortable clothing. Ironically enough, given their albeit distant connection to peace and discipline, such clothes are aspects of what radical Islam cites as attributes of the undisciplined infidel. That hippie fashion had no bench-mark was one of the reasons for its success. By the 1970s it was all but formalized—it could simply play itself out in a wide tie with clashing psyche-delic colours that was a creative amalgam of Japanese Edo textiles and In-dian saris. The Indian Orient is somewhere in its makeup, glaring predominant or as some background ghost. These fashions were permeable, and could be expanded and contracted to suit the occasion and the person, and had its register in every aspect of clothing, from sunglasses to hair to jewellery. One of the more scurrilous clichés about hippies about which I will refrain to com-ment is that they were averse to bodily hygiene. But what is true is that the hippie generation did not have much of a hand in perfume.

PERFUME

Perfumes can be dated back to ancient Egypt and Mesopotamia, refined by the Romans and Persians. Early approximations can also be found in India. In other words, perfume is largely an oriental invention. But like silks, cotton and certain designs, they reached an altogether new level with European in-tervention. The first stage occurred in the thirteenth to eighteenth centuries, the second with industrialization, urbanization and mass marketing. Perfume began to be packaged at the beginning of the eighteenth century when in 1706 *Eau de Cologne* was marketed from the German city of the same name. Cultivating flowers for floral essences originated around the 1300s, making regions like Grasse in France and Calabria in Italy centres of production. But as anyone who has smelt a perfume would be willing to admit, perfumes would be sickly and monotonous if their sole source were flowers. Including the fact that a greater portion of the flowers harvested in Europe for such pur-poses had their distant origin in Persia and China, the list of other important ingredients for perfumes that came from the Orient are too plentiful to name. To begin with, in addition to ethanol, scents can be moderated using refined, odourless coconut or jojoba oil.

Perfume is divided into different categories, such as floral, woody, leathery or musky. Also known as ambered, named after ambergris, oriental has its own category—typically containing ambergris, labdanum, vanilla and tonka bean and possibly accented with incense resins and camphorous oils—but the list of ingredients is far longer. Here is a random, short list: sandalwood, agar wood, bergamot, ginger, vetiver root, coumarin, cinnamon, cloves, cori-ander, caraway, cocoa, nutmeg, mace, cardamom, patchouli, mango, passion fruit, ylang-ylang blossom, frankincense, myrrh, and Peru balsam. Some are melded into 'nonoriental' perfumens, whereas others, like clove and vanilla, are a scent's dominant note.

Perfumes in the 1970s and 1980s were important marketing tools for couture houses. It is a common exercise to start a brand with a fragrance. Its profit share is higher than any other part of a fashion range and it is the most effective in conveying a brand's general image. In the case of Chanel, Dior and YSL, fragrances are important ways of placing themselves with consumers who cannot afford their clothes. Because of perfume is in itself impalpably mysterious—its name is from the Latin *per fumus*, 'through smoke'—it draws heavily from oriental associations, if not from within the bottle, then in name, packaging and marketing imagery. And given that the olfactory sense eludes verbalization, existing only as a sensation and an association, it lends itself to all forms of transoriental licence. Fragrances can be said to be loaded with different compulsions: one is a personal signature, another is as seduction and another is the promise of something beyond. These qualities can of course all be interconnected, but they are also separate because they also define different varieties of perfume and the desires they connote (and elicit). Chanel No 5, possibly the most successful perfume of all time, contains relatively few orientalist notes, while vampish seduction of the Salome variety is embodied in Dior's *Poison*, and escape is provided by Dior's *Dune*, whose actual scent is not especially oriental.

The most famous orientalist perfume, combining seduction and escape, is YSL's *Opium*. Its name could not be more suggestive. Its bottle and packaging carried a vaguely bamboo motif. Its case, designed by Pierre Dinand, recalled the Japanese *inro*, the perfume container traditionally worn under a kimono. Launched in 1977, it was immediately met with surprise and indignation by some who believed it condoned drug use. A particularly voluble outcry came from America's Chinese community, who called for the name to be changed. For its New York launch Saint Laurent hired a tall ship called *Peking*, which was decked out in gold, red and purple banners and adorned with a massive Buddha covered in cattleya orchids. Later ad campaigns, such as those over the last decade or more, have featured women in vulnerable sexual positions, leaving unchallenged the phallocentric myth of the Orient as an earthly paradise of endless pleasures of the flesh.

The perfume house that draws most consistently from orientalist scents and allusions is Guerlain. In name or smell, Guerlain has long offered an indiscriminate kaleidoscope of references to the Orient, from Arabia, Japan, India to South Asia. When founded in 1828, like most other perfumers Guerlain specialized in florals and colognes. *Jicky*, which appeared in 1889, is said to be the first modern perfume and the benchmark in a style now known as '*fougère*' (named after *Fougère Royale*, by Paul Parquet, joint owner of the

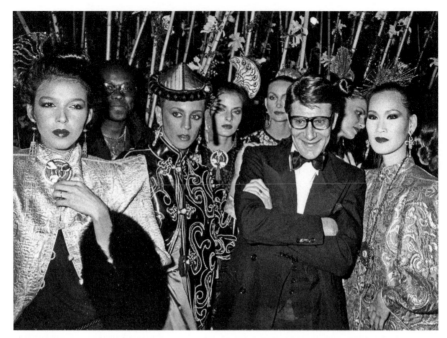

Figure 38   Launch of *Opium* perfume. Yves Saint Laurent and models, 20 September 1978, © Photo by Ron Galella/WireImage.

house of Houbigant), which is a herbaceous style that simply means 'fern-like'. *Jicky* was of the first perfumes to use the synthetic odorants of vanil-lan and coumarin, and contains distinctive notes of civet, the small, arboreal animal from tropical Africa and Asia best known for excreting musk. The Ja-poniste titled *Mitsouko* (1919), the first orientalist fragrance to have a pro-vocatively orientalist name, contains the relatively unoriental notes of iris and peach. But the first 'truly' orientalist fragrance arrived shortly after. *Shali-mar* (1925), named after the gardens built by Shah Jahan in memory of his wife of the same name, is rich and luscious, thanks to the plentiful portion of vanillan. Its dense, heady composition of both the sharp and the cloying makes it seem almost more than a perfume but a mixture that provides a rite of passage into an exotic wilderness. It is considered the perfume house's 'flagship' fragrance. More recently, in 1979, Guerlain introduced *Nahéma*. Meaning 'daughter of fire', she is one of two sisters in a story told by Schehe-razade. It was created with Catherine Deneuve in mind, who played a role in the movie *Benjamin* not dissimilar from the Arab heroine. The publicity image finds Deneuve in a gold cage surrounded by roses. Ten years later appeared the jasmine and sandalwood-dominant *Samsara*, the name referring to the Hindu cycle of birth, death and recreation.

As for Guerlain's men's range, *Habit Rouge* (1965), with its thick vanillan base, is widely thought of as the first oriental fragrance for men, surpassing *Vétiver* (1959) for the title; while the more understated title of the contemporary *L'Homme* (2008) contains recognizable notes of green tea. The blurb on the Guerlain Web site is what might be called orientalism on speed:

Habit Rouge incarnates the magnificent and unpredictable hunter, a man who is enamored of refinement and capable of all manner of audacity. He lives his life fervently and distinguishes himself with an allure that combines sophistication and sensuality. An oriental that is by turns citrusy, warm and accented with vanilla, Habit Rouge expresses the genius of contrast and well-mastered emotions.[15]

This is risible stuff, and what for the beauty of the fragrance itself, this verbiage does everything to warn you off it. This is the colonizer with a square jaw, with a private-school education who presides with stern aplomb over his subservient colonial coolies. With Lothario-like ideas like magnificent and unpredictable hunters running amuck, one is tempted to say to ask whether orientalism in the fashion world has at all evolved at all. Perhaps it hasn't. Its connotative fabric only becomes denser as more fictional material is added to it.

The life, or lives, of perfume confirms what has already been shown in fashion and dress since the 1400s, namely that there is more than one category of oriental. Perfume's evolution in the nineteenth century occurs at the same time that florals were becoming absorbed into lace and crinoline of dresses. By the end of the nineteenth century, Europe had assumed ownership of many of the so-called non-Western components to fragrances. The 'oriental category' per se—so entrenched is the style that a perfume can be categorized as 'an oriental'—within the perfume industry suffices to illustrate the life of the floating concepts of transorientalism. Even the ingredients themselves—from Asian spice to Middle Eastern plants—are brought into the ambit of what they portend instead of what they simply 'really' are, what they *might be*, as opposed to cultural facts. Indeed, from the twentieth century onward, orientalism is a place in Euro–American marketing in which the geographical Middle East and Asia pale before the endless possibilities of suggestions in which past and present histories are enmeshed. Orientalism is the vast and deep reservoir for all kinds of presumption. I will end this section with a selective list of perfumes that avail themselves of orientalist idioms: Bourjois, *Kobako* (c. 1936); Marquay, *Prince Douka* (1951); Annik Goutal, *Eau d'Hadrien* (1961); Pierre Balmain, *Ivoire* (1980); Givenchy, *Organza* (1996); Donna Karan, *Black Cashmere* (2002); Bond No 9, *Chinatown* (2005); Hermès, *Un Jardin sur le Nil* (2005); Penhaligon's, *Lily and Spice* (2006). Others, such as Estée Lauder, 'Private Collection': *Lavender White Moss* (2009), is not an oriental fragrance but a more than vaguely Egyptianizing package: the glass is a thick block; the cavity for the liquid is vessel-shaped, like an ancient barque; the stopper in gold with white and blue-lapis inspired faux-gems is Egyptian deco.

THE NEW JAPANESE REVOLUTION IN FRENCH COUTURE

In his own time, Louis XIV's insatiable thirst for grandiose architecture and finery may have had a crippling effect on his country, but the French have much to thank him for. Louis's legacy made Paris the undisputed city of style, and luxury goods—which were commodities based on perception as much as worth—comprise a sizable portion of the French economy. In fashion, perception is everything. This was the motivation of Japanese designers, from Kenzo onward, who believed that their success was incomplete without Parisian approval.

The most thorough account of this neo-japonism is given by Yuniya Kawamura, who emphasizes France's extraordinary hold on fashion and style since the era of Louis XIV's court. Since the 1970s, Italian and American clothing industries enjoyed untold success, but Paris would always be the city where the biggest ideas and greatest talent in fashion were considered to gravitate and germinate. Before the 1970s, Paris fashion was still preoccupied with itself, distrustful of any foreign interpolation. The influx of Japanese designers changed that. Kenzo, Rei Kawakubo (Comme des Garçons), Issey Miyake, Yohji Yanomoto and Hanae Mori are the most successful of a group now hailed as bringing about a new wave of fashion in the 1970s to the 1990s, and of integrating orientalist styling into very substance of haute couture. The generation after that includes Junya Watanabe, Matsaki Matsunisha, Hiromichi Nakano and Yuji Yamada. The Japanese new wave suggests that not all secondary entries arrive as farce. By the second half of the twentieth century, Japonism was firmly etched into the French range of styles but not so as to appear overly unfamiliar, quaint or outlandish. On another point one can only speculate: the floating, unspecific nature of the Japoniste sign was what separated itself from the more grisly connections of accusations of postwar guilt. Guilt and anger were emotions still fresh in the era of the Vietnam War. But it seems that Japanese–French fashions as they emerged at this time were relatively free of negative connotations. One reason, as Gayatri Spivak speculates, is the extent to which Japanese culture is imbibed and defined by Euro–American cultural history. In these years Japan wanted yet again to reassert itself as the best of Asian nations, which meant foregrounding Asian-ness and offering something else that was therefore paradoxically not quite Asian.[16]

In this rather unquantifiable terrain of the familiar–unfamiliar, as Kawamura suggests, Kenzo and the designers in his wake began to use marginality as an asset: 'Japanese designers began to use their "race" card to be acknowl-edged by the French. . .'.[17] This was part of a much larger chapter in which orientals and postcolonials enter into Western life to remake themselves while simultaneously moulding and massaging their own cultural identity to personal advantage. It is a discourse whose ethical and aesthetic ramifica-tions are still to be thought through thoroughly. It is a double game where the other plays out his or her role as other within a revisionist environment. The quintessence of this manoeuver is for Spivak summed up in the figure of Rei Kawakubo, whose fashions are 'the-same-yet-not-the-same, different-but-not-different'.[18] While Kawakubo rejects anchorage to culture ('I have always felt it important not to be defined by tradition or custom or geography'[19]), it is a disavowal that is made possible by the manner in which Japan markets spe-cific Asian characteristics of itself to the West. It is the Western response to consume signs of difference, particularly when they are in the shape of com-modities. It is also the contemporary Western inclination to embrace its other with a mind to correcting former colonialist injustice. This is done on the un-spoken condition that the other never fundamentally foregoes his or her other-ness; the other plays out this otherness for the revisionist pantomime within the global Euro–American system. This dynamic holds as much for novelists and artists as it does for orientalist fashions.

But it seems that various marginal groups not only grasp this dynamic differently but are not unified in their willingness to monopolize on it, to sac-rifice their belief in indigenous cultural values for recognition by the West. Kawamura describes how unabashedly some of the Japanese fashion de-signers flouted their Japanese-ness before the Parisian scene: Mori drew on a panoramic history of Kyoto with silk sashes and dresses designed with Mt Fuji, and Kenzo bombarded his public with flowers in which the fields of Grasse melded with the blossoms of Japan. On the other hand, as we have seen, Kawakubo was resistant to the 'Japanese designer' label. Yamomoto made much of his individual status as a 'creator', and Miyake has distanced him-self from a single culture and situates himself within a global one.[20] Seen as a group, these conflicting standpoints proved immensely useful in promoting the Japanese movement as one that was heterogeneous and alive. So much so that by the 1980s French fashion critics were remarking on their 'Oriental rivals'.[21] Japan, meanwhile, proved enormously efficient in consuming their own—Japanese prosperity in the 1980s had secured itself the dubious hon-our as a leader in fashion consumption as opposed to production[22]—so long as it had undergone the Parisian rite of passage. Between 1970 and 1990, Japanese designers not only overhauled Paris fashions but asserted their influence on the Belgian designers, like Dries van Noten, emerging from the 1980s and galvanizing prospective designers from Korea and Africa to do the same, changing Western fashion from within.

Kenzo is the Christopher Columbus of the Japanese fashion revolution. First venturing to Paris in 1964, Kenzo later found a place as an industry designer with Louis Féraud. When branching out with limited means on his own, their bold combinations of nonoriental checks and plaids with more recognizably Japanese florals and patterns distinguished his first collections. Whether this is legend or fact, such combinations were both expedient and tactical. The piecemeal character of the design came from cheaper fabric off-cuts, which were then creatively married. Drawing with indiscriminate energy on all facets of fashion, the spirit of eclecticism that drew from other ethnic traditions in addition to his own,[23] Kenzo's fashions are still appended to a Japanese armature. This is particularly evident in the highly rectilinear nature of his designs, which contrastingly support curvaceous lines, bright patterns and lustrous textures. That Kenzo, as a non-Westerner was so disposed to the promiscuous borrowing from other fashions had been called a democratic approach to influence—compare this to the occasional and rather stock accusation of the Westerner plundering from worlds not his.

This idea of a relatively stable 'traditional' Japanese armature is also present in the three designers who cam in Kenzo's wake, Kawakubo, Miyake and Yanomoto, especially when one thinks of Miyake's concept of 'A Piece of Cloth' that began in the mid-1970s, his 'handkerchief' dresses in 1970, Comme des Garçons's 'Wrapped Collection' of 1983, or Yamomoto's cavernously thick layers of cloth the year after. These designers embraced that Japanese fashion has a different sense of space from that of the West, being far more architectonic—in the sense of structure—and works from a whole downwards to the smaller elements (the limbs, the head), whereas Westerner fashion is always conscious of the local elements and how they aggregate to the whole. All emphasize freedom of form and movement, whether using large swathes of cloth, down to Miyake's signature crumpled pleats, which afford easy movement in a casing whose constriction is entirely visual.

Kawakubo's designs had a considerable effect in rethinking women's clothing and the women's body. At a time when deconstruction was alive in both philosophy, art and architecture, Kawakubo was expressing ideas about the body that challenged space, continuity and expectation with openings and pathways in garments that went nowhere, irrationalities like extra sleeves, and imbalances that addressed a mobile rather and ideal body ('Perfect symmetry is ugly . . . I always want to destroy symmetry'[24]). Caroline Evans and Minna Thornton comment that Kawakubo's 'starting from zero' ethic of working was a mechanism of creating slippages in conventions. This amounted to a 'making strange' of the female body that, like Westwood, she caused one to rethink female sexiness, which means both her idea of herself and the presumptions of others. They state: 'Kawakubo allows one to "re-see" the body and its possibilities. Emphasising the continuity of the female body, even its contiguity, in space, calls into the practice of "seeing the body in bits" that has been identified as intrinsic to the representation of the female body in patriarchal culture.'[25] Thus, the rhetoric of starting from nothing identifies with an effort to clear the slate of history and to make clothing whose references are random; a 'decontextualisation' on par with that of Vionnet.[26] Like the designs of Yamomoto and Miyake, her designs spill over into unisex, defying gender presumptions altogether. One recalls the pre-Meiji era when the line and logic of clothing was the same for men and women; only the fabric designs may have varied.

As such, Kawakubo's work is often called a minimalism. It begins with the elemental 'pure' forms of fabric and space and is built upward according to her intuition. This is mystical stuff, of course, but highly effective in granting her work an ahistorical air. From another angle, her work has been characterized as 'post-Hiroshima', meaning a new beginning, but also a radical if not brutal reconfiguration of form, the echo of trauma restated as beautiful art. A favourite technique of Kawakubo, which at the time was maybe only popular in the syntax of jeans, was chic ragged—prewearing and tearing the clothes, giving garments an imprint of time that they never experienced. This can be construed as the signs of discomfort; it could also be the natural effects of wear with time. Time is an important quantity in her work and with her peers. Like Kenzo, everything is free game: from Japanese peasant clothing to Heian or Edo pomp. Kawakubo sees Japanese-ness as a vast storehouse of signs to be remoulded into or against canonical presumptions of other fashions outside it. Thus is reflected in this image of an ensemble that matches a marked Japanese flag T-shirt with plaid pants seemingly assembled from hacked fragments. In a sense both cultural signatures have been subject to tame desecrations while ensuring that their recognizability remains intact.

But the attitude to history of these Japanese designers is not necessarily a postmodern one that, in an unsympathetic reading, views history as a grab bag of elements to be recycled at a whim. The famous statement of Theodor Adorno, in his essay 'Cultural Criticism and Society', that 'After Auschwitz all lyric poetry is barbarism' is relevant here, as it calls for a seismic rethinking of the beauty and aesthetic interest. That fashion has been on the margins of this debate is not least because it was regarded with suspicion bordering on contempt by cultural critics like Adorno and his Frankfurt school colleagues. Yet it is reasonable to speculate that without 'Hiroshima'—which has as much metonymic resonance as Auschwitz—the work of Miyake and that of many of his peers might not have been possible. The reorganization of history is one factor of a definitive break with the past; the reorganization of form is another. They are both hysterical measures, as is the attempt at a new dawn in optimistic colours and uncomplicated lines. In the words of Mark Holborn,

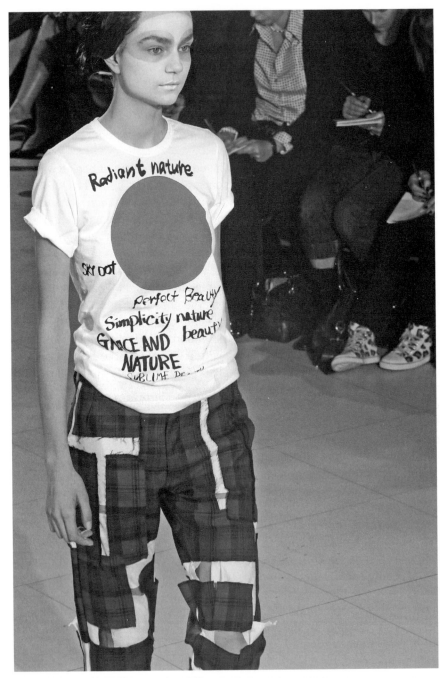

Figure 39 A model presents a creation by Japanese designer Rei Kawakubo for Comme des Garçons during the Spring/Summer 2007 ready-to-wear collections in Paris, 2 October 2006, © Pierre Verdy/AFP/Getty Images.

'Miyake's creativity exists not in detachment from the shadows of Japanese history, but in an inescapable response to such experience'.[27] 'The benign breeze from the Miyake Design Studio in fact originates in the dark ages of modern Japan.'[28] This is not only in terms of a symbolic, psychological response but of a material one. The American occupation after the war meant that the Japanese were literally bombarded with popular culture, which offered different perspectives and the promise of a new and better way of life. Miyake and his peers are comfortable, receptive observers of popular culture, which they bring together with myths and legends, celebrated in fashion shows of spectacular theatricality, a creative mise en scène that would be have its creative progeny in Alexander McQueen and John Galliano.

What the re-envisioning of Japan exerted by Japanese designers of this era occurred within fashion but not in society. They did not so much explode what orientalism means within fashion as enrich its repertoire. This is a view supported by Dorinne Kondo in her invaluable study of Japanese fashion in Paris.

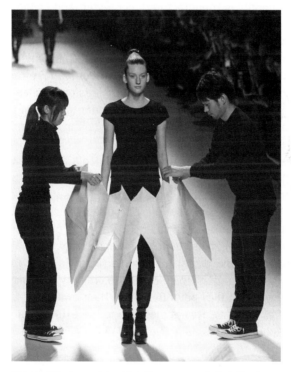

Figure 40 A model walks the runway during the Issey Miyake ready-to-wear Autumn/Winter 2011/2012 show during Paris Fashion Week at Pavillon Concorde on March 4, 2011 in Paris, © Photo by Antonio de Moraes Barros Filho/ WireImage.

She observes that the challenges of designers like Miyake and Kawakubo to orientalist typologies of race and gender occurred within a commodified structure created by elite, postcolonial corporatization.[29] Kondo is highly insightful in showing how Japanese-ness was, and continues to be, refigured according to an indeterminate, shifting set of coordinates. Art plays a continual part in these designers' strategies, on the level of the pieces themselves to enlisting artists like Cindy Sherman to photograph them.[30] Their sculptural attitude to garments and their stepping into areas of art and conceptual fashion in turns means that their relationship to Japan the country and Japan the idea is being invented over and again. Their idioms and iconography are analogous to touristic conceptions of Kyoto which lies poised as a symbol of 'a blurry, elegiac past'.[31]

Fashion's disengagement from ideology makes it available to cultural diagnosis, but this freedom is also arguably the condition of its limits. Kawakubo may have contested assumptions of gender, but only partially and temporarily. For Kondo the Japanese revolution revealed the limited capacity of fashion to exert social change.[32] Yet it also brought to notice how fashion is the locus where cultural identity is manufactured, contested and confirmed. We might go so far as to infer that the Japanese aesthetic that gives primacy to the artificial over the natural is what for this to occur; it also exposes an inner truth to all cultural reflections, namely that cultures rely on innumerable fictions to support its image of unity. From Japan's renovations and retraditionalizing in the Meiji era, reinstating real and typologized ideas of Japanese tradition and infusing it with that of others in recent times bears testament to the ability of Japan to remap and reorder its aesthetic priorities in a way that both caters to foreign will, but also reshapes that will.

The kinds of historical and cultural displacements of the new Japanese design mean that it was prophetic of the 'contemporary' within both contemporary art and fashion. Confusingly, the 'contemporary' has supplanted that of 'postmodern' as a descriptor for our period. One of its key characteristics in fashion is the radical permeability of style and the spillage of fashion as a practice and an idea into other genres, especially dance, experimental performance, sculpture, installation and digital multimedia. Inspired by the rich history of kabuki theatre (*kabuku* means 'to be out of the ordinary'), Miyake's designs are unusual for the way that they potentially have their own kind of life on display, independent of being worn. This is also due to the extraordinary sensitivity to sculptural metaphor, which is as active outside the garment itself as within.

POSTMODERN AND CONTEMPORARY COUTURE

Toward the beginning of his meditation on Japan, *Empire of Signs*, Barthes writes:

I am not lovingly gazing toward an Oriental essence—to me the Orient is a matter of indifference, merely providing a reserve of features whose manipulation—whose invented interplay allows me to 'entertain' the idea of an unheard-of symbolic system, one altogether detached from our own. What can be addressed, in the consideration of the Orient, are not other symbols, another metaphysics, another wisdom (thought the latter might appear thoroughly desirable); it is the possibility of a difference, a mutation, a revolution in the propriety of symbolic systems. . . . Today there are doubtless a thousand things to learn about the Orient . . . but it is also necessary that, leaving aside the vast regions of darkness . . . a slender thread of light search out not other symbols but the very fissure of the symbolic. . . . The author has never, in any sense, photographed Japan. . . . Japan has starred him with any number of 'flashes'; or, better still, Japan has afforded him a situation of writing. This situation is the very one in which a certain disturbance of the person occurs, a subversion of earlier readings. . .[33]

When transposed into the realms of fashion, Barthes outlines what is the ideal state of transorientalism: 'a reserve of features whose manipulation—whose invented interplay' allows for a 'detachment' from the regular symbolic system into an elsewhere that promises a fertile pastures of creation. Barthes is also dodging the increasingly more turgid responsibilities of good faith and better knowledge that haunt the postimperialist with an exhortation that the Orient be kept alive in all its intangibility to provide a scene for 'writing'. This is anyway what many artists and designers in love with the Orient have done for several hundred years: the creative voice that assumes no authority over a place; it knows little or nothing about but craves indulgence from it to feed his fancies. One must at this point give due credence to Spivak's hostility to Barthes's formulation. Barthes's suggestion of the slackened line between representation and origin is pertinent to what she calls 'transnational' fashion, although Barthes's disburdening of political conscience is for her highly moot.[34] To be sure, however, as we have seen with both Asian and European designers, if a decision is to be made between cultural criticism and invention, the latter will win out. Fashion is, after all, an industry.

Transorientalism in fashion is not to be understood as a name for absolution from the moral responsibilities. It does however draw much sustenance from the history of fashion in which the Orient was, in certain theatres, a willing player in shaping and manipulating an image congenial to the oriental phantasm. On the other hand, as we will see below, the prolongation of the orientalist urge in couture—I will avoid the word *stereotype* here as it is a source of enormous invention—nourishes an idea of norms and clichés in countries that have evolved and that are bent on restoring some degree of autonomy to their fashions, designs and other practices besides. In the 1990s there has been a steady stream of exhibitions on orientalism which include the Costume Institute of the Metropolitan Museum in New York (1994), *Japonisme et la Mode* at the Palais Galerie costume museum two years later, *Touches d'Exotisme* at the Fashion and Textile Museum in Paris (1998) and a survey of Japanese taste, *Japonisme* at the Brooklyn Museum of Art in New York (1999), and *China Chic: East Meets West* at the Fashion Institute of Technology, New York. While American and Europe were being historical and anthropological, other countries were reassessing their traditions, also with the mind to freeing constricting stereotypes.

Sounding a bleaker note, Hal Foster remarks that 'contemporary design is part of a greater revenge of capitalism on postmodernism—a recouping of its crossings of arts and disciplines, a routinization of its transgressions'.[35] The statement not only does calls to account the globalization's disavowal of difference for the sake of a fictional 'normalizing' whole, but it brings into healthy reassessment the extent of the transgressive import of contemporary orientalist fashion. What is certain is that when we turn to the orientalisms from Saint Laurent to Galliano, transgression exists as the narrative twinge of some line of force that is now part of a laconic register of emotions and histories. But fashion's absorption of ideas into its aesthetic folds, which may be said to parallel capitalism's absorption of forms of resistance, is also witnessed a sublimation, especially after 9/11. Here the East looms up as a place to be tamed and as a renewed threat. Chadors, burqas and hijab have been dealt a new onslaught. But as with the psychology of horror movies, many of us enjoy vicarious fear when we know we are safe. So, on the other pole, orientalism has been given new sustenance by the upheavals in the East. Sex, death and exoticism have always been drivers for fashion since it 'began' in the eighteenth century. Orientalism enshrines all of these factors. The ongoing military presence of America and Europe in the East—Iraq, Afghanistan, Syria—is enough for the Euro–American capitalist imagination to indulge again in ideas of power—the satisfactions that emanate from greater safety and economic superiority. For the most part, attention by fashion and cultural theorists for more than a decade has been on the efforts by colonialized and 'oriental' states to situate themselves in the complex, muddy territory of globalization.

An important marker in the transoriental era after Poiret is Saint Laurent's peasant collection of 1976, in which an entire array of folk themes was translated into high-level couture. While this was not orientalism, it spelt a process whereby designers were freely adapting cultural languages, remoulding and reinscribing them. This set the pattern, if you like, for the next three or more decades. Writing about the this collection, Entwistle argues that the peasant collection exemplified the volatility of the fashion industry. Exotic themes have become a leitmotif of new fashions through the incorporation of themes such as jungle and tropical imagery, 'exotic' peoples and cultures, elements of 'folk' and 'ethnic' costume, and recycled items from earlier fashions. Frequently exotic motifs from tourist destinations or from post-colonial cultures form the basis of fashion derivations.[36]

For her, the lust for exoticism is an outward sign of the West's assertion of its superiority over other cultures.[37] Fashion is a powerful yet politically surreptitious form of stating ownership of an idea or principle. In the introduction I suggested that orientalism was fashion's device to claim to dominion. This claim is at once blatant and entirely hidden. In the age after colonization, orientalist references cannot have the same purchase, since there is no longer dominion, or empire. Or rather, empire does exist, yet intangibly.

In more ways than one Yves Saint Laurent can be said to embody the transition from the orientalism as based in ownership and transorientalism in which ownership is assumed, asserted, dreamed up, lost and re-won.[38] Born in Algiers in 1936, he worked for the house of Dior before falling afoul of it due to his intemperance. After 1963 he returned to North Africa, ensconced in Marrakech during the 1968 student riots in Paris. He would continue to sojourn to Morocco, and in 1980 he and his partner, Pierre Bergé, bought the Jardin Majorelle, which was in a state of ruin. Bergé himself dilated on this orientalist connection with his own hagiography. The genius of Saint Laurent, he wrote, was to 'delve into the Orientalist bric-à-brac and with the legitimacy of a magician make his own world emerge out of it'.[39] A periodical from 1997 gushed: 'Yves Saint Laurent is headed for China, but it isn't the somber China of Deng Xiapong. Yves Saint Laurent's Orient has bright colours, slit trousers and daring bustiers'.[40] Although from very different sources, they share a common theme—that of Saint Laurent as a latter-day Prospero who, with the rare and arcane gifts of transformation, turned dross into something legitimately warranting the epithet of creation. Extrapolating, one might be forgiven for saying that it was only the Western-Prospero creator who could really bring the Orient into the being.

As Lise Skov indicates, this legitimacy stems from the presumptions about field of production and the authority that Paris has over the fashion industry.[41] While this holds true for some such Japanese designers, it is less relevant to countries that are using fashion to assert their own cultural terms of reference, and for the economies of China and India for whom it is becoming more incongruous to pay lip service to an economy a fraction of its size and growth. It is very hard to generalize about such vast cultures, many sectors of whose different concepts of fashion's status and its performative function make the prospect of Paris-centrism incongruous. In her words, 'The contrast between Western exoticism and Asian modernism is striking, and should prompt some self-critical reflections. . .' The globalization of Asian fashion brings home the view that 'fashion emerges in a field of tension'.[42]

To put it another way: the locus of empire is more in the designed and fabricated objects themselves than in a geographical place. The question of orientalism's status in fashion in the last few decades has to take into account the enormous economic evolution of India and China and smaller states like Korea and Taiwan. Sometimes called the Asian Economic Miracle, in the West it precipitated a mixture of consternation and admiration. Asian chic rose up again in the 1990s with an energy that seemed to recognize a newly solidified, stable Asia. But what was the tenor of this recognition? Carla Jones and Ann Marie Leshkowich argue that this economic boom resulted in a yet another reductionism by Western marketing and design. Asia was reduced to a series of symbols—clothing, implements, bibelots—witch had a metonymic value that discouraged any connection between actual origins. They cite Galliano's 1997 collection for Dior that featured bright reinterpretations of the Chinese cheongsam or the way that American homeware chains like Pottery Barn marketed rice bowls and chopsticks. When the Asian economy underwent recession in 1998 and 1999, Euro–America's marketing of an undifferentiated Asia continued undeterred. Jones and Leshkowich attribute the motivation for this phenomenon as a conscious and subconscious action to emasculate, or trivialize, the Asian threat to Western superiority by reducing it to a series of inert symbols. This action came to the fore most forcibly in fashion and dress.[43] Their argument makes some sense, but it loses traction when one thinks of the rise of the Japanese economy in the decade before. It is also overly conspiratorial, not accounting for the already heterogeneous migrant cultures within Europe and America. It also does not look forward to the continued appropriations of Asia and orientalism in fashion to the present. I emphasize my own point that orientalism is a structural variable within fashion itself, as integral to fashion as a system, an idea and an industry in which the Orient and the West are specious—yet tenacious—co-dependent constructs that exist in parallel to nature and culture.

It is a view supported by Valerie Steele and John S. Major in the summation of *China Chic*, whose punctuation point is Hong Kong's return to China in 1997. Hong Kong is itself an interesting point of analysis for anything pertaining to orientalism, since for over two centuries it constituted the most important port for British trade. Its culture now testifies to the embrace of both 'Chinese-ness' and the 'West'. It is a comfortable hybrid, and proudly so. Steele and Major cite various examples of the ways that designers have made use of references—Gaultier Mongolia, Karan Maoist China—and argue that it is obfuscatory to subject such inspiration to overly rigid ideological objection. We may add to this Hermès' announcement that 1997 was 'The Year of Africa', after four years of already using designs of the warrior race of the Sahara, the Taureg. Hermès has an entire 'Taureg line' of scarves, leather bags with cross closures, buckles, bracelets and rings, and its jewellery is made by Taureg smiths in Agadez. In what perhaps is a ploy at absolution, to sanitize its usury, Hermes publishes pictures from its exotic workshops and descriptions of the local artisans from far off places to promote products that sell for many times the artisans' yearly earnings.[44]

These are emotive facts. Steele and Major acknowledge wholeheartedly that cultural purloining potentially reduces references to 'empty symbols of exoticism', but what they also insist is just as indisputable: the criticism that lifted references in fashion are imbued with insufficient empathy or knowledge 'could be made *whatever* designers are inspired by in *anything* beyond their daily lives'.[45] This is a very plain, commonsense and courageous plea not to try to mix anthropology and politics too smoothly with fashion. 'Relatively few fashion designers have more than a cursory knowledge of the history of western dress'.[46] This is not to pledge moral immunity, but to identify, as Kant would say, different categories of understanding. Also, in defence of this, one can cite Jennifer Craik when she states: 'Fashion statements appear to mark a moment, but the fashion body is never secure or fixed. The body is constantly re-clothed and re-fashioned in accordance with changing arrangements of the self.'[47]

What Jones and Leshkowich more convincingly establish is how oriental/Asian women continue to be typecast as mysterious and erotic, which only shows that the symmetry between the oriental–feminine paradigm as against the masculine West continues its centuries-long lineage. This is even made more complex in imagery of the female sweatshop worker, which ostensibly sets out to emancipate her: 'Representations of docile factory women, even as they call attention to very real circumstances of exploitation, confirm longstanding Western stereotypes of the subservient Asian woman.' In other instances, as confirmed by Arthur Golden's extraordinarily successful *Memoires of a Geisha*, the Asian woman is a nostalgic relic of an indeterminate past. She is beautiful, oppressed, waiting silently in her kimono, brutalized by a society lacking the West's enlightened vision.[48] Compelling as this argument is, it must also consider the objectification of women at all levels of the fashion industry and the media. We must also ask what differences exist, within the fashion industry (and elsewhere), between African, Middle Eastern woman and the Asian woman. For 9/11 has made for many the Middle Eastern woman a figure of alarm, while models like Iman and Naomi Campbell walk a line between exoticism and 'white-black'. The gendering of the Orient as feminine is theoretically

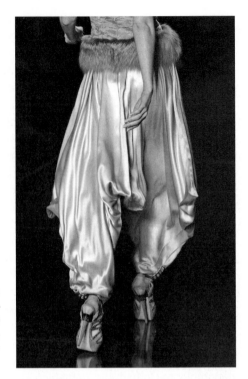

Figure 41 A model presents a creation by British designer John Galliano for Christian Dior during the autumn/winter 2009 ready-to-wear collection show in Paris, on 6 March 2009. © François Guillot/AFP/ Getty Images.

incontestable, but like the sex–gender distinction in gender studies, feminism and psychoanalysis, once it seeks an objective correlative, it runs into all kinds of problems.[49]

For the rest of this section I will concentrate on as good a case study as any: John Galliano's 2009 couture and prêt-à-porter range for Dior, one of his last for the house before he was dismissed. This range unequivocally looked back to the 1920s and to Poiret: harem pants, gold brocade, high-key florals, horizontal folds and ikat patterns. Galliano stated that for this collection he had looked to paintings by Delacroix and back to Dior himself. The comment posted on Geniusbeauty.com is revealingly transorientalist, especially to the extent that Orient is a free-associative universe: 'The East was always a source of inspiration for Christian Dior and he travelled a lot through Asian countries. And John Galliano seems to wander more in his fantasies.'[50] It is instructive and even amusing comment, not only for the admission that Galliano's grasp of the Orient is from 'fantasies' but also how the Orient is remains generalized and indiscriminate: 'Asian countries'. A passing validation is in suggesting that Dior himself had had a more first-hand experience—'he travelled a lot'. What is important to emphasize here is the tertiary level of Galliano's inspiration. It had no serious experiential, empirical links to the cultures in question.

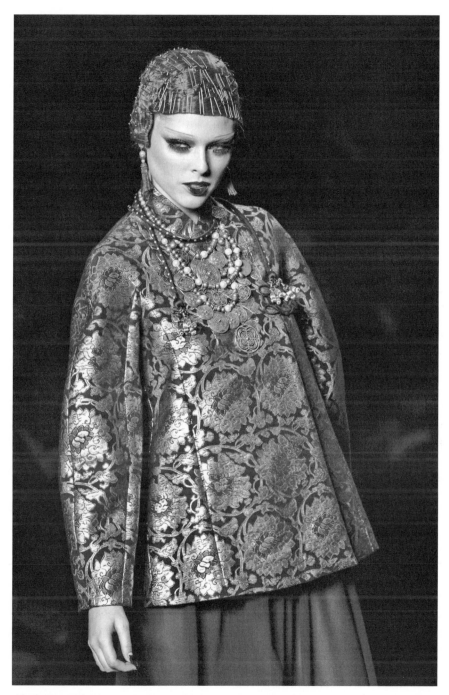

Figure 42   A model presents a creation by British designer John Galliano for Christian Dior during the autumn/winter 2009 ready-to-wear collection show in Paris, on 6 March 2009, © François Guillot/AFP/Getty Images.

REORIENTING AND SELF-ORIENTALIZING THE ORIENT

While the halls of haute couture indulge in baroque freedoms, defining and maintaining the oriental fetish, other countries have mixed reactions to Western appropriations. The fate of clothing in the broad reach of the many countries that at one time were associated with the Orient has been either to re-adopt and re-enact tradition as a form of resistance, and as a mainstay of its own cultural norms, or to meld casually into the normalizing fog of the global environment. Binaries are often good places to start a critical discussion, but the issue is a lot more complex with numerous coordinates. Some countries, such as India, are at pains to carve out autonomy and thus to name their own standards for Indian dress. Others, such as Africa, are maintaining and nurturing traditions anew for their consumption by richer countries. In other cases, Western adoption of foreign styles remains a tender issue.

This can be illustrated using the very contemporary example of the abuses of Australian Aboriginal art within art as well as textiles. Aboriginal is what I have elsewhere called 'the last bastion of the primitive'—in which 'primitive' here can be used interchangeably with 'exotic'—the last place where the roving Euro–American eye casts itself, hungry for a new world to reinvigorate the old.[51] When traditional Aboriginal art began to grow in popularity in the early-mid 1980s, it became intimately associated with a particular mission in the Western Desert, Papunya Tula, and to a lesser extent the region just north of it, the Kimberly Ranges. To this day, dots and concentric circles remain synonymous with Aboriginal art at the expense of countless other styles belonging to different groups. When these designs became widespread, and with indiscriminate use—tea towels, mousepads, T-shirts—debate raged amongst Aboriginal elders and their people as to the suitability of this exposure. These designs, which became prodigally spattered over airplanes, as they were on scarves, shirts and ties, derived from deeply sacred rituals whose inner sources and truths were the confined to a select group of tribal elders and custodians. Their promiscuous use for the sake of taking advantage of yet another exotic novelty—such as the generic dot designs on the Qantas stewardess's uniforms—was, and to many still is, an abomination. To the most private nonassimilationist of the indigenous peoples, it represents a galling double standard. While sacred imagery can be used with middling respect to those from whom it originated, in the same country enforceable laws yet make it a punishable offence to desecrate the national flag (but not the Aboriginal one). But the prevalence of these designs suggests that they are densely entrenched, and the more religious indigenous peoples are too much in a minority to be able to mount any form of effective resistance.

Taking a more tempered view, Margaret Maynard argues that the cultural appropriation that took place within Australia is far different from the kind

typified by Poiret. The lines of influence and benefit are far more fluid and reciprocal. It is a view based on the fact that Aboriginal art was effectively 'born'
in the 1970s and 1980s, that is it was introduced into the perimeter of art,
the Western, modern construct, from its former status as a mechanism of
spiritual transmission. Maynard forcefully suggests that this evolution meant
that Aboriginal art was by definition in a state of transformation, from paintings on stone to those on canvas, or patterns on sand to patterns on cloth.
The dot motif that saturates the market is avowedly selective yet is an amenable symbol Aboriginal cultural heritage. This kind of metonymic detachment
of motifs and styles comes with its problems, some of which she cites, but
she also claims that dots are as prevalent elsewhere and are a means by
which the black and white can make links. The late 1970s was a period in
which there was so much collaboration and crossfertilization that 'it is virtually impossible to separate out the strands of influence'.[52] This is neither to
denigrate the specificity of Indigenous motifs and their meanings, which have
fallen prey to countless copies that have debased their integrity, something
that has gained momentum with the rising popularity of Aboriginal art by the
1990s. But the very heterogeneous evolution of Aboriginal styles in fashion
makes the line between authentic and inauthentic impossible to draw. 'So it
would seem' she concludes,

> that ethnicity, national imagery and perhaps indigenous imagery, too, can never
> be 'essential' but must be regarded as moving through cultures and through art
> forms and be seen as expandable and subjective notions, looking back to shared
> cultural or historical markers but always in process and never static.[53]

The other important lesson to be learned is that Aboriginal designs are never
too remote from politics.

The same can be said of most, if not all, traditions that were renegotiated
in the postcolonial era, in which particular articles were singled out as having
a deep national significance and used as tools for dissent. As mentioned earlier, the most famous example of this is Gandhi's dhoti and *chadar* (shawl).
As Emma Tarlo explains, dress in India was never a simple matter, and many
found themselves juggling their sartorial identities. Gandhi's is the most famous instance of a history of cultural ambivalences in dress, dating back at
least to the Moghul period, that enforced its own styles on the Hindus who, to
maintain their private dignity, removed the clothing before entering their own
homes.[54] Nor was Gandhi's example greeted with universal approval. His attempt to introduce the *sola topi* hat into national dress was rejected out of
hand.[55] More successful was his advocacy of the *khadi*, the traditional cloth
wrapping, especially since it was versatile enough for it to able to be Europe-
anized. One could register more than one level of belonging a once.[56] In Kenya

in the late 1960s, the Mau Mau rebellion objected to Western dress, emboldening Eliad Mathu, the first African to be elected to Parliament, to tear off his jacket in reclamation of his indigeneity. Entwistle observes that the Bengali language has eschewed coining words for 'fashion' and 'style'. Instead, they use the English words, as a way of announcing the place whence they originated, namely not from India.

Later, in the 1990s in Korea the *hanbok*—the traditional skirt and dress jacket—made its re-entry into official dress, worn as a third option in formal circles to the suit, asserting the presence of Korean rural life.[57] The story of the *hanbok* is a little like the kimono insofar as it was a response to outside stimuli before it moulded itself into the rhetoric of tradition. Born from both Japanese and Western influence, the *hanbok* emerged out of the colonial era (1905–1945), before which the common clothing for women was a long skirt (*ch'ima*) and a very short jacket (*cheongori*). The 1990s version is yet another modification of this already recent construction. Retaining only the former shape, it is usually wool or cotton instead of silk, more muted in colour and may use modern fasteners such as zippers. Rebecca Ruhlen in her essay aptly titled 'Korean Alterations' concludes that 'the new hanbok styles were part of a repertoire for the performance and consumption of national identity, available to all Koreans but used especially by activists'.[58] She outlines the extent of the *hanbok*'s involvement as a signifier of Korean domestic and economic self-assertion, even where the 'lifestyle' *hanbok* is extolled over the unhealthy ostentation of women's Western dress.[59]

Other countries witnessed a similar orchestrated evolution in traditional dress. After recovering from the war, Vietnam created a garment consisting of wide pants, a vest-like blouse with mandarin collar and knotted buttons especially for the tourist market hungry for local authenticities. It has subsequently become reabsorbed back into Vietnamese society.[60] In Indonesia, older traditions are being revived, remarked and 'resold' back to its urban populations. Indonesian designers are effectively exoticizing Indonesia to itself.[61] Or in a more sinister way, the West (America) seeks to encourage countries in political jeopardy like Afghanistan to turn to an idea of stable tradition as a means of instrumenting broader political stability. As the Philosopher Slavoj Zizek remarked in his book in response to the 9/11 disaster:

Hamid Karzai of Afghanistan is already a 'democratic leader externally imposed on a people'. When Karzai, Afghanistan's 'interim leader' installed by the Americans in 2001, appears in our media, he always wears the same clothes, which cannot fail to look like an attractive modernized version of traditional Afghan attire (a woollen cap and a pullover beneath a more modern coat, etc.)—his figure thus seems to exemplify his mission, that of combining modernization with the best of the old Afghan traditions . . . no wonder, since his attire is the work of a top

Western fashion designer! As such, Karzai is the best metaphor for the status of Afghanistan itself today.[62]

This is one extreme case, but it is nevertheless part of set of cultural family relations in which identity is a highly choreographed affair—stage-managing the natural–traditional.

In about the same time as Korea, India witnessed a renewed enthusiasm for the sari, a reflection of growing nationalism and the confidence gained from economic growth. Nasa Khan remarks that the sari has burgeoned into its own design subculture, including the *nouvelle saree*. It is subject to numerous liberties; one designer has the sari tucked into *churidars*, or tight trousers. The sari is now something of a national signature and incorporates both traditional and nontraditional designs.[63] Another garment that has enjoyed a renaissance in the last few decades is the voluminous, baggy kurta suit, an involved interplay of pants which can be either a capacious shalwar, a *pyjama* or tighter *churidar*, an upper garment which is either like a tunic (*kameez*) or a shirt (kurta) and generous cotton stole (*duputta*). These too have both contemporary and traditional fabric variants. In a reversal of oriental inflection in Western fashion, it might be said that these were traditional, emphatically non-Western clothes that drew on the West for inspiration.

This was already evident in the Indian grasp of Western fashions of the 1970s. While the West was making its own versions of shalwars and pyjamas, or just importing them, India was importing fashions from the West. Bell-bottoms, or flares, for which the era is notorious, were coordinated with long shirts, or kurtas.[64] There was also a perceptible exchange between East and West at this time in jewellery-wearing, which became more abundant and thicker. Now that the 1970s made cheap 'big' jewellery popular and advanced the principle of quantity over quality, India continues to be a producer of affordable 'spiritual' and folksy jewellery: wooden bangles, massive earrings and beads in drunken profusion.

This journey back and forth across borders is best exemplified by the instance of Diana Spencer, who appeared in shalwar-kameez in Pakistan in May 1997. Worn by North Indian and Pakistani women for hundreds of years, this prosaic garment was refined then ratified to become chic by a world celebrity from the West. Its irony, as Jones and Leshkowich argue, is that it is the West that locates what is precious about India's own heritage. In a vaguely amusing tangle of codes, Indian 'women could be imitating Western fashions even as they were aid to be wearing their own traditional clothing'.[65] This reversal, or tangle, spells an invidious and agonistic relationship to cultural inheritance and ownership that is rendered yet more complicated if one considers the different kinds of Indian designers and markets, not least those connected with Britain. Parminder Bhachu's analysis of transnational fashion markets mirrors very much the kinds of manufacture of several hundred years before, when India and China were receptive, through coercion or entrepreneurship, to what Europe wanted and altered their 'authenticities' accordingly. The shalwar-kameez is a case in point and has taken on its own life, with modifications in Britain by British–Indian designers that is appealing to both European and Indian markets, although in different ways.[66] Non-Indians also now wear the salwar-kameez. In Britain it raises no eyebrows.

India's efforts, managed and spontaneous, to instate a separate fashion economy have had mixed results, not least because of its outwardly looking, upwardly mobile youth who are reaping the benefits of the world's largest democracy. The need for sartorial identity is a vexed issue. To use the words of Joytsna Singh,

> orientalist revivals of 'tradition' appear frequently in post-colonial articulations of Indian nationalism as it mediates between a 'real' and imagined India. The trajectory of Coryate's discovery of the fabled India/Indes—following the footsteps of Tamburlaine—to William Jones's Hindu golden age and Kehru's evocations of ancient India *Ram Rajya* is uneven. So is the trajectory from tradition to modernity. The recurring desire for a monolithic definition of India proves elusive, while colonial tropes continue to cast their long shadow on an India in search of its identity.[67]

Although her subject is literature, her words can as easily be applied to the circumstances of fashion. The overlap between real and imagined is one that is becoming harder and harder to situate, as India continues to manufacture and rebrand its identity for inside and outward consumption.

A similar reinvention, or reformulation, of tradition has occurred in African nations, notably in Senegal, for which its textile designs have long been signs of national character and are profitable exports. But as Leslie Rabine explains, the binary of tradition and modernity elides the fact that the region of the Senegal and Gambia Rivers, which flow to the Atlantic and have been trade routes since the tenth century, has witnessed immeasurable amounts of exchange:

> In the production and exchange of Senegalese fashion, 'tradition' signifies rather the layers of an alternative model of historicity and change. For the time of Arabic Islamization beginning in the ninth century, through the tragic encounters with the slave trade, colonialism, neo-colonialism and globalized capital, the Senegalese have continued to build a rich, and uniquely hybrid culture, incorporating and transforming other cultures, including those of migrating African ethnic groups. Influences from elsewhere are not perceived to fill an absence, as in Kikuyu Kenyan and Black American African fashion, but to be threaded into an ongoing cultural project that for centuries has been building even as it is unravelling, tragically, to do so. This history then, with its differently centred global circuits, follows a different logic from a universalizing model of necessary capitalist expansion.[68]

An example of 'knotted' evolution, as she calls it, is the *pagne* or *séru ràb-bal* in Wolof, the native language. It can refer to a basic dress that begins with a rectangle of cloth but also to cloth in general which is adapted onto the body. It can be worn underneath a *boubou*, caftan, *ndoket* or *marinière*. The latter is a shorter version of an *ndoket*, whose French word is *camisole*. A *boubou* is a more imposing version of a caftan and follows the non-Western principle of nontailored construction; a three-metre bolt of cloth with a head opening and sewn to the sides, with the exception of the armholes. The *bou-bou* is a more overt signature of 'tradition', the plain surface for brilliant knot-dying techniques, while the *marinière* is more contemporary and resembles a blouse. Of mixed ancestry, these clothing forms have now become impor-tant cultural mainstays following the social horrors of the 1980s onward. Rabine suggests that tradition in the streets of Dakar is not of the anthropo-logical variety driven by genealogies based on verifying cultural authenticity—something of a Western dream anyway—but one of cultural assertion of dif-ference from the West that nonetheless embraces the country's diverse flux of histories and influences. Fashion was one of Senegal's mainstays in its re-building process around 1990, the most amenable and accessible vector for reinstating an idea of national integrity.[69]

Most Senegalese fashions abroad revolve around the Sotiba print, around which there are different notions of authenticity. Much like the way that con-centric-circle dot design is branded quintessentially Aboriginal, the Sotiba de-signs are unhesitantly named 'authentic African', while on home soil it is called touristic. Unlike many touristic forms, like Aboriginal art tea towels, however, it is not a reductio ad absurdum produced in sweatshops far from their place of origin. Rather, they are produced according to the lines that we say in earlier chapters, for example of China using Indian Tree of Life de-signs or producing *brisé* fans exclusively for Europeans. Sotiba fabrics have an extraordinarily broad market, including most other African states as well as France, Japan and Brazil. With chameleon-like adaptability, the designs change for their clients. The Americans expect masks, drums and cowry shells, while the designs destined for Benin and Togo are bolder and colourful.[70] They are willing to offer out a vision of African-ness while catering to the expectation of the respective markets of what that may look like. With Senegal itself, tailors in Kaolack and Banjul comb Western magazines for inspiration, be it neck-lines or kinds of sleeves, but the outcome is still quintessentially 'African'.[71] Urban Senegalese in particular avail themselves of Western genera such as jeans but during any special occasion will always resort back to the *mbubb* or *grand boubou*.[72]

In many respects, the economies of free adaptation within a recognizable framework are a contemporary transorientalist model for what is outside of the Euro–American sphere. Such economies enact the webs of influence that are natural to the evolution of any country whose borders have changed over centuries. Territories with a history of expansion, contraction and contestation are naturally susceptible to outside expectations, and how these might be moulded for their own gain. And to a singular degree it is the layered and mobile state of being that provides a satisfactory image of postcolonial cultural identity. Here authenticity is organized less along examples and things and more according to an economy of ideas and expectations that are built along continually shifting lines of external expectation and internal self-assertion. In short, clothing and dress can reflect matters of deep political interest in oriental, or formerly deemed oriental, countries.

This is only too evident in China which, after its cultural revolution in 1949, faced with the problem of its national dress. Like all revolutionary transitions that seek to make the impression of a clean break with the past, clothing played a central role positioning Maoist China to the rest of the World, especially the two Cold War powers of Russia and the United States. Mao himself was sure to advertise his renunciation of the standard suit in favour of an austere jacket that suggested a worker's uniform. Antonia Finnane notices that a string of famous travellers like Simone de Beauvoir and Alberto Moravia were all struck by the same thing, namely the austerity of the clothing in China to the extent that it made its population appear androgynous. Even the hair was kept short or was otherwise free of the embellishments that typically differentiate the sexes. The reactions of European visitors from this time range from appreciation to dismissive, according to their political leaning.[73] In stark comparison to the Indian reinvention of itself through dress items like the sari, China all but abolished traditional dress, relegating it to museums and history books. It was as if, in one fell swoop, Mao had effected a swift and brutal de-orientalization.

Such draconian austerity experienced a brief sigh of respite in 1956 when the Party allowed dress to experience 'one hundred flowers blooming'. This pseudofestival allowed for floral dresses and various modified versions of the *keipo*, better known as the *qipao,* the long, body-hugging one-piece dress that, in the 1920s, had become associated with Chinese national dress; the manufactured, tardy equivalent of the Japanese kimono. Known alternatively in the Cantonese as the *cheongsam*, its name comes from *zansae*, which means both long shirt and dress. The qipao was also known as the 'banner gown' after the women who were associated with Manchu banner regiments.[74] The male equivalent is *changshan*, a looser flowing gown that can be worn with a complementary shirt or tunic. The *qipao*'s origins are obscure, although located from the region between Shanghai and Hong Kong, and it is almost certainly a Chinese riposte to the modern postwar dress with its simple fine lines that was coming out of Europe. Its simplicity was also conducive to all

kinds of textile decoration, from old-style, to plain, to made-up, to cloud designs built into the fabric weave. The *qipao* was also suited to East–West
mixes and matches inclined to combinations with bolero jackets[75] and ac-
cessorized with stockings, gloves, hats, purses and Western-style high heels.
Shoes with platforms, heels and other elevating devices occurred long back
in high-class Chinese dress, but the high heels in the Western fashion drew
attention to themselves in shape, material and manner of production. Dorothy
Ko insists that in China at this time 'the West' was far less a specific country or geography and far more a generic, discursive category[76]—much like
the West's erratic grasp of Asia. In the 1920s 'the West' was an especially
desirable category that connoted a progress and liberation in contrast to the
repressive retrogressive practices of China's past. Women at this time were
also inclined to 'French' nail polish and make-up styles that were more Western than Chinese.[77] The side slits of the *qipao* were of particularly Western
inspiration to glamorize the sheer stockings and the shape of the leg created
by high heels.[78]

While it took a little over a decade in the 1920s and 1930s to sow the seeds
of its 'tradition', the *qipao*'s reappearance in Maoist China ended as suddenly
as it appeared and was viewed as an aberration. The party preferred stolid
neutrality. After Mao's death these strictures have become increasingly more
relaxed, especially in present times when China is producing more Western-
style clothing than the West. Encouraged in no small way by the Internet, China's fashions have become as diverse and internationalized, albeit regulated
and tamed, as any industrial country. But the astronomical production and the
rate of growth to other developing nations have seen it jettisoning the need to
assert constructions of nationality.

Although it lived on in neighbouring states such as Taiwan, Singapore and
Hong Kong, where it remains the closest thing to national dress, from a Chinese perspective the *qipao* is now a relic left to movies, usually associated
with Shanghai, 'the Paris of the East', the city with which the garment is now
mythically married. (In 1998 there was even appeared a special collector's
'Qi-Pao Barbie'.[79]) But as Finnane shows, the resurrection of the *qipao* in the
1950s was not because of resonances of the last imperial dynasty but owing
far more to early modern China's repudiation of the Confucian separation of
the sexes. It was a way of bringing women closer to the status of men, its
simplicity of line connoting a more masculine order. The 'Four Modernizations'
after the 1980s that led to the industrial machine we know today, has swept
away many of the inhibitions of the past. This said, some rural parts of China
maintain cottage, home-production of clothes, and much production is destined only for Western consumers, leaving the domestic supply oddly inconsistent with gross production.[80]

The discussion so far highlights the differing ways in which the erstwhile (or still) Orient has reacted to global dress. In the words of Carla Jones and Ann Marie Leshkowich, in their book *Re-Orienting Fashion: The Globalization of Asian Dress*, 'The extent to which Asian dress is reorienting fashion versus re-Orientalizing Asia rests fundamentally on the factors of who is performing, with what intentions, under what circumstances, and before what audience'.[81] It is this multivalence that defines the transorientalist order. The 're-Orientalizing' can be for reasons of economic interest, nostalgia or in the interests of political dissent. In this regard identity and difference are *performed*, a notion that introduces the intentional, theatrical and assertive into the equation. These integers are different notions from the osmotic evolution of fashion and dress over time. The rhetoric of globalization that says that almost anything can be made available to almost anyone almost anywhere builds counter-movements that go to the heart of the early definition of fashion described by Simmel: the paradoxical process of belonging and differentiation, a simultaneous movement that both signals integration into a code and departure from others.

Orientalism in fashion and dress is an indispensible part of this process, but it occurs differently in different countries. When it is used within formerly oriental countries it is predominately for nationalistic purposes, to construct a meaning of people and their belonging to a smooth and palatable continuity with place and history. In the West, orientalism in fashion and dress is used to manifest what is close to the opposite purpose. Transorientalism is the usual–unusual in which exotic fascination is part of the semantic code that no longer needs fascination to be enacted. Unlike orientalist dress, Western dress is not used for nationalist or ideological purposes, since it is seen as normative and global. This has come under some stress with the debates around burqas and hijab.

THE BURQA WARS

When we ask about the West's antipathy to burqas, we have to go somewhere deep into the Christian psyche and to the history of revelation. Islam's idea of revelation has to do with prophets, but never the equivalent of Christ himself. Muhammad was the messenger of God, not his worldly scion. To a degree, burqas reignite this ancient anxiety emphasizing the state of something hidden. The hysteria burqas can spawn reached a somewhat understandable but still irrational pitch after 9/11. Exacerbated by the 'Danish cartoon controversy' of July 2005,[82] burqas and turbans—that is the reduction ad absurdum of Middle Eastern clothing—were marked out as indicators of the terrorist threat by those in the more suspicious and igno-rant circles.

A wider perspective on the particular nature of the today's fraught re-sponse to the burqa may also be located in the evolution of fashions since World War II. The fashions that came out of the 1960s had an unmistakably futuristic edge about them: bright colours, big geometric shapes and shiny synthetic fabrics. Polka dots were legion. Metallic fabrics and jumpsuits paid homage to the possibilities of space travel. The discomforts of plastic were a sacrifice for sleekness. André Courrèges made sci-fi fashion an institution. Out of trauma or out of the accelerations of technological progress, fashion has been dissociative of the past. There are historical registers, but these are part of a signifying stockpile, much as orientalism is the name of a (nebulous) grouping among myriad floating signifiers. Western fashion, when not want-ing to be different, is by degrees akin to a uniform: suits, sneakers, jeans, T-shirts. On the other hand, it is instructive to see how technology has led us into an unconscious love affair with uniforms: airline fashions are most cit-able here.[83] Burqas are therefore jarring to such principles on several levels. They communicate belonging but are not a uniform. Unlike monks' cassocks and the habits of nuns, burqas circulate more widely and the belonging that they spell out is more diverse than monasticism. And rather than be part of a timeless present or an imprecise future, they emphasize continuity with the past. Finally, as was stated already, they are not fashion and are a lot more than just dress.

Banning the burqa has a long history. The mixed response to France's law forbidding its public use that came into effect in April 2011 can be traced back to France's colonial past. During the Algerian war, the French enforced the unveiling of women, received by the native population as an affront tan-tamount to rape. It is because of this moment in its history that the veil now has a special place in Algeria and is a symbol of its identity. Veils and the associated measures of covering the body and the face continue to have an ambivalent status in both East and West. For veiling is not simply a matter of faith; it has to do with the distinctions that Islam is at pains to make with the infidel West. When hijab or burqas are worn in the East, there is still a re-sidual understanding of its irritation to Western mores. To the secular West-erner, one does not normally wear one's religion on one's sleeve. Religion is a private affair about which most people remain respectfully discrete. An ex-ception may be orthodox Jews, but they still wear the Western uniform, the black suit.

The status of what Tarlo calls 'visibly Muslim'[84] becomes a problem, how-ever, when the non-Islamic state expects a certain degree of conformity and assimilation from its citizens. The irony is that it is an expectation in Western democracies that clothing reflect freedom. For this reason, the burqa is perennially the locus where the stark differences between cultural values become apparent. Assimilation usually begins with learning the language. But the ideas of 'shared' and 'common' values are always liable to experience friction with democratic values of tolerance and multiculturalism.

This came to a head in France in June 2008, when its highest administrative court denied citizenship to a Moroccan woman, Faiza Silmi, who had been living on French soil for the last eight years with four children who were all French citizens. Silmi had recently decided to wear the *niqab*, a head-to-toe veil with only a small slit for the eyes. The court ruled that although the defendant had 'a good command of the French language, she has nonetheless adopted a radical practice of her religion incompatible with the essential values of the French community and notably with the principle of equality between the sexes'.[85] It was believed that this was not in violation of the other standard of freedom of religious expression. Robert Paxton cites an argument by the law professor Danièle Lochak who suggests that if this logic is taken to its logical conclusion, it disqualifies all men who engage in domestic violence from French citizenship.[86] Yet at over five million, Muslims are a populous group in French society. Numerically speaking, observers of Islam are second only to Catholics. All countries have Islamic migrants, but France is a special case because its Muslim population is drawn from places with a particularly high incidence of Islamic fundamentalism. This statistic is critical when applied to the high French thresholds of what it means to assimilate.[87]

At this point one cannot resist the temptation to draw a parallel with the sanitary paper masks used by Japanese, Taiwanese and others of East Asia. In fact, the Western indifference to them serves to highlight a thinly veiled hypocrisy: the variance to facial covering is not a matter of security so much as to a creed, and perhaps to gender as well. Non-Muslims do not identify with the protection sought by Muslim women, although by virtue of the paramount discourse of science, they identify with viral contagion, even if they do not see fit to protect themselves in this way. The former threat is internalized as ideological; the latter is biological and therefore supposedly factually neutral.

With different motivations, for almost a century the Turkish government has consistently discouraged women from covering their heads and faces. After the secularist reforms that occurred between 1924 and 1937, a new law came into force in 1982, a more stringent form of 1961, which expressly prohibited the *basörtü*, or headscarf. After a wave of student indignation, where they refused to yield to the new law, it was relaxed in May 1984. The compromise was to shorten the length of the scarf and to permit a turban, a smaller scarf tied at the back of the head. Elisabeth Özdalga explains that this gave rise to series of hair-splitting arguments that amounted to questions about the difference between it meant to tie a scarf at the front or the back, and the thresholds of proper length. In 1987 the restrictions were lifted, but only to resurface in 1996.

The inconsistent compromise that the ban on veiling be lifted from universities but not from public offices only serves to demonstrate the divisions within Turkey and the Islamic community at large. Because it continues to loom on the political horizon, as well as erratic lines between prohibition and permission, women for whom some form of head covering is integral to their identity are left perpetually uncertain as to their capacity to manoeuvre in their careers.[88] In April 2011 the *Wall Street Journal* reported that while sixty per cent of the female population continues to wear scarves, the very few female members of parliament are disallowed from wearing them, since they are holding a government job.[89] Özdalga points out that the secularism issue

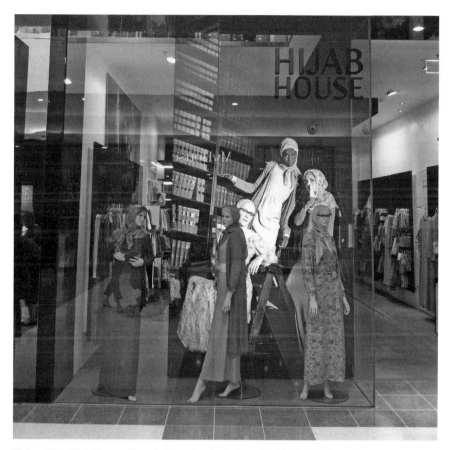

Figure 43   Hijab House. Store in Merrylands, Sydney, April 2011, © Photo Heidi Abraham.

in Turkey is not a matter of friction between two different social systems, which is how it is soften painted. Rather it is one of 'two different ideologies, one coloured by rationalism, the other marked by romanticism'. As is normal with politics, arguments of a sacred nature are used to stir and steer the workings of realpolitik and of political self-interest.[90] More positively, however, greater Islam may learn something from how in Turkey 'Islamic opposition may integrate itself into a modern democratic system'.[91]

Western countries outside of France, such as Britain, the United States and Australia, have in many instances removed references to Islamic dress and rebadged it 'modest' or 'faith-friendly'.[92] As Lewis and Tarlo both stressed, there is a rising interest in 'modest fashion' amongst Muslim women through-out the world and a growing Internet economy. Lewis notices that this practice is not confined to Muslims but also pertains to Jewish and Mormon women whose clothing is central to their faith. The Internet has been integral to the circulation and cultivation of such clothing.[93] More noticeably than ever it is not only a religious attribute but also inhabits the different category of com-prising its own specialized fashion system. For the non-Islamic eye is not at-tuned, and certainly many do not care to be, to the fact that hijab come in many different variants. One has only to visit the Web site of a major outlet like the 'The Hijab Shop' to see this.[94] This site is an easy-access reminder of the diffusion of styles on a single theme. It is lends the lie to the belief that hijab and jilbab are static and uniform, made by men for imprisoning the female form.

The assertion of wearing hijab as a culture with its own integrity, and the private rights that accrue to this has not deterred the media from continually stepping in to encourage the interpretation of covered women as, in Tarlo's words, a sign 'for lack of integration, oppression and threat'.[95] Tarlo appropri-ately observes that accusations in France, and elsewhere, that hijab is a sign of anachronistic oppression and division elicits the counterclaim that uncov-ered women are subject to their share of oppressions, and far more diverse ones at that. Covering the body is way of resisting pressures propagated by the media such as body image, which may lead to low self-esteem and eat-ing disorders.[96] Finally, she draws on Erving Goffman's work on social interac-tion in 1960s America that shows how stigmatized groups such as Jews and blacks accentuated outward signs of their difference—Hassidic Jewish dress or the Afro—and invested them with greater meaning.[97] She also emphasizes the discord between what women wearing hijab wish to convey and how it is interpreted.[98] An historical and maybe more extreme analogy is Chinese foot binding. The Western view of it as the inhumane nadir of female oppression was not necessarily shared by he Chinese women themselves, who took pride in their small feet and which were signs of their gentility, prestige, beauty and femininity.[99]

There appear to be two levels of discord that 'oriental' dress generates in the West. One is driven by misunderstanding, the other by titillation. Although they share the same foundation, as I have tried to argue, they are not account-able to the same opprobrium. When the titillatory is internalized by the Ori-ent itself, 'self-mirroring' risks undermining the capacity for autonomy. Yet, to use words like *autonomy* is to fall into the trap that there is a clear distinction between cultural being and cultural representation, thing-in-itself and thing-in-appearance, a philosophical distinction that fashion shatters. What the study, it is hoped, shows beyond doubt is how the West exists in the East as much as East in the West. They 'live' in one another and their 'own' identity is cre-ated by acts of constant slippage and renewal. Transorientalism is that point at which these renegotiations, paradoxes and misprisions are exposed. It is the moment of exposing the imaginary remainder of the undisclosed. Orien-talism, with its metonym the harem, is the name for what in the West prefers to remain sublimated, a mystery, even if that mystery has an empty centre. In the East, that mystery is itself a very live commodity: to sell to the West and to keep their own imaginations alive about how to reconfigure, on a constant basis, local tradition.

Conclusion: The Revenge of China

Dolce color d'orientale zaffiro [Sweet hue of oriental sapphire].

—Dante Alighieri, *Purgatorio*, Canto I

I began this book with a personal anecdote, and so I will end with one. Around the same time that I was completing the section on hippies, I visited a Ralph Lauren outlet store to buy a smart shirt for my five-year-old son to wear for my next exhibition opening. While browsing, I could not ignore the men's Polo line in navy blue blasted with a white horizontal batik pattern (Figure 44). I didn't give it a second thought, but once I had removed the hat of everyday personal taste and replaced it with that of the theorist and historian, I wryly saw a connection I had been making about contemporary orientalisms. I later returned to the shop and purchased the shirt. It has the unmistakable Polo insignia on the left breast, but ostentatiously enlarged, a style I quite dislike. I wore it all the same, but with ironic good humour, since it articulates everything that I have wanted to express about transorientalism.

Here is a textile style that originated in India and Indonesia and which became one of the heraldic symbols of the alternative, anti-establishmentarians of the Protest Era. It then resurfaces in a garment from a design house that peddles an image of privilege, prim self-satisfaction and private-school education. In receding memory, batik was worn by the Western spiritual sons and daughters of Gandhi and Saibaba, who eschewed meat in the name of cruelty to animals and educated their children on communes so their minds would not be corrupted by a world of corporate rapacity. Now batik is being used by the very symbolic forces that once ridiculed it, and under the brand of one of the most financially successful fashion companies in history, valued in 2007 at over four billion dollars. Almost two centuries ago Britain made the *buta* its own; now, Ralph Lauren has single-handedly transformed the flavour of a Royal Ascot opening day into an American style. This relatively humble shirt is an example of both *absorption* and *inflection*: absorption because the batik design has lost its transgressive connotations and has been brought down to the denominator of conventional clothing; inflection because it temporarily invigorates that convention, although the powerful armature of the Polo shirt remains intact.

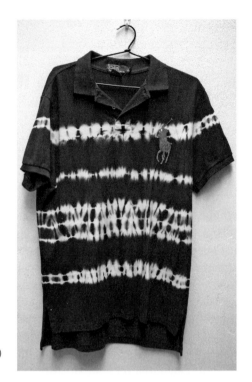

Figure 44   A Ralph Lauren tie-die (print) Polo, 2011. Photo courtesy of the author.

As a final observation, some Ralph Lauren clothes are made in Peru, the Philippines and Taiwan, but this shirt was made in China—even more convenient for what I needed to write about. Since it began its economic reforms in the 1980s, China is now by far the biggest clothing manufacturer in the world. According to China's statistics bureau, in 2007 retail sales in clothing were in excess of 150 billion dollars.[1] Once producers, Europe and America are now consumers, making short-term profits from cheap foreign labour. But more recently this has affected their job market. In the US millions of jobs are at stake. This is an ongoing and, it seems, unresolvable political issue, for it must straddle the attractiveness of the cheaper foreign markets with the long-term goals of domestic sustainability.[2]

There are several ironies emanating from China's dominance that are as unsubtle as the scale of industry is large, one of them being that one of the mainstays of British domestic economic growth in the nineteenth century was clothing and textiles. Another is that orientalist-inspired clothing, subtle or overt, like that of my new favourite shirt, comes from a place that four hundred years ago was considered an oriental crucible. Not only are the zones of influence splayed out of recognition, so are those of production. If there can be said to be a stable centre of authority in fashion, it is perhaps still Paris, but it is an unstable super-ego for the fashion world. Its actual influence on everyday clothing is questionable. From an orientalist perspective, in China brute industry wins over enchantment.

The image of the West is not the same kind of invention as that of the Orient. Whereas the West is more in control of its own image, the Orient has long occupied a *fanciful space of enchantment* in the Western psyche. Since at least the last two centuries it has evolved as very much a Western creation. And from the point of view of fashion, even more so than media such as cinema or television, it is a creation that the East is more than willing to re-absorb. What is startling about contemporary international trends in fashion is the way in which the orientalisms derived from Middle Eastern and Asian sources have come to be accepted by Middle Eastern and Asian contemporary designers, a cultural flip-flop that has incited comment in rising economies such as India.

The high level of visibility and circulation of fashion, clothing and dress make desires and social organizations easier to gauge. With orientalism in fashion and dress, the knotted, multivalent histories of colonizer and colonized that Said speaks about in *Culture and Imperialism* come directly to the fore. As this book has shown in a litany of cases, fashion has been one of the central meeting grounds between East and West, so central in fact that, apart from scholarly articles and museum catalogues, it begs the question as to why this book was not written sooner. But then again, fashion is still struggling with its own marginalization within the academy. This book is more than a history and a synthesis of ideas; it is another forcible demonstration of the importance of fashion to understanding points of meeting. With orientalism this is exceptionally exigent, since the points of meeting entailed trade, struggle, perception and fabrication. It is both a material object and a signifier through which whole societies could redefine themselves by dissembling for resistance or reintegration.

Orientalism, as I have attempted to show, is an essential part of fashion's complex and protean composite, on an astonishing number of levels: from cotton, the textile we take for granted, to silk, the eternal luxury textile; from floral motifs to paisley; from dressing gowns to tie-dye. These coordinates are so diverse and reach into so many areas that they almost make orientalism redundant—except that the idea of the Orient holds it together. The taste for motley otherness is seemingly self-propelled and self-perpetuating. The 'Orient', a hallucination, is called upon by couture to sex-up a garment, or it pretends to inhabit the realm of facts, such as the hysteria behind burqas and hijab. This book has attempted to bring these frameworks around orientalist fashion and dress into perspective. It has sought to acknowledge and to gauge the levels of ethical accountability in the appropriation of orientalist styling, from arbitrary tokenism to out-and-out masquerade. But it has also defended the right of in situ improvisation, of practicality and of aesthetic enthusiasm—we wear a kimono-style dressing gown because it appealed to us in the shop at the time, or we wear a sarong during a beach trip, or we wear a spicy fragrance on our bodies to allure others and for our own delicious self-satisfaction.

The Orient lives on everywhere, including in the Orient itself. This is one of the components of transorientalism, which acknowledges that orientalism operates on a number of cultural levels and for differing purposes. Transorientalism also acknowledges that orientalism is an idea that is as true and factual as it is make believe. As I sit clothed in a T-shirt made in China and write listening to Zeava Ben sing 'What Will Be?' in Hindi to an electronic backbeat on the Claude Challe mix for the *Buddha-Bar* CD series, after earlier listening to Rameau's *Les Indes Galantes*, Mozart's 'Turkish' violin concerto and an aria from Rossini's *The Italian in Algiers*, sipping the green tea I bought at Tokyo Mart in a comfortable Sydney suburb just after a visit to my father nearby, I get reports on my iGoogle page of arrests in France for unlawful wearing of the burqa, and of NATO air strikes causing the death of Qaddafi's youngest son, and later hear the solemnly triumphant voice of America's Hawaiian-born president of Kenyan heritage announce the killing of Osama Bin Laden. But nothing is strange. I am still here. I am busy enjoying the comforts of my own eclectic orient while a large section of the 'real' Orient has no time for such dalliances. They are experiencing, and recreating, their own version.

After quoting the line from Dante reproduced above, Borges adds: 'Dante suggests the colour of the East, the Orient, by a sapphire that includes the Orient in its name. He thus implies a reciprocal play that may well be infinite.'[3] In writing this book, I have been regularly compelled to this as the best definition of orientalism by far. Fashion confirms this, and also gives this conundrum, with its tangled perspectives, sharper contours.

Notes

INTRODUCTION

1. Gérard de Nerval, '*Voyage en Orient*', in Jean Guillaume and Claude Pichois, eds., *Œuvres complètes*, vol. 2 (Paris: Gallimard Pléiade, [1851] 1984), 608.
2. Joanne Eicher, ed., 'Introduction', in *Dress and Ethnicity* (Oxford: Berg, 1995), 1.
3. These include John Sweetman, *The Oriental Obsession: Islamic Inspiration in British and American Art and Architecture, 1500–1920* (Cambridge: Cambridge University Press, 1988); John MacKenzie, *Orientalism: History, Theory and the Arts* (Manchester: Manchester University Press, 1995); and more recently Zeynep Inankur, Reina Lewis and Mary Roberts, eds, *The Poetics and Politics of Place: Ottoman Istanbul and British Orientalism* (Istanbul: Pera Museum, 2011). See also my review of this book, 'Contested Pleasures', *Oxford Art Journal* 34/2 (2011): 295–7.
4. Gayatri Chakravorty Spivak, *Nationalism and the Imagination* (London: Seagull Books, 2010), 44–5.
5. Elizabeth Wilson, *Adorned in Dreams: Fashion and Modernity* (London: Virago, 1985), 117.
6. Richard Berstein, *The East, the West, and Sex: A History of Erotic Encounters* (New York: Knopf, 2009); Ronald Hayms, *Empire and Sexuality* (Manchester: Manchester University Press, 1990).
7. Théophile Gautier, *Histoire du romantisme* (Paris: Les Introuvables, 1993), 79; see also Mary Gluck, *Popular Bohemia: Modernism and Urban Culture in Nineteenth-century Paris* (Cambridge, MA: Harvard University Press, 2005), 26–32.
8. Ann Marie Leshkowich and Carla Jones, 'What Happens When Asian Chic Becomes Asian Chic in Asia?', in Nirmal Puwar and Nandi Bhatia, eds., *Fashion Theory: Orientalism and Fashion* 7/3–4 (Special Double Issue on Fashion and Orientalism, 2003), 281–99.
9. Bernard Smith, *European Vision and the South Pacific*, 2nd edn. (Sydney: Harper and Row, 1984), ix–x; see also Rex Butler, 'Australian Art History and Revisionism', in *A Secret History of Australian Art* (Sydney: Craftsman House, 2002), 101–2.
10. Reina Lewis, *Rethinking Orientalism: Women Travel and the Ottoman Harem* (London: I. B. Tauris, 2004), 213; Gail Ching-Liang Low, *White Skins/Black Masks: Representation and Colonialism* (London, Routledge, 1996).

11. This topology was reached independently of that formed by Joanna Entwistle in her chapter 'Exotic Impulses in Techniques of Fashion', which is worth quoting:

> In this chapter, three forms of exoticism are considered. First, certain techniques of dress and decoration in non-western cultures (for example, the customs associated with the sari in India or veil in some Islamic cultures; body decoration in Africa or Oceania). Second, adaptions of traditional dress combined with elements from western fashion systems in post-colonial cultures and displaced cultures in western societies (for example adaptions of the sari and the veil). And third, 'exotic' elements in western fashion borrowed and adapted from other fashion systems (for example 'Indian' influences in the 'hippie' look; the toga and use of draped fabric more generally; 'peasant' motifs in high fashion).

    Joanna Entwistle, *The Fashioned Body* (Cambridge: Polity, 2000), 18. These are schemata that complement mine and from which I inevitably draw.
12. James Stevens Curl, *Egyptomania: The Egyptian Revival: A Recurring Theme in the History of Taste* (Manchester: Manchester University Press, 1994), 113.
13. Jennifer Craik, *The Face of Fashion: Cultural Studies and Fashion* (London: Routledge, 1994), 17.
14. Craik, *The Face of Fashion,* 17–43.
15. Entwistle, *The Fashioned Body*, 42.
16. H. Hoodfar, 'Return of the Veil: Personal Strategy and Public Participation in Egypt', in N. Radcliffe and M.T. Sinclair, eds., *Working Women* (London: Routledge, 1991), cit. Entwistle, *The Fashioned Body,* 75.
17. J.C. Flügel, *The Psychology of Clothes* (London: Hogarth, 1930).

CHAPTER 1: EARLY ORIENTALISM AND THE BARBARESQUE

1. Entwistle, *The Fashioned Body* 105.
2. See also Valerie Steele, *Paris Fashion: A Cultural History*, 2nd edn (Oxford: Berg, 1998), 19.
3. Nerval, 'Les Nuits de Ramazan', in *Voyage en Orient*, 632.
4. Hugh Honour, *Chinoiserie* (London: John Murray, 1961), 36.
5. Antonia Finnane, *Changing Clothes in China* (Sydney: University of New South Wales Press), 9.

6. Julian Raby, 'The Serenissima and the Sublime Porte: Art in the Art of Diplomacy, 1453–1600', in Stefano Carboni, ed., *Venice and the Islamic World*, exhibition catalogue (New York: Metropolitan Museum of Art, 2007).
7. See Sweetman, *The Oriental Obsession*, 11.
8. Sweetman, *The Oriental Obsession,* 5.
9. Niels Steensgaard, *The Asian Trade Revolution of the Seventeenth Century* (Chicago: University of Chicago Press, 1973), 160–2.
10. Edmund Herzig, 'The Iranian Raw Silk Route and European Manufacture', in Maureen Fennel Marouzi, ed., *Textiles: Production, Trade and Demand* (Aldershot: Ashgate, 1998), 73–89.
11. Walter Denny, 'Oriental Carpets and Textiles in Venice', in Stefano Carboni, ed., *Venice in the Islamic World,* exhibition catalogue (New York: Metropolitan Museum of Modern Art, 2007), 189–90.
12. Carlo Poni, 'Fashion as Flexible Production: The Strategies of the Lyons Silk Merchants in the Eighteenth Century', in C. F. Sabel and J. Zeitlin, eds, *World of Possibilities: Flexibility and Mass Production in Western Industrialisation* (Cambridge: Cambridge University Press, 1997), cit. Luca Molà, *The Silk Industry of Renaissance Venice* (Baltimore and London: Johns Hopkins University Press, 2000), 303.
13. Raby, 'The Serenissima and the Sublime Porte', 113. Raby quotes the sixteenth-century French ambassador to Turkey de Busbecq-Forster-Daniell: 'No nation in the world has shown greater readiness than the Turks to avail themselves of the useful inventions of foreigners, as is proved by their employments of cannons and mortars, and many other things invented by the Christians.'
14. Molà, *The Silk Industry of Renaissance Venice*, 303–4.
15. See also Mildred Davison, 'Printed Cotton Textiles', *The Art Institute of Chicago Quarterly* 52/4 (1 Dec. 1958), 83.
16. Giorgio Riello and Tirthankar Roy, 'Introduction', in Giorgio Riello and Tirthankar Roy, eds, *How India Clothed the World* (Leiden: Brill, 2009), 9.
17. K. N. Chaudhuri, 'Trade as a Cultural Phenomenon', in Jens Christian Johansen et al., eds, *Clashes of Cultures: Essays in Honour of Niels Steensgaard* (Odense: Odense University Press, 1992), 210. See also Beverly Lemire, 'Fashioning Global Trade', in Rielleo and Roy, eds, *How India Clothed the World*, 365–6.
18. Alice Beer, *Trade Goods: A Study of Indian Chintz* (Washington, DC: Smithsonian Institution Press, 1970), 31, 34.
19. See also Davison, 'Printed Cotton Textiles', 84, 87.
20. Joyce Appleby, *Economic Thought and Ideology in Seventeenth-century England* (Princeton, NJ: Princeton University Press, 1978), 166.

21. John Pollexfen, *A discourse of trade, coyne, and paper credit* (1697), 99, cit. Appleby, *Economic Thought and Ideology*, 167.

22. Appleby, *Economic Thought and Ideology*, 167. See also 197–8.

23. Jyotsna Singh, 'Introduction', *Colonial Narratives, Cultural Dialogues: 'Discoveries' of India and the Language of Colonialism* (London: Routledge, 1996), 3.

24. During the period 1827–1833 East India cotton exported 2,835,500 yards to England's 6,915,577 yards, whereas between 1841–50 East India exported 4,776,590 to England's 107,675,091. Joseph Inikori, 'English Versus Indian Cotton Textiles', in Riello and Roy, eds, *How India Clothed the World*, 106 and passim.

25. H. V. Bowen, 'British Exports of Raw Cotton from India to China', in Riello and Roy, eds, *How India Clothed the World*, passim.

26. Dawn Jacobson, *Chinoiserie* (London: Phaidon, 1993), 54.

27. Honour, *Chinoiserie*, 50.

28. See also Sweetman, *The Oriental Obsession*, 48; Edith Standen, 'English Tapestries "After the Indian Manner" ', *Metropolitan Museum Journal* 15 (1980), 119–42.

29. John Evelyn, *Diary*, ed. E. S. Beer (London: Oxford University Press, 1959), 464–5.

30. Samuel Pepys, *Diary*, cit. Esmond de Beer, 'Charles II's Own Fashion: An Episode in Anglo–French Relations, 1666–1670', *Journal of the Warburg Institute* 2/2 (Oct. 1938), 105.

31. Pepys, cit. de Beer, 'Charles II's Own Fashion', 107.

32. Chamberlayne, *Angliae Notitia*, 25–6, cit. de Beer, 'Charles II's Own Fashion', 108.

33. De Beer, 'Charles II's Own Fashion', 108.

34. See Diana de Marly (1974), 'King Charles II's Own Fashion: The Theatrical Origins of the English Vest', *Journal of the Warburg and Courtauld Institutes* 37 (1974), 380.

35. Cit. Honour, *Chinoiserie*, 79.

36. Thomas Dallam, cit. Gerald MacLean, *The Rise of Oriental Travel* (Basingstoke: Palgrave Macmillan, 2004), 39–40.

37. Evelyn, *Diary*, 464–5.

38. Evelyn, *Diary*. See also Honour, *Chinoiserie*, 79.

39. De Beer, 'Charles II's Own Fashion', 114.

40. Ina Baghdiantz McCabe, *Orientalism in Early Modern France: Eurasian Trade, Exoticism, and the Ancien Régime* (Oxford: Berg, 2008), 254.

41. Madeleine Jarry, *Chinoiserie* (New York: Vendome Press, 1981), 40.

42. Michael Curtis, *Orientalism and Islam* (Cambridge: Cambridge University Press, 2009), passim.

43. Curtis, *Orientalism and Islam*.

44. Nicholas Dew, *Orientalism in Louis XIV's France* (Oxford: Oxford University Press, 2009), 4 and passim.

45. Andrea Stuart, 'Court Masques', in Christopher Breward and Caroline Evans, eds, *Fashion and Modernity* (Oxford: Berg, 2005), 88–91.

46. Françoise Boucher, *A History of Costume in the West* (London: Thames and Hudson, [enlarged edition] 1996), 285.

47. Norbert Elias, *La societé de cour* (Flammarion, 1985), p. 158ff.

48. McCabe, *Orientalism in Early Modern France*, 5–6.

49. Cit. Ian Dunlop, *Louis XIV* (London: Pimlico, 2001), 130.

50. Honour, *Chinoiserie*, 62–3. See also Jacobson, *Chinoiserie*, 31.

51. Joan DeJean, *The Essence of Style: How the French Invented High Fashion, Fine Food, Chic Cafés, Style, Sophistication, and Glamour* (New York: Free Press, 2005), 243.

CHAPTER 2: 1690–1815

1. Denis Diderot, *Oeuvres Complètes*, vol 4 (Paris, Garnier Fréres, 1875), 205.

2. Louis Antoine Fauvelet de Bourienne, *Mémoires*, vols. 1–2 (10 vols., Paris, 1831), 292, cit. Paul Strathern, *Napoleon in Egypt* (London: Vintage, 2007), 182.

3. Kate Berridge, *Waxing Mythical: The Life and Legend of Madame Tussaud* (London: John Murray, 2006), 37.

4. See also Caroline Weber:

In October 1773, Rose Bertin, an unmarried twenty-four year old woman from Picardy, defied this law [*merchandes des modes*, the guild that only allowed the all-male mercer's guild and their wives to practice tailoring] by setting up shop as a *marchande des modes* on the rue Saint-Honoré. Exotically named the Grand Mogol, in reference to a putatively luxury-loving grandee, her boutique boasted large windows filled with displays that were designed to divert foot traffic from the Palais Royal. With their artistic arrangements of bonnets, shawls, fans, spangles, furbelows, silk flowers, gemstones, laces and other accessories, the displays set up a bewitching siren's song. Once lured inside, ushered through the door by a liveried footman, potential customers found themselves in a setting as luxurious as an aristocrat's salon: gilded mouldings adorned the ceilings, full-length mirrors and fine oil paintings hung on the walls, and expensive furniture was scattered about among the piles of damasks, silks, brocades, and baubles that announced the place's true purpose. This purpose, indeed, would

have been hard to overlook, for, along with its piles of fabrics and ornaments, the Grand Mogol boasted indoor fashion displays of complete,
one-of-a-kind ensembles, covered from neck to hemline in luscious
frippery.

Queen of Fashion: What Marie Antoinette Wore to the Revolution (New
York: Henry Holt, 2006), 103.
5. Champfort, *Maximes et pensées; Caractères et anecdotes* (Paris: Gallimard, 1795, 1965), 86.
6. Erin Mackie, *Market à la Mode. Fashion, Commodity and Gender* (Baltimore: John Hopkins University Press, 1997), 40–1.
7. Adam Nicholson, *Men of Honour. Trafalgar and the Making of the English
Hero* (London: Harper, 2005), 105.
8. Beverly Lemire, *Dress, Culture and Commerce: The English Clothing Trade
Before the Factory 1660–1800* (London: Macmillan, 1997), 34–8. See
also K.N. Chaudhuri, *The Trading World of Asia and the East India Company 1660–1760* (New York: Cambridge University Press, 1978).
9. Daniel Defoe, cit. Christopher Breward, *The Culture of Fashion* (Manchester: Manchester University Press, 1995), 125–6.
10. Denny, 'Oriental Carpets and Textiles in Venice', 190.
11. Elizabeth Wilson, *Adorned in Dreams* (London: Virago, 1985), 68.
12. As S. Arasaratham explains,

> There is evidence of this happening not infrequently in the seventeenth
> and eighteenth centuries. Their extended kinship ties over a number of
> villages enabled them to take refuge in other villages for long periods.
> They appear to have been capable of collective action . . . From the
> 1760s such migratory movements, away from the reaches of power,
> were happening in response to the changes introduced by the English.

'The Handloom Industry in Southeastern India 1750–1790', in Mazzaoui,
ed., *Textiles: Production, Trade and Demand*, 192.
13. For a good concise account see Pamela Ulrich, 'Fustian to Merino: The
Rise of Textiles Using Cotton before and after the Gin', *Agricultural History* 68/2; 'Eli Whitney's Cotton Gin, 1793–1993: A Symposium' (Spring,
1994), 219–31.
14. Natalie Rothstein, 'The Elegant Art of Woven Silk', ed. Edward Maeder, *An
Elegenat Art*, exhibition catalogue (Los Angeles: Los Angeles Museum of
Art and Abrams Publishers, 1983), 79.
15. Louis-Sébastien Mercier (1781–9), *Tableau de Paris*, ed. Jean-Claude
Bonnet (Paris: Mercure de France, 1994), v.2, 125.
16. Diderot, *Oeuvres Complètes*, 6.

17. Jennifer Jones, 'Repackaging Rousseau: Femininity and Fashion in Old Regime France', *French Historical Studies* 18/4 (Autumn 1994), 944.
18. McCabe, *Orientalism in Early Modern France*, 254.
19. See also De Jean, *The Essence of Style*, 238, and McCabe, *Orientalism in Early Modern France,* 249.
20. Beverly Lemire, 'Fashioning Global Trade', in Riello and Roy eds., *How India Clothed the World*, 373.
21. Lemire, 'Fashioning Global Trade', 375.
22. See McCabe, *Orientalism in Early Modern France,* 252:

> A fan also commemorates the event. At one ball given by Monsieur, the Princess Adelaide was dressed as a sultana and Jean Bérain had designed a Chinese buffet. The Ponchartins gave a ball for the Princess Adelaide in a room *ornée à la chinoise* with the 'Rulers of the Orient' as a theme. It is possibly such an event that a fan held at Greenwich Museum commemorates. The fan displays a number of items of lacquered furniture, porcelains, silks, and Indian cottons, all items brought back by the *Amphirite*. The fan illustrates a man dressed as a Persian displaying cottons, and a lady dressed *à la Turque* buying a Chinese fan. Chinese men have black lacquer boxes spread before them. Two men who look Indian carry exotic goods; one has a large porcelain vase on his head and the other is draped in a cotton cloth.

23. Cit. in Carol Dorrington-Ward ed., *Fans from the East* (New York: Viking, 1978), 47.
24. Bruno Kisch, 'Europerien auf China-Porzellan', *Artibus Asiae* 6/3–4 (1937), 272–82.
25. A. Hyatt Mayor, 'Chinoiserie', *The Metropolitan Museum of Art Bulletin* 36/5 (May 1941), 113.
26. Honour, *Chinoiserie*, 85: 'Porcelain vases were either mounted in gilt metal or arranged *en masse* in a very un-Chinese fashion; lacquer cabinets were placed on great gilded stands bulging with putti and swags of fruit.'
27. See also Mildred Davison, 'A "Vernis-Martin" Fan', *Bulletin of the Art Institute of Chicago (1907–1951)* 24/4 (Apr. 1930), 50–51.
28. See Katie Scott, 'Playing Games with Otherness: Watteau's Chinese Cabinet at the Château de la Muette', *Journal of the Warburg and Courtauld Institutes* 66 (2003), 189–248.
29. See also Maria Gordon-Smith, 'The Influence of Jean Pillement on French and English Decorative Arts Part One', *Artibus et Historiae* 21/41 (2000), 171–96.
30. Dawn Jacobson, *Chinoiserie* (London: Phaidon, 1993), 75.

31. See also Sweetman, *The Oriental Obsession*, 32.
32. Terry Castle, *Masquerade and Civilization: The Carnavalesque in Eighteenth-century English Culture and Fiction* (London: Methuen, 1986), 82, 107.
33. Champfort, *Maximes et pensées,* 140.
34. See Terry Castle, 'Eros and Liberty at the English Masquerade, 1710–90', *Eighteenth-Century Studies* 17/2 (Winter 1983–1984), 156–76.
35. Cit. Philippa Scott, *Turkish Delights* (London: Thames and Hudson, 2001), 89.
36. See also Diana De Marly, 'King Charles II's Own Fashion: The Theatrical Origins of the English Vest', 381.
37. Mary Obelkevich, 'Turkish Affect in the Land of the Sun King', *The Musical Quarterly* 63/3 (Jul. 1977), 368.
38. Matthew Head, *Orientalism, Masquerade and Mozart's Turkish Music* (London: Royal Music Association, 2000), 27.
39. Head, *Orientalism, Masquerade and Mozart's Turkish Music,* 90–1.
40. Benjamin Perl, 'Mozart in Turkey', *Cambridge Opera Journal* 12/3 (2000), 227.
41. Head, *Orientalism, Masquerade and Mozart's Turkish Music,* 95–6.
42. *Receuil de Cent Estampes représentent différentes Nations du Levant tirées sur les tableaux peints d'après Nature en 1707 et 1708 par les orders de M. de Ferriol, Ambassade du Roi à la porte et gravés en 1712 et 1713 par les soins de Mr le Hay.* See Aileen Ribeiro, *The Dress Worn at Masquerades in England, 1730 to 1790, and its Relation to Fancy Dress in Portraiture* (New York: Garland Publishing, 1984), 217.
43. Fatma Müge Göçek, *East Encounters West. France and the Ottoman Empire in the Eighteenth Century* (Oxford: Oxford University Press, 1987), 25–38.
44. See Perrin Stein, 'Amédée Van Loo's *Costume turc*: The French Sultana', *The Art Bulletin* 78/3 (Sep. 1996), 417–38.
45. Ribeiro, *The Dress Worn at Masquerades in England,* 222.
46. Castle, *Masquerade and Civilisation*, 60–2.
47. Castle, *Masquerade and Civilisation,* 57–8.
48. Mary Wortley Montagu, *Complete Letters*, v. 1, 1708–1720, ed. Robert Halsband (Oxford: Oxford University Press, 1965), 326–7.
49. Montagu, *Complete Letters,* 328.
50. Srinivas Aravamudan, 'Lady Mary Wortley Montagu in the Hammam: Masquerade, Womanliness, and Levantinization', *ELH* 62/1 (1995), 80.
51. See Aileen Ribeiro, ' "The Whole Art of Dress": Costume in the Work of John Singleton Copley', in Carrie Rebora et al. eds., *John Singleton Copley* (New York: Metroolitan Museum of Art, 1995), 107.
52. Isobel Grundy, ' "The Barbarious Character We Give Them": White Women Travellers Report on Other Races', *Studies in Eighteenth Century Culture* 2

(1992), 73–86; Cynthia Lowenthal, 'The Veil of Romance: Lady Mary's Embassy Letters', *Eighteenth Century Life* 14 (1990), 66–82; Elizabeth Bohls, *Women Travel Writers and the Language of Aesthetics 1716–1818* (Cambridge: Cambridge University Press, 1995); see also Katherine Turner, 'From Classical to Imperial: Changing Visions of Turkey in the Eighteenth Century', in Steve Turner ed., *Travel Writing and Empire: Post-colonial Theory in Transit* (London: Zed Books, 1999), 113–28.

53. Aravamudan, 'Lady Mary Wortley Montagu in the Hammam', 93. Gill Perry, 'Women in Disguise: Joshua Reynolds', in Gill Perry and Michael Rossington eds., *Feminity and Masculinity in Eighteenth-Century Art and Culture* (Manchester: Manchester University Press, 1994), passim.

54. See also Jacobson, *Chinoiserie*, 94, 110.

55. Paul Poiret, *En habillant l'époque* (Paris: Grasset, 1930), 110.

56. See also Wendy Frith:

> Montagu's experience in Turkey, albeit mediated by her class, culture and gender, provided a means whereby she could begin to articulate a critique of, and a resistance to, the prevailing attitudes towards women in West, as well as to the West's self-glorification, dependent as it was upon the representation of the East as backward and unenlightened.

'Sex Smallpox and Seraglios', in Perry and Rossington, *Feminity and Masculinity in Eighteenth-Century Art and Culture*.

57. Morag Martin, *Selling Beauty: Cosmetics, Commerce and French Society, 1750–1830* (Baltimore: Johns Hopkins Press, 2009), 142–5.

58. As he wrote in *Emile*: 'Give to a young girl of taste who despises la mode some ribbons, some gauze, some muslin, and some flowers; without diamonds, pompons or lace she will make herself an outfit which will make her a hundred times more charming than all the brilliant rags of Duchapt [a celebrated hatmaker].' Cit. Jennifer Jones, 'Repackaging Rousseau', 945.

59. Clare Cage, 'The Sartorial Self: Neoclassical Fashion and Gender Identity in France, 1797–1804', *Eighteenth-Century Studies* 42/2 (2009), 197.

60. Mercier, 'Salon de peinture', *Tableaux de Paris* 1, 1236: 'Que le peintre s'abstienne donc désormais de peinde des perruques poudrées et des robes noires. L'habillement des Hottentots serait cente fois moins étranger au pinceau, et ne le repousserait pas d'une manière aussi dure, aussi discordante.'

61. McCabe, *Orientalism in Early Modern France,* 272.

62. See also McCabe, *Orientalism in Early Modern France,* 6.

63. Daniel Roche, *The Culture of Clothing: Dress and Fashion in the 'Ancien Régime'*, trans. Jean Birrell (Cambridge: Cambridge University Press, 1994), 140.
64. Roche, *The Culture of Clothing,* 149.
65. Berridge, *Waxing Mythical,* 170–1.
66. Richard Holmes, 'The Great de Staël', *New York Review of Books*, 28 May 2009, 14.
67. See also Steele, *Paris Fashion,* 59–60.
68. Richard Sennett, *The Fall of Public Man* (Cambridge: Cambridge University Press, 1977), 67–9. See also Entwistle, *The Fashioned Body,* 102.
69. Steele, *Paris Fashion,* 39.
70. Cit. Berridge, *Waxing Mythical,* 171.
71. Ernest John Knapton, *Empress Josephine* (Cambridge, MA: Harvard University Press, 1963), 32.
72. Aileen Ribeiro, *Ingres in Fashion* (New Haven, CT: Yale University Press, 1999), passim and 86, 100, 104, 188–92. Some of the paintings in question include *Alix-Geneviève de Seytres-Caumont, Comtesse de Tournon*, 1812 (Philadelphia Museum of Art); *Marie Marcoz, Vicomtesse de Senommes*, 1816 (Musée des beaux-Arts, Nantes).
73. Jean Alazard, *Ingres et ingrisme* (Paris, 1950), 30, cit. Ribeiro, *The Dress Worn at Masquerades in England,* 98.
74. Cit. Berridge, *Waxing Mythical,* 174.
75. Maya Jasanoff, *Edge of Empire: Conquest and Collecting in the East, 1750–1850* (London: Harper, 2006), 278 and passim.
76. See also Charlotte Jirousek, 'More than Oriental Splendour: European and Ottoman Headgear, 1380–1580', *Dress, the Annual Journal of the Costume Society of America* 21 (1995); Jirousek, 'Ottoman Influences in Western Dress' (2004), 244–7, Suraiya Faroqhi and Christopher Newmann eds., *Ottoman Costumes: From Textile to Identity* (Istanbul: Eren), 244–7.
77. See also Susannah Worth and Lucy Sibley, 'Maja Dress and the Andalusian Image of Spain', *Clothing and Textiles Research Journal* 12 (1994), 51–60.
78. Worth and Sibley, 'Maja Dress and the Andalusian Image of Spain'.
79. Judith Lopez and Jane Farrell-Beck, 'What Colored the Transition from Madder to Alizarine?', *Clothing and Textiles Research Journal* 10 (1992), 37.
80. Honoré de Balzac, *Les Chouans* (Paris: Livre de Poche, 1845, 1997), 279: 'elle avait jeté, dans un des cartons, un elegant poignard, jadis porté par une sultane et dont elle voulut se munir en venant sur le theatre de la guerre, comme ces plaisants qui s'approvisionnent d'albums pour les idées qu'ils auront en voyage; mais elle fut alors moins séduite par la perspective d'avoir du sang à répandre, que par le plaisir de porter

un joli *cangiar* orné de pierreries, et de jouer avec cette lame pure comme un regard.'

CHAPTER 3: 1815–1871

1. Jorge Luis Borges, 'Translators of *The Thousand and One Nights*', in Esther Allen et al., trans., Eliot Weinberger, ed. *Selected Non-Fictions* (New York: Penguin, [1934–6] 1999), 94.
2. Richard Martin and Harold Koda, *Orientalism: Visions of the East in Western Dress*, Museum of Modern Art exhibition catalogue (New York: Abrams, 1994), 46.
3. There was also Barthélemy d'Herbelot's *Bibliothèque Orientale* of 1697. In Sweetman's words,

   with a preface by Galland [it constituted] a rich alphabetically arranged conspectus of Eastern cultures . . . including entries on Islamic cities, customs, costume and history, though with little on art and architecture and no illustrations or examples.

   The Oriental Obsession, 46.
4. John Beer, 'Fragments and Ironies', in John Beer, ed., *Questioning Romanticism* (Baltimore: Johns Hopkins University Press, 1995), 262.
5. See Marylin Butler, 'Orientalism', in David B. Pirie, ed., *The Romantic Period* (Harmondsworth: Penguin, 1994), 426.
6. Cit. Nicholas Drew, *Orientalism in Louis XIV's France* (Oxford: Oxford University Press, 2009), 3.
7. Roger Benjamin, *Orientalist Aesthetics: Art, Colonialism and French North Africa, 1880–1930* (Berkeley: California University Press, 2003), 58.
8. Sally Price, *Primitive Art in Civilized Places* (Chicago: University of Chicago Press, 1989), 46–7.
9. Sennett, *The Fall of Public Man,* passim.
10. Entwistle, *The Fashioned Body*, 121.
11. Walter Benjamin, *Charles Baudelaire: A Lyric Poet in the Era of High Capitalism*, Harry Zohn, trans. (London: Verso, 1983), 34. See also Mary Gluck, *Popular Bohemia*, 8; Mark Gluck, 'Dressing Up: Bohemia, Commerce and the Creation of the Artist's Life', in Adam Geczy and Vicki Karaminas, eds., *Fashion and Art* (Oxford: Berg, 2012).
12. I use the word *overtly* here to distinguish from more mainstream uses of orientalist styles and of luxury fabrics such as cottons and silks, and particularly cashmere, which will be discussed later in this chapter.

13. Mayor, 'Chinoiserie', 111.
14. Charles Lamb, 'Old China', *The Collected Essays of Charles Lamb in Two Volumes*, vol. 1 (London: J. M. Dent and Sons, [1823] 1929), 287.
15. Elizabeth Wilson, *Bohemians: Glamorous Outcasts* (London: I. B. Tauris, 2000), passim. See also Sandra Barwick, 'Bohemia, True and Blue', *A Century of Style* (London: Allen and Unwin, 1984), passim.
16. Mary Gluck, 'The Primitive Artist', *Popular Bohemia*, 187. With regard to 'ironic' bohemia, on page 15 she states:

> The second, less familiar, version, I have called "ironic bohemia", since it is concerned with the parodic gestures and ironic public performances of experimental artists and aimed to differentiate the artist of modernity from his middle-class counterparts.

17. Mary Gluck, *Popular Bohemia,* 28.
18. See also Rula Razek, *Dress Codes: Reading Nineteenth Century Fashion* (Stanford, CA: Stanford Honors Essay in Humanities, no. 43, 1999), 21–38.
19. Jerome K. Jerome, *Three Men in a Boat* (Harmondsworth: Penguin, [1889] 1957), 60.
20. Gautier, cit. Joanna Richardson, *Théophile Gautier: His Life and Times* (London: Max Reinhardt, 1958), 51.
21. Cit. Richardson, *Théophile Gautier: His Life and Times,* 76.
22. Ernest Hébert, cit. Richardson, *Théophile Gautier: His Life and Times,* 273.
23. Théophile Gautier, *Baudelaire*, Claude-Marie Senninger and Lois Cassandra Hamrick, eds (Paris: Klincksieck, [1867] 1986), 115, 146.
24. See also Penelope Byrde, *Nineteenth Century Fashion* (London: B. T. Batsford Ltd, 1992), 103.
25. Eugène Fromentin, *Une année dans le Sahel* (Paris: Plon, 1877), 144–5:

> Coiffé de foulards noirs et bleus, et peut-être un peu moins déshabillé que ne l'est une femme mauresque dans son intérieur, ele portait un corset de drap bleu richement doré sous un cafetan bleu sans manche, et contre l'usage du pays, une sorte de ceinturon d'or à fermoir massif retenait autour de sa taille un peu grêle un *fouta* très ample de couleur écarlate. Son costume, ainsi composé de trois couleurs, mais où le rouge ardent écrasait tout, exagérait encore, par ce contact extrêmement vif, la pâleur morne de sap eau. Elle avait les yeux bordés d'antimoine, les mains enluminées de *henné*, les pieds aussi; ses talons, rougis par la teinture, << ressemblaient à deux organges >>.

26. Fromentin, *Une année dans le Sahel*, 85.

27. Fromentin, *Une année dans le Sahel*, 161–2.

28. For what is perhaps the best account of French orientalist painting in the nineteenth century, see R. Benjamin, *Orientalist Aesthetics: Art, Colonialism and French North Africa, 1880–1930*.

29. Delacroix, cit. Tom Prideaux, *The World of Delacroix, 1798–1863* (Netherlands: Time-Life International, 1966), 107.

30. Eugène Delacroix, 'Souvenirs d'un voyage dans le Maroc', *Journal,* vol. 1: 1822–1857 (Paris: José Corti, 2009), 276.

31. Ibid., 277.

32. Cit. Graham Robb, *Rimbaud* (New York: Norton, 2000), 327–8.

33. Nerval, *Voyage en Orient*, 587:

> << Vous venez bien me voir en habit noir! . . . >> me dit-il.
>
> La replique était juste; pourtant je sentais bien que j'avais eu raison. Quoi que l'on fasse, et si loin que l'on puisse aller dans la bienveillance d'un Turc, il ne faut pas croire qu'il puisse y avoir tout de suite fusion entre notre façon de vivre et la sienne. Les coutumes européennes qu'il adopte dans certains cas deviennent une sorte de terrain neutre où il nous accueille sans se livrer lui-même; il consent à imiter nos mœurs comme il use de notre langue, mais à l'égard de nous seulement. Il ressemble à ce personage de ballet qui est moitié paysan et moitié signeur; Il montre à l'Europe le côté *gentleman*, il est toujours un pur *Osmanli* pour l'Asie.
>
> Les préjugés des populations font ailleurs de cette politique une nécessité.

34. Richard Berrong, *In Love with a Handsome Sailor: The Emergence of Gay Identity in the Novels of Pierre Loti* (Toronto: University of Toronto Press, 2003), passim.

35. Hélène de Burgh, *Sex, Sailors and Colonies: Narratives of Ambiguity in the Works of Pierre Loti* (Bern: Peter Lang, 2005), passim.

36. Caroline Karpinski, 'Kashmir to Paisley', *The Metropolitan Museum of Art Bulletin*, New Series 22/3 (1963), 116–20.

37. Bessie Bennett, 'The Shawl: A Costume Accessory', *Bulletin of the Art Institute of Chicago* 29/4 (1907–1951), 48–9.

38. Chitralekha Zutshi, ' "Designed for Eternity": Kasmiri Shawls, Empire, and Cultures of Production and Consumption in Mid-Victorian Britain', *Journal of British Studies* 48 (2009), 422–3. See also Elizabeth Mikosch, 'The Scent of Flowers: Kashmiri Shawls in the Collection of the Textile Museum', *Textile Museum Journal* 24 (1985), 12.

39. Penelope Byrde, *Nineteenth Century Fashion*, 29.

40. Rudolph Ackermann, *The Repository of Arts, Literature, Commerce, Manufactures, Fashions and Politics*, 397, cit. Byrde, *Nineteenth Century Fashion*, 29.

41. Zutshi, "Designed for Eternity", 425.

42. Zutshi, "Designed for Eternity", 429.

43. See also Robert Penn Cuff, 'The Permanent Values of Thackeray's *Vanity Fair'*, *Peabody Journal of Education* 27/2 (1949), 95–6.

44. Walter Benjamin, *The Arcades Project*, Howard Eiland and Kevin McLaughlin, trans. (Cambridge, MA: Belknap Press, 1999), 55. See also Susan Hiner, ' "Cashmere Fever": Virtue and the Domestication of the Exotic', *Accessories to Modernity: Fashion and the Feminine in Nineteenth-century France*, Philadelphia: University of Pennsylvania Press, 77–106.

45. Ibid.

46. Hiner, *Accessories to Modernity,*86.

47. Hiner, *Accessories to Modernity*, 79–80 and passim.

48. Hiner, *Accessories to Modernity*, 98.

49. See Ribeiro, *Ingres in Fashion*, 188, 247.

50. Hiner, *Accessories to Modernity*, 99.

51. Christa Thurman and Jessica Batty, 'Long Shawl', *Art Institute of Chicago Museum Studies* 29/2 (2003), 28:

> Shawls were first woven in France in 1804; ultimately the French became the best producers of shawls by utilizing the Jacquard attachment, introduced by Joseph Marie Jacquard in the first decade of the nineteenth century, but not widely accepted by the shawl industry until the late 1820s. When mounted onto a loom, the Jacquard attachment eliminated the need for one of the weaver's assistants, the drawboy who sat atop the loom and helped create complex patterns by raising selected warp threads. Jacquard's patent used punched cards strung together to control the design, each card forming one row of the woven pattern and arranged so that the needles of the shaft lifting the warp threads would pass through the holes, in turn allowing the shuttle to travel across and thereby form the pattern. The Jacquard attachment, once it was embraced, increased the pace of weaving. While it did away with the need for a drawboy, it created jobs for card punchers and card lashers who put the cards in proper sequence. These were skilled jobs because the designs had to be read correctly by the card punchers, and the correctness of the finished shawl depended more on their work than on the weaver's.

52. Bennett, 'The Shawl', 49.

53. Cit. Byrde, *Nineteenth Century Fashion*, 51.

54. John Hibberd, 'Paris Fashions in Kleist's "Berliner Abendblätter"', *The Modern Language Review* 94/1 (1999), 127.

55. Saloni Mathur, *India by Design: Colonial History and Cultural Display* (Berkeley: University of California Press, 2007), 5.

56. See also Sweetman, *The Oriental Obsession*, 167. See also 175:

> Jones's chapters concerned the 'Mohammedan' design are valuable on a number of counts. In the first of them, on Arabian decoration, the multifarious origins of Muslim art are set against the speed of development of a style 'complete in itself', a fact that has continued to preoccupy modern historians of the subject. In the following chapters a serious attempt is made to differentiate and evaluate various national styles: Turkish (3 plates), Moresque (8 plates), Persian (6 plates) and Indian (9 plates). In all, 454 Islamic motifs are illustrated in colour. In the all-important chapter on 'Moresque' ornament, the processes by which the Moors deploy a pattern on a surface are examined. Every ornament 'arises quietly and naturally from the surface decorated'; there is a balanced distribution of straight, inclined and curved elements; all lines flow from a parent stem; natural forms are never directly copied, but conventionalised into two-dimensional elements. Colours are used so as to be 'best seen in themselves, and add most to the general effect.'

57. Cit. Breward, *The Culture of Fashion*, 169.

58. Émile Zola, *Au Bonheur des dames* (Paris: Le Livre de Poche, [1883] 1980), 7–8. See also Steele, *Paris Fashion*, 147–50.

59. Clay Lancaster, 'Oriental Contributions to Art Nouveau', *The Art Bulletin* 34/4 (1952), 301–2.

60. See Sweetman, *The Oriental Obsession*, 187–8; Zutshi, "Designed for Eternity", 437.

61. See also John MacKenzie, *Orientalism: History, Theory and the Arts* (Manchester: Manchester University Press, 1995), 195.

62. Sarah Nichols, 'Arthur Lasenby Liberty: A Mere Adjective?', *The Journal of Decorative and Propaganda Arts* 13 (1989), Stile Floreale Theme Issue, passim.

63. Razek, *Dress Codes*, 12:

> 'Seen in this light' she comments, 'the highly constructed bustle dress—anchored with fine, light chains placed under the knees—literally caged a woman in her clothing, containing her sexualized body much as the body of Saartje Bartman was finally contained: in a glass case in the French Museum of Natural History, on display'.

64. *Illustrated London News*, 30 July 1853, 63, cit. Penelope Byrde, *Nine-teenth Century Fashion*, 55.
65. Cit. Ribeiro, *Ingres in Fashion*, 39.
66. Gayle Fischer, ' "Pantalets" and "Turkish Trowsers": Designing Freedom in the Mid-Nineteenth-Century United States', *Feminist Studies* 23/1 (1997), 124.
67. Fischer, ' "Pantalets" and "Turkish Trowsers" '.
68. Fischer, ' "Pantalets" and "Turkish Trowsers" ', 128. See also Marjorie Garber, *Vested Interests: Cross-Dressing and Cultural Anxiety* (New York: Routledge, 1992), 314.
69. Fischer, ' "Pantalets" and "Turkish Trowsers" ', 129.
70. Charlotte Jirousek, 'Ottoman Influences on Western Dress', in S. Faroqhi and C. K. Neumann, eds, *Ottoman Costumes: From Textile to Identity* (Istanbul: Eren, 2004), 243–4.
71. See also Diana de Marly, *The History of Haute Couture, 1850–1950* (London: B. T. Batsford Ltd, 1980), 72–3, and Steele, 'Women in Trousers', *Paris Fashion*, 162–7.

CHAPTER 4: 1868–1944

1. Cit. Barbara Harlow and Mia Carter, eds, *Imperialism and Orientalism: A Documentary Sourcebook* (Oxford: Blackwell, 1999), 210.
2. Stéphane Mallarmé, *La Dernière Mode*, in Henri Mondor and G. Jean-Aubry, eds, *Œuvres completes* (Paris: Pléiade, [1874–5] 1954), 712:

    La Civilisation! lisez << l'époque où a disparu Presque toute puissance créatrice . . . dans la Bijouterie comme dans le Mobilier >>; et, dans l'un comme dans l'autre, nous sommes forces ou d'exhumer ou d'importer. Importer quoi? Les bracelets de verre filé d'Inde et les pendants d'oreilles en papier découpé de la Chine? Non; mais, souvent, le goût naïf qui preside à leur confection.

3. See also R. Benjamin: '. . . when French painters "went native", Agerians "went modern" ', *Orientalist Aesthetics*, 9.
4. Patricia Highsmith, 'Djemal's Revenge', *Selected Stories* (New York: Norton, 2001), 13.
5. See also MacKenzie, *Orientalism*, 124.
6. Cit. Edmund de Waal, *The Hare with the Amber Eyes* (New York: Farrar, Strauss and Giroux, 2010), 47.
7. Marcel Proust, 'Mme Swann at Home', *A la recherché du temps perdu*, vol 1., C.K. Scott Moncrieff and Terence Kilmartin, trans. (Harmondsworth: Penguin, 1989), 662.

8. Lancaster, 'Oriental Contributions to Art Nouveau', 299.
9. Cit. Virginia Spate and David Bromfield, 'A New and Strange Beauty: Monet and Japanese Art', in *Monet and Japan*, exhibition catalogue (Canberra: National Gallery of Australia, 2001), 24–5.
10. Anne Hollander, 'Kimono', *Feeding the Eye* (Berkeley: University of California Press, 1999), 129.
11. See esp. Ilsa Goldstein-Gidoni, 'Kimono and the Construction of Gendered and Cultural Identities, *Ethnology* 38/4 (1999), 351–70.
12. Julia Sapin, 'Merchandising Art and Identity in Meiji Japan: Kyoto *Nihonga* Artists' Designs for Takashimaya Department Store, 1868–1912', *Journal of Design History* 17/4 (2004), 317.
13. Sapin, 'Merchandising Art and Identity in Meiji Japan', 322–3.
14. Sapin, 'Merchandising Art and Identity in Meiji Japan', 324.
15. See also Yuniya Kawamura, *The Japanese Revolution in Paris Fashion* (Oxford: Berg, 2004), 93–4.
16. Alan Kennedy, *Japanese Costume: History and Tradition* (Paris: Adam Biro,1990), 6.
17. Kennedy, *Japanese Costume*.
18. Toby Slade, *Japanese Fashion: A Cultural History* (Oxford: Berg, 2009), 41.
19. Slade, *Japanese Fashion*, 52.
20. Slade, *Japanese Fashion*, 68.
21. Slade, *Japanese Fashion*, 93.
22. Slade, *Japanese Fashion*, 95–6.
23. Slade, *Japanese Fashion*, 96.
24. Keiichiro Nakagawa and Henry Rosovsky, 'The Case of the Dying Kimono: The Influence of Changing Fashions on the Development of the Japanese Woolen Industry', in Mary-Ellen Roach-Higgins et al., eds, *Dress and Identity* (New York: Fairchild, 1995), 467.
25. Nakagawa and Henry Rosovsky, 'The Case of the Dying Kimono', 468–9.
26. Ryusaku Tsunoda et al., 'Return to the East', in *Sources of Japanese Tradition* (New York: Columbia University Press, 1958).
27. Nerval, *Voyage en Orient*, 349:

> Habiller une femme jaune à l'européenne, c'eût été la chose la plus ridicule du monde. Je me bornai à lui faire signe qu'il fallait laisser repousser les cheveux coupés en rond sur le devant, ce qui parut l'etonner beaucoup; quant à la brûlure du front et à celle de la poitrine, qui resultait probablement d'un usage de son pays, car on ne voit rien de pareil en Égypte, cela pouvait se cacher au moyen d'un bijou ou d'un ornement quelconque; il n'y avait donc pas trop de quoi se plaindre, tout examen fait.

28. Nerval, *Voyage en Orient*, 587:

Le pacha me quita un instant, sand doute pour aller remplir ses devoirs religieux; ensuite, il revint et me dit: "Nous allons diner 'l'européenne." En effet, on apporta des chaises et une table haute, au lieu de retourner un tabouret et de poser dessus un plateu de metal et des cousins autour, comme cela se fait d'ordinaire. Je sentis tout ce qu'il y avait d'obligeant dans le procédé du pacha, et toutefois, je l'avouerai, je n'aime pas ces coutumes de l'Europe envahissant peu à peu l'Orient; je me plaignis au pacha d'être traité par lui en touriste vulgaire.

'Vous venez bien me voir en habit noir! . . .' me dit-il.

La replique était juste; pourtant je sentais bien que j'avais eu raison. Quoi que l'on fasse, et si loin que l'on puisse aller dans la bienveillance d'un Turc, il ne faut pas croire qu'il puisse y avoir tout de suite fusion entre notre façon de vivre et la sienne. Les coutumes européennes qu'il adopte dans certains cas deviennent une sorte de terrain neuter où il nous accueille sans se livrer lui-même; il consent à imiter nos mœurs comme il use de notre langue, mais à l'égard de nous seulement. Il ressemble à ce personage de ballet qui est moitié paysan et moitié signeur; Il montre à l'Europe le côté *gentleman*, il est toujours un pur *Osmanli* pour l'Asie.

29. Ussama Makdisi, 'Ottoman Orientalism', *The American Historical Review* 107/3 (2005), 18.
30. Bernard Lewis, *The Emergence of Modern Turkey*, 3rd edn (Oxford: Oxford University Press, 2002), 100–1. Lewis also cites M. Canard, 'Coiffure européene et Islam', *Annales de l'Institut d'Études Orientales* (Algiers), 8 (1949–50), 200.
31. B. Lewis, *The Emergence of Modern Turkey*, 102.
32. B. Lewis, *The Emergence of Modern Turkey*, 101.
33. Nora Seni, 'Fashion and Women's Clothing in the Satirical Press of Istanbul at the End of the 19th Century', in Sirin Tekeli, ed., *Women in Modern Turkish Society* (London: Zed Books, 1995), passim; Reina Lewis, *Rethinking Orientalism*, 192ff.
34. R. Lewis, *Rethinking Orientalism*, passim.
35. R. Lewis, *Rethinking Orientalism*, 192.
36. Barbro Karabuda, *Good bye to the Fez: A Portrait of Modern Turkey*, trans. from the Swedish by Maurice Michael (London: Denis Dobson, 1959), 47.
37. Karabuda, *Good bye to the Fez*, 48.
38. B. Lewis, *Modern Turkey*, 267.
39. Cit. B. Lewis, *Modern Turkey*, 269.
40. Thomas Mann, *Der Zauberberg* (Frankfurt am Main: Fischer Verlag, [1924] 1977), 348–49:

Auch er hatte sein Äusseres ein wenig karnevalistich aufgemuntert, indem er nämlich zu dem klinischen Kittel, den er auch heute trug, da sein tätigkeit ja niemals ruhte, einen echten türkischen Fez, karminrot, mit schwarzer troddel, die ihm über das Ohr baumelte, aufgesetzt hatte,—Kostum genug für ihn, dies beides zusammen; es reichte hin, seine ohnehin merkante Erscheinung ins durchaus Wunderliche und Ausgelassene zu steigern.

41. For a far more nuanced and detailed discussion, see R. Lewis, *Rethinking Orientalism*, 194ff.
42. With the establishment of *La Chambre syndicale de la confection de la couture pour dames et fillettes*.
43. See also Adam Geczy, 'Modernity: Three Defining Moments in the Crossover of Art and Fashion', in Adam Geczy and Vicki Karaminas, eds, *Fashion and Art* (Oxford: Berg, 2012).
44. Poiret, *En habillant l'époque*, 64.
45. See Steele, *Paris Fashion*, 107–8:

    Fashion costumes, of course, were a natural theme for the fashion illustrator. Another series of prints, *Les Filles de l'empire céleste* (1850), featured the charms of the "exotic" East, and Anaïs [Colin] did dozens of other pictures on costumes of different countries: Spanish, Swiss and Italian folk dresses, Turkish, Syrian and Persian costume, a hopelessly inaccurate version of the Indian sari, one fairly accurate version of a Japanese kimono and another that combined Chinese and Japanese clothing elements into something that would have been unrecognizable to a person of either country. Héloïse [her sister] did similar series, in which, for example, flowers provided the motif: Chinese girls with camellias, Indians (their saris are better) with Dahlias, Middle Eastern women with roses, medieval women with marguerites, and so on.

46. Peter Wollen, *Reading the Icebox: Reflections on Twentieth Century Culture* (London: Verso, 1993).
47. Yvonne Deslandres and Dorothy Lalanne, *Paul Poiret, 1879–1944* (London: Thames and Hudson, 1987), passim.
48. Nancy Troy, *Couture Culture: A Study of Modern Art and Fashion* (Cambridge, MA: MIT Press, 2003), passim.
49. Valerie Steele, *Fashion and Eroticism* (Oxford: Oxford University Press, 1985), 232–33.
50. Troy, *Couture Culture*, 128.
51. Cit. de Marly, *The History of Haute Couture*, 86.

52. Poiret, *En habillant l'époque*, 138; translation mine.
53. See also Wollen, 'Fashion/Orientalism/The Body', *Raiding the Icebox: Reflections on Twentieth-century Culture*, 1.
54. Wollen, *Raiding the Icebox*, 1.
55. Nikolay Rimsky-Korsakoff, *My Musical Life*, Judah A. Joffe, trans., Carl van Vechten, ed. (New York: Tudor Publishing, 1935), 248.
56. Poiret, *En habillant l'époque*, 137.
57. Poiret, *En habillant l'époque*.
58. Cit. Troy, *Couture Culture*, 113.
59. Cit. Wollen, *Raiding the Icebox*, 2.
60. John Gage, *Colour and Culture: Practice and Meaning from Antiquity to Abstraction* (London: Thames & Hudson, 1993), 31.
61. David Batchelor, *Chromophobia* (London: Reaktion Books, 2000), 21–2.
62. Eirik Hanssen, 'Symptoms of Desire: Colour, Costume, and Commodities in Fashion Newsreels of the 1910s and 1920s', *Film History* 212 (Special Issue: Early Colour Part 2, 2009), 112.
63. Troy, *Couture Culture*, 109.
64. Rosalind Krauss, 'Giacometti', in William Rubin, ed., *Primitivism' in 20th Century Art: Affinity of the Tribal and the Modern* (New York: MOMA, 1984).
65. Petrine Archer-Straw, *Negrophilia: Avant-Garde Paris and Black Culture in the 1920s* (London: Thames and Hudson, 2000), 60–74.
66. Archer-Straw, *Negrophilia*, 66.
67. Personal correspondence, 16 April, 2011.
68. Wollen, *Raiding the Icebox*, 13
69. Cit. Troy, *Couture Culture*, 128.
70. Proust, 'The Captive', *A la recherché du temps perdu*, vol 3., C. K. Scott Moncrieff and Terence Kilmartin, trans. (Harmondsworth: Penguin, 1988), 412.
71. Proust, 'The Captive', 401.
72. Proust, 'The Captive', 375–6.
73. Gilles Lipovetsky, *L'empire de l'éphémère* (Paris: Gallimard, 1987), 95.
74. Michelle Tollini Finamore, 'Fashioning the Colonial at the Paris Expositions, 1925 and 1931', in Nirmal Puwar and Nandi Bhatia, eds, *Fashion Theory*, 348–51 and passim. Finamore makes a scholarly case for the orientalist presence in fashion during this period; my distinction is simply that it was less obvious and less flamboyant than other periods, a view supported by Lipovetsky and others.
75. Miriam, Hansen, 'Pleasure, Ambivalence, Identification: Valentino and Female Spectatorship', *Cinema Journal* 25/4 (1986), 22.

CHAPTER 5: 1944–2011

1. Quentin Bell, *On Human Finery* (London: Hogarth, 1976), 27.
2. Phoebe Philo, *W* magazine, cit. Justine Picardie, 'The Beautiful and the Damned', *Harper's Bazaar* Australia (November 2008), 50.
3. Philo, cit. Picardie, 'The Beautiful and the Damned', 50.
4. Sanjay Sharma and Aswani Sharma, 'White Paranoia: Orientalism in the Age of Empire', in Puwar and Bhatia, eds, *Fashion Theory* 7/3–4, 308.
5. Sharma and Sharma, 'White Paranoia', 310.
6. Hyunshin Na, 'Echoes of the East: Patternworks International Best Solution to a Patternmaking Problem Award, 2004', *Clothing and Textiles Research Journal*. 25/2 (2007), 202.
7. Nirmal Puwar, 'Multicultural Fashion . . . Stirrings of Another Sense of Culture and Memory', *Feminist Review* 71 (2002), 74–6 and passim.
8. Audrey Wipper, 'African Women, Fashion, and Scapegoating', *Canadian Journal of African Studies/Revue Canadienne des Études Africaines* 6/2 (Special Issue: The Roles of African Women: Past, Present and Future, 1972), 334.
9. Wipper, 'African Women, Fashion, and Scapegoating', 331.
10. Wipper, 'African Women, Fashion, and Scapegoating', passim.
11. It also featured other traditional Indian instruments obscure to Western ears: the *tabla*, *dilruba*, *swordmandal* and *tambura*.
12. Jane Pavitt, *Fear and Fashion in the Cold War* (London: V&A Publishing, 2008), 8, 11.
13. Leslie Rabine, *The Global Circulation of African Fashion* (Oxford: Berg, 2002), 53–5.
14. Sheila Rowbotham, *Edward Carpenter: A Life of Liberty and Love* (London: Verso, 2008), 236–7.
15. http://www.guerlain.com/int/en/base.html#/en/home-parfum/cata logue-parfums/men-fragrances/men-fragrances-habit-rouge/habit-rouge-eau-de-parfum.html
16. Gayatri Chakravorty Spivak, *A Critique of Postcolonial Reason: Toward a History of the Vanishing Present* (Cambridge, MA: Harvard University Press, 1999), 339ff.
17. Kawamura, *The Japanese Revolution in Paris Fashion*, 95.
18. Spivak, *A Critique of Postcolonial Reason*, 340.
19. Cit. Spivak, *A Critique of Postcolonial Reason*, 341.
20. Kawamura, *The Japanese Revolution in Paris Fashion*, 96.
21. Kawamura, *The Japanese Revolution in Paris Fashion*, 106.
22. Kawamura, *The Japanese Revolution in Paris Fashion*, 108.
23. Cf. Kawamura, *The Japanese Revolution in Paris Fashion*, 115:

He realized that the 'exotic' elements were attractive to the French public, so he began to look elsewhere for other ethnic cultures. He also used straight lines and square shapes which are derived from kimono that do not have any curves.

24. Cit. Kawamura, *The Japanese Revolution in Paris Fashion*, 133.
25. Caroline Evans and Minna Thornton, *Women and Fashion: A New Look* (London: Quartet Books, 1989), 159.
26. Evans and Thornton, *Women and Fashion*, 161.
27. Mark Holborn, *Issey Miyake* (Cologne: Taschen, 1995), 20.
28. Holborn, *Issey Miyake*, 20.
29. Dorinne Kondo, *About Face: Performing Race in Fashion and Theatre* (London: Routledge, 1997), 151.
30. See also Kondo, *About Face*, 121.
31. Kondo, *About Face*, 81.
32. Kondo, *About Face*, 149–52.
33. Roland Barthes, *Empire of Signs*, Richard Howard, trans. (London: Jonathan Cape, [1970] 1982), 3–4.
34. Spivak, *A Critique of Postcolonial Reason*, 414:

To place the export-based garment industry in transnationality, then, allow me to use a bland everyday happening that I put in a frame for a seminar in feminist cultural studies, to explain that transnationality did not primarily mean people moving from place to place, although labor export was certainly an important object of investigation.

The example is Gayatri Spivak on a winter's day at an opening in New York's New Museum. I was wearing a jacket over a sari, and, to layer myself into warmth I was wearing, under the jacket, a full-sleeved cotton top, rather an unattractive duncolored cheap thing, 'made in Bangladesh' for the French Connection. By contrast, the sari I was wearing, also made in Bangladesh, was an exquisite woven cloth produced by the Prabartana Weavers' collective under the coordination of Farida Akhter and Farhad Mazhar. Until I saw these weavers at work, I had no idea how the *jamdanis* that I had so admired in my childhood and youth were fabricated. It is complicated teamweaving and simultaneous embroidery at speed, hard to believe if you haven't actually seen it, certainly as delicate and difficult as lacemaking. As a result of the foreign direct investment related to the international garment industry, the long tradition of Bangladeshi handloom is dying. Prabartana not only subsidizes and 'develops' the weavers' collective, but it also attempts to undo the epistemic violation suffered by the weavers by recognizing them as artists. This is not merely a reversal, but also a displacement of Ackerman's *Compendium*; there is no allegory-referenced transcoding here. Thus I was standing in the museum wearing the contradiction of transnationalization upon my body, an exhibit, though no one knew it. No persons or groups had moved much to make this possible. There *can* be labor migrancy associated with transnationalization, but in fact it is not necessary—with postfordism and export processing zones. The demographic determining factors for labor migrancy lie elsewhere, and are beyond the scope of these concluding pages.

35. Hal Foster, 'Architecture and Design', *Design and Crime and Other Diatribes* (London: Verso, 2002), 25.
36. Entwistle, *The Fashioned Body*, 38.
37. Entwistle, *The Fashioned Body*, 36.
38. See also Valerie Steele and John S. Major, *China Chic: East Meets West* (New Haven: Yale University Press, 1999), 78–9:

    Yves Saint Laurent was probably the supreme exponent of exotic fashion. Over the course of his very long and successful career, he created extraordinarily beautiful fashions inspired by Africa, the Middle East, India, Russia, and China. A year after Saint Laurent's world-famous Ballets Russes Collection of 1976, he produced another major collection inspired by imperial China, which in turn launched the next wave of fashionable chinoiserie.

39. Pierre Bergé, 'Du côté de l'Orient', in *Yves Saint Laurent—Exotisme* (Marseilles: Musées de Marseille, 1994), 17.
40. *Woman's Wear Daily*, 1997, cit. Steele and Major, *China Chic*, 79.
41. Lise Skov, 'Fashion-Nation', in Sandra Niessen, Carla Jones and Ann Marie Leshkowich, eds, *Re-Orienting Fashion: The Globalization of Asian Dress* (Oxford: Berg, 2003).
42. Skov, 'Fashion-Nation', 240–1.
43. Carla Jones and Ann Marie Leshkowich, 'Introduction: The Globalization of Asian Dress; Re-orienting Fashion or Re-Orientalising Asia?', in Sandra Niessen et al., eds, *Re-Orienting Fashion*, 18–19.
44. Kristyne Loughran, Jewelry, Fashion, and Identity: The Tuareg Example, *African Arts* 36/1 (Memorial to Roy Sieber, Part 1), 57.
45. Steele and Major, *China Chic*, 69–70.
46. Steele and Major, *China Chic*, 70.
47. Craik, *The Face of Fashion*, 225.
48. Jones and Leshkowich, 'Introduction', 20–1.

49. This parallel between orientalism and femininity and the sex–gender distinction has, oddly enough, never been explored. The sex–gender distinction identifies that while sex can be equated to a series of biological attributes, those attributes cannot always be corroborated to gender. One can 'feel' like a woman but have the biology of a man. This misalliance in the subject's psychopathological make-up can sometimes be 'corrected', but what of the transsexual or transvestite who dresses as a woman but is happy keeping certain traces of sexual masculinity? The sex–gender distinction is a sine qua non of gender studies in locating the limits of essentialism. The shifting plates of identification can be strongly applied to orientalism—especially in its contemporary incarnations. Transorientalism suggests that orientalism is a series of shifting plates and parallax points of view.

50. http://geniusbeauty.com/fashion-and-wear/paris-fashion-week-dior/

51. Adam Geczy, 'Djamu Gallery: Notes on Exhibiting Aboriginal Art', *Postwest* 14 (University of Western Sydney, 1999), 10.

52. Margaret Maynard, 'Grassroots Style: Re-evaluating Australian Fashion and Aboriginal Art in the 1970s and 1980s', *Journal of Design History* 13/2 (2000), 144.

53. Maynard, 'Grassroots Style', 149.

54. Emma Tarlo, *Clothing Matters: Dress and Identity in India* (Chicago: University of Chicago Press, 1996), 24.

55. Tarlo, *Clothing Matters*, 121.

56. Tarlo, *Clothing Matters*, 120.

57. Entwistle, *The Fashioned Body*, 28–9.

58. Rebecca Ruhlen, 'Korean Alterations: Nationalism, Social Consciousness and "Traditional" Clothing', in Niessen et al., eds, *Re-Orienting Fashion*, 120.

59. Ruhlen, 'Korean Alterations', 128.

60. See Ann Marie Leshkowich and Carla Jones, 'What happens When Asian Chic Becomes Asian Chic in Asia?', in Puwar and Bhatia, eds, *Fashion Theory*, 287–8.

61. Leshkowich and Jones, 'What happens When Asian Chic Becomes Asian Chic in Asia?', 290–2.

62. Slavoj Zizek, *Welcome to the Desert of the Real* (London: Verso, 2002), 115.

63. Nasa Khan, 'Asian Women's Dress: From Burqah to Blogs—Changing Clothes for Changing Times', in J. Ash and E. Wilson, eds, *Chic Thrills* (London: Pandora Press, 1992), 62.

64. Khan, 'Asian Women's Dress', 63–4.

65. Jones and Leshkowich, 'Introduction', 20.

66. Paminder Bhachu, 'Designing Diasporic Markets: Asian Fashion Entrepreneurs in London', in Niessen et al., eds, *Re-Orienting Fashion*. See also

Sandra Niessen, 'Afterword: Re-Orienting Fashion Theory', *Re-Orienting Fashion*, 248.

67. Singh, *Colonial Narratives/Cultural Dialogues*, 186.

68. Rabine, *The Global Circulation of African Fashion*, 29.

69. Rabine, *The Global Circulation of African Fashion*, 29–34 and passim.

70. Rabine, *The Global Circulation of African Fashion*, 135–48.

71. Deborah Heath, 'Fashion, Anti-Fashion, and Heteroglossia in Urban Senegal', *American Ethnologist* 19/1 (1992), 21.

72. Heath, 'Fashion, Anti-Fashion, and Heteroglossia in Urban Senegal'.

73. Antonia Finnane, 'What Should Chinese Women Wear?', in Antonia Finnane and Anne McLaren, eds, *Dress, Sex and Text in Chinese Culture* (Melbourne: Monash Asia Institute, 1999), 4.

74. Hazel Clark, 'The Cheung Sam: Issues of Fashion and Cultural Identity', in Steele and Major, *China Chic*, 155.

75. See also Steele and Major, *China Chic*, 48.

76. Dorothy Ko, 'Jazzing into Modernity: High Heels, Platforms and Lotus Shoes', in Steele and Major, *China Chic*, 145.

77. Ko, 'Jazzing into Modernity', 149.

78. Clark, 'The Cheung Sam', 150–3; in Steele and Major, *China Chic*, 155–65.

79. Clark, 'The Cheung Sam', *China Chic*, 164–5.

80. Finnane, *Changing Clothes in China*, 21–6.

81. Jones and Leshkowich, 'Introduction', 8.

82. Also known as the Jyllands-Posten Muhammad cartoons controversy, the Danish newspaper Jyllands-Posten posted a series of twelve editorial cartoons ridiculing Islam, in which Islamic dress played a significant part. These were greeted with livid consternation and violence, including bombing the Danish embassy in Pakistan and incendiary attacks on Danish embassies in other Middle Eastern countries. The Danish Prime Minister at the time stated that it was the country's worst disaster since World War II.

83. See also Pavitt, *Fear and Fashion in the Cold War*, 49 and passim.

84. Emma Tarlo, *Visibly Muslim: Fashion, Politics, Faith* (Oxford: Berg, 2010), passim.

85. Katrin Bennhold, 'A Veil Closes France's Door to Citizenship', *The New York Times* (19 July 2008), passim.

86. Robert Paxton, 'Can You Really Become French?', *New York Review of Books* (April 2009), 53.

87. Paxton, 'Can You Really Become French?', 55.

88. Elisabeth Özdalga, *The Veiling Issue: Official Secularism and Popular Islam in Modern Turkey* (Richmond, VA: Curzon, 1998), 34–49.

89. Ayla Albayrak, 'Moustaches Yes, Headscarves No: Signs of Change in Turkish Politics', *Wall Street Journal* (15 April 2011), http://blogs.wsj.com/emergingeurope/2011/04/13/yes-to-moustaches-no-to-headscarves/

90. Özdalga, *The Veiling Issue*, 89.
91. Özdalga, *The Veiling Issue*, 93.
92. See also Tarlo, *Visibly Muslim*, 57.
93. See http://www.fashion.arts.ac.uk/research/projects-collaborations/ modest-dressing and see also the podcasts of the symposium at the London College of Fashion on 15 June 2011: http://www.religionandsociety.org. uk/publications/podcasts/show/mediating_modesty_reina_lewis
94. http://www.thehijabshop.com
95. http://www.thehijabshop.com
96. Tarlo, *Visibly Muslim*, 67.
97. Tarlo, *Visibly Muslim*, 67–8. See also Erving Goffman, *Stigma: Notes on the Management of Spoiled Identity* (Harmondsworth: Penguin, [1963] 1968).
98. Tarlo, *Visibly Muslim*, 68.
99. Dorothy Ko, *Teachers of the Inner Chambers: Women and Culture in Seventeenth-century China* (Stanford: Stanford University Press, 1994), 149–71. See also Steele and Major, *China Chic*, 41.

CONCLUSION

1. Steven Zhao, 'Analysis of Chinese Clothing Consumption in Market in 2007 and 2008', http://www.buzzle.com/articles/analysis-of-chinese-clothing-consumption-in-market-in-2007-and-2008.html
2. Although out of date, the following article is instructive and indicative of what is now a long-term problem: Barbara Nordquist, 'International Trade in Textiles and Clothing: Implications for the Future', *Clothing and Textiles Research Journal* 35/3 (1985), 35–39.
3. Borges, '*Purgatorio* I, 13', in Eliot Weinberger, ed., *Selected Non-Fictions*, 292.

Bibliography

Abu-Lughod, Ibrahim, *Arab Rediscovery of Europe: A Study in Cultural Encounters*, Princeton, NJ: Princeton University Press, 1963.

Albayrak, Ayla, 'Moustaches Yes, Headscarves No: Signs of Change in Turkish Politics', *Wall Street Journal* (15 April 2011), http://blogs.wsj.com/emergingeurope/2011/04/13/yes-to-moustaches-no-to-headscarves/

Appleby, Joyce, *Economic Thought and Ideology in Seventeenth-century England*, Princeton, NJ: Princeton University Press, 1978.

Aravamudan, Srinivas, 'Lady Mary Wortley Montagu in the Hammam: Masquerade, Womanliness, and Levantinization', English Literary History 62/1 (Spring, 1995), pp. 69–104.

Archer-Straw, Petrine, *Negrophilia: Avant-Garde Paris and Black Culture in the 1920s*, London: Thames and Hudson, 2000.

Ashcroft, Bill, et al., eds, *The Postcolonial Studies Reader*, London: Routledge, 1995.

Ballets Russes: The Art of Costume, exhibition catalogue, Canberra: National Gallery of Australia, 2010.

Balzac, Honoré de, *Les Chouans*, Paris: Librairie Générale Française, [1845] 1997.

Barthes, Roland, *Empire of Signs*, Richard Howard, trans., London: Jonathan Cape, [1970] 1982.

Barwick, Sandra, *A Century of Style*, London: Allen and Unwin, 1984.

Batchelor, David, *Chromophobia*, London: Reaktion Books, 2000.

Beaulieu, Jill, and Roberts, Mary, eds, *Orientalism's Interlocutors: Rewriting the Colonial Encounter*, Durham, NC: Duke University Press, 2002.

Beer, Alice, *Trade Goods: A Study of Indian Chintz*, Washington, DC: Smithsonian Institution Press, 1970.

Beer, John, 'Fragments and Ironies', in John Beer, ed. *Questioning Romanticism*, Baltimore: Johns Hopkins University Press, 1995.

Bell, Quentin, *On Human Finery*, London: Hogarth, 1976.

Benjamin, Roger, *Orientalist Aesthetics: Art, Colonialism and French North Africa, 1880–1930*, Berkeley: University of California Press, 2003.

Benjamin, Walter, *The Arcades Project*, Howard Eiland and Kevin McLaughlin, trans., Cambridge, MA: Belknap Press, 1999.

Benjamin, Walter, *Charles Baudelaire: A Lyric Poet in the Era of High Capitalism*, Harry Zohn, trans., London: Verso, 1983.

Bennett, Bessie, 'The Shawl: A Costume Accessory', *Bulletin of the Art Institute of Chicago* 29/4 (1907–1951), pp. 48–9.

Bennhold, Katrin, 'A Veil Closes France's Door to Citizenship', *The New York Times* (19 July 2008), http://www.nytimes.com/2008/07/19/world/europe/19france.html?pagewanted=all

Bergé, Pierre, 'Du côté de l'Orient', in *Yves Saint Laurent—Exotisme*, Marseilles: Musées de Marseille; Réunion des Musées Nationaux, 1994.

Berrong, Richard, *In Love with a Handsome Sailor: The Emergence of Gay Identity in the Novels of Pierre Loti*, Toronto: University of Toronto Press, 2003.

Berstein, Richard, *The East, the West, and Sex: A History of Erotic Encounters*, New York: Knopf, 2009.

Blum, Dilys, 'Fans', *Philadelphia Museum of Art Bulletin* 84/358–359 (1988), pp. 1–36.

Bohls, Elizabeth, *Women Travel Writers and the Language of Aesthetics, 1716–1818*, Cambridge: Cambridge University Press, 1995.

Boisdeffre, Pierre de, *Pierre Loti: Ses maisons*, St-Cyr-sur-Loire: Christian Pirot, 1996.

Borges, Jorge Luis, 'Translators of *The Thousand and One Nights*', *Selected Non-Fictions*, Esther Allen et al., trans., Eliot Weinberger, ed., New York: Penguin, [1934–6] 1999.

Boucher, Françoise, *A History of Costume in the West*, London: Thames and Hudson, 1996.

Breskin, Isabel, '"On the Periphery of a Greater World": John Singleton Copley's "Turquerie" Portraits', *Winterthur Portfolio* 36/2–3 (2001), pp. 97–123.

Breward, Christopher, *The Culture of Fashion*, Manchester: Manchester University Press, 1995.

Breward, Christopher, and Evans, Caroline, eds, *Fashion and Modernity*, Oxford: Berg, 2005.

Brook, Timothy, *Vermeer's Hat. The Seventeenth Century and the Dawn of the Global World*, New York: Bloomsbury, 2008.

Burgh, Hélène de, *Sex, Sailors and Colonies: Narratives of Ambiguity in the Works of Pierre Loti*, Bern: Peter Lang, 2005.

Butler, Marylin, 'Orientalism', in David B. Pirie, ed., *The Romantic Period*, Harmondsworth: Penguin, 1994.

Butler, Rex, *A Secret History of Australian Art*, Sydney: Craftsman House, 2002.

Byrde, Penelope, *Nineteenth Century Fashion*, London: B. T. Batsford Ltd, 1992.

Cage, Clare, 'The Sartorial Self: Neoclassical Fashion and Gender Identity in France, 1797–1804,' *Eighteenth-century Studies* 42/2 (2009), pp. 193–215.

Cannadine, David, *Ornamentalism: How the British Saw Their Empire*, Oxford: Oxford University Press, 2001.

Castle, Terry, 'Eros and Liberty at the English Masquerade, 1710–90', *Eighteenth-century Studies* 17/2 (Winter 1983–1984), pp. 156–76.

Castle, Terry, *Masquerade and Civilisation: The Carnivalesque in Eighteenth-century English Culture and Fiction*, London: Methuen, 1986.

Carter, Michael, *Fashion Classics: From Carlyle to Barthes*, Oxford: Berg, 2003.

Çelik, Zeyneb, *The Remaking of Istanbul: Portrait of an Ottoman City in the Nineteenth Century*, Berkeley: University of California Press, 1986.

Chaudhuri, K. N., *Trade and Civilisation in the Indian Ocean*, New York: Cambridge University Press, 1985.

Chaudhuri, K. N., 'Trade as a Cultural Phenomenon', in Jens Christian Johansen et al., eds, *Clashes of Cultures: Essays in Honour of Niels Steensgaard*, Odense: Odense University Press, 1992.

Chaudhuri, K. N., *The Trading World of Asia and the East India Company, 1660–1760*, New York: Cambridge University Press, 1978.

Chaudhuri, K. N., *The Economic Development of India Under the East India Company, 1814–58*, Cambridge: Cambridge University Press, 1971.

Chaudhury, Sushil, 'European Companies and the Bengal Textile Industry in the Eighteenth Century: The Pitfalls of Applying Quantitative Techniques', *Modern Asian Studies* 27/2 (1993), pp. 321–40.

Cheang, Sarah, 'Selling China: Class, Gender and Orientalism at the Department Store', *Journal of Design History* 20/1 (2007), pp. 1–16.

Chow, Karen, 'Popular Sexual Knowledges and Women's Agency in 1920s England: Marie Stopes's "Married Love" and E. M. Hull's "The Sheik"', *Feminist Review* 63(1999, Negotiations and Resistances), pp. 64–87.

Çizgen, Engin, *Photography in the Ottoman Empire, 1839–1919*, Istanbul: Haset Kitalevi, 1987.

Clark, Hazel, 'The Cheung Sam: Issues of Fashion and Cultural Identity', in Valerie Steele and John S. Major, *China Chic*, New Haven, CT: Yale University Press.

Colchester, Cloe, ed., *Clothing the South Pacific*, Oxford: Berg, 2003.

Craik, Jennifer, *The Face of Fashion: Cultural Studies and Fashion*, London: Routledge, 1994.

Cuff, Robert Penn, 'The Permanent Values of Thackeray's *Vanity Fair*', *Peabody Journal of Education* 27/2 (1949), pp. 94–101.

Curl, James Stevens, *Egyptomania: The Egyptian Revival: A Recurring Theme in the History of Taste*, Manchester: Manchester University Press, 1994.

Currie, Kate, *Beyond Orientalism: An Exploration of Some Recent Themes in Indian History and Society*, Calcutta: K. P. Bagchi and Co., 1996.

Curtis, Michael, *Orientalism and Islam*, Cambridge: Cambridge University Press, 2009.

Dalby, Liza, *Kimono: Fashioning Culture*, New Haven: Yale University Press, 1994.

Daniel, Norman (1960), *Islam and the West: The Making of an Image*, Edinburgh: Edinburgh University Press.

Davis, Fred, *Fashion, Culture and Identity*, Chicago: University of Chicago Press, 1992.

Davison, Mildred, 'Printed Cotton Textiles', *The Art Institute of Chicago Quarterly* 52/4 (1 Dec. 1958), pp. 82–9.

Davison, Mildred, 'A "Vernis-Martin" Fan', *Bulletin of the Art Institute of Chicago, 1907–1951* 24/4 (Apr. 1930), pp. 50–1.

De Beer, Esmond, 'Charles II's Own Fashion: An Episode in Anglo–French Relations, 1666–1670', *Journal of the Warburg Institute* 2/2 (Oct. 1938), pp. 105–115.

De Marly, Diana, *The History of Haute Couture, 1850–1950*, London: B. T. Batsford Ltd, 1980.

De Marly, Diana, 'King Charles II's Own Fashion: The Theatrical Origins of the English Vest', *Journal of the Warburg and Courtauld Institutes* 37 (1974), pp. 378–82.

De Marly, Diana, *Worth: Father of Haute Couture*, London: Elm Tree Books, 1980.

DeJean, Joan, *The Essence of Style: How the French Invented High Fashion, Fine Food, Chic Cafés, Style, Sophistication, and Glamour*, New York: Free Press, 2005.

Delacroix, Eugène, *Journal* (2 vols.), Paris: Corti, 2009.

Denny, Walter, 'Oriental Carpets and Textiles in Venice', in Stefano Carboni, ed., *Venice in the Islamic World*, exhibition catalogue, New York: Metropolitan Museum of Art, 2007, pp. 189–90.

Deslandres, Yvonne, and Lalanne, Dorothy, *Paul Poiret, 1879–1944*, London: Thames and Hudson, 1987.

De Waal, Edmund, *The Hare with the Amber Eyes*, New York: Farrar, Strauss and Giroux, 2010.

Drew, Nicholas, *Orientalism in Louis XIV's France*, Oxford: Oxford University Press, 2009.

Dickson, T. Elder, and Irwin, David, 'Paisley Shawls', *The Burlington Magazine* 105/718 (1963), p. 34.

Diderot, Denis, *Oeuvres Complètes*, vol. 4. Paris: Garnier Fréres, 1875.

Dorrington-Ward, Carol, ed., *Fans from the East*, New York: Viking, 1978.

Dunlop, Ian, *Louis XIV*, London: Pimlico, 2001.

Egyptomania: Egypt in Western Art 1730–1930, exhibition catalogue, Ottowa: National Gallery of Canada, 1994.

Eicher, Joanne, *Dress and Ethnicity*, Oxford: Berg, 1995

Elias, Norbert, *La societé de cour*, Paris: Flammarion, 1985.

Entwistle, Joanne, *The Fashioned Body*, Cambridge: Polity, 2000.

Evans, Caroline, *Fashion on the Edge*, New Haven: Yale University Press, 2003.

Evans, Caroline, and Thornton, Minna, *Women and Fashion: A New Look*, London: Quartet Books, 1989.

Evelyn, John, *Diary*, E. S. Beer, ed., London: Oxford University Press, 1959.

Faroqhi, Suraiya, and Neumann, Christopher, *Ottoman Costumes: From Textile to Identity*, Istanbul: Eren, 2004.

Finnane, Antonia, *Changing Clothes in China*, Sydney: University of New South Wales Press, 2007.

Finnane, Antonia, and McLaren, Anne, eds, *Dress, Sex and Text in Chinese Culture*, Melbourne: Monash Asia Institute, 1999.

Fischer, Gayle, ' "Pantalets" and "Turkish Trowsers": Designing Freedom in the Mid-Nineteenth-Century United States', *Feminist Studies* 23/1 (1997), pp. 110–40.

Flügel, J. C., *The Psychology of Clothes*, London: Hogarth, 1930.

Foster, Hal, 'Architecture and Design', *Design and Crime and Other Diatribes*, London: Verso, 2002.

Fromentin, Eugène, *Une année dans le Sahel*, Paris: Plon, 1877.

Gage, John, *Colour and Culture: Practice and Meaning from Antiquity to Abstraction*, London: Thames and Hudson, 1993.

Garber, Marjorie, *Vested Interests: Cross-Dressing and Cultural Anxiety*, New York: Routledge, 1992.

Gautier, Théophile, *Baudelaire*, Claude-Marie Senninger and Lois Cassandra Hamrick, eds, Paris: Klincksieck, [1867] 1986.

Gautier, Théophile, *Histoire du romantisme*, Paris: Les Introuvables, 1993.

Geczy, Adam, 'Contested Pleasures', *Oxford Art Journal* 34/2 (2011), 295–7.

Geczy, Adam, 'Djamu Gallery: Notes on Exhibiting Aboriginal Art,' *Postwest* 14 (University of Western Sydney, 1999).

Geczy, Adam, and Karaminas, Vicki, eds, *Fashion and Art*, Oxford: Berg, 2012.

Gere, Charlotte, 'European Decorative Art at the World's Fairs, 1850–1900', *The Metropolitan Museum of Art Bulletin, New Series* 56/3 (1998–99), pp. 1, 16–56.

Gide, André, *Voyage au Congo*, Paris: Gallimard, 1927.

Glickman, Lawrence, ' "Make Lisle the Style": The Politics of Fashion in the Japanese Silk Boycott, 1937–1940', *Journal of Social History* 38/3 (2005), pp. 573–608.

Gluck, Mary, *Popular Bohemia: Modernism and Urban Culture in Nineteenth-century Paris*, Cambridge, MA: Harvard University Press, 2005.

Glynn, Prudence, *In Fashion: Dress in the Twentieth Century*, London: Allen and Unwin, 1978.

Göçek, Fatma Müge, *East Encounters West: France and the Ottoman Empire in the Eighteenth Century*, Oxford: Oxford University Press, 1987.

Göçek, Fatma Müge, and Balaghi, Shiva, *Rise of the Bourgeoisie, Demise of Empire: Ottoman Westernisation and Social Change*, New York: Oxford University Press, 1996.

Goffman, Erving, *Stigma: Notes on the Management of Spoiled Identity*, Harmondsworth: Penguin, [1963] 1968.

Goldstein-Gidoni, Ilsa, 'Kimono and the Construction of Gendered and Cultural Identities, *Ethnology* 38/4 (1999), pp. 351–70.

Gordon-Smith, Maria, 'The Influence of Jean Pillement on French and English Decorative Arts, Part One', *Artibus et Historiae* 21/41 (2000), pp. 171–96.

Gordon-Smith, Maria, 'Jean Pillement at the Court of King Stanisław August of Poland (1765–1767)', *Artibus et Historiae* 26/ 52 (2005), pp. 129–63.

Gordon-Smith, Maria, 'Jean Pillement at the Imperial Court of Maria Theresa and Francis I in Vienna (1763 to 1765)', *Artibus et Historiae* 25/50 (2004), pp. 187–213.

Griffith University's Tokyo Vogue, exhibition catalogue, Brisbane: Griffith University, Queensland College of Art.

Grundy, Isobel, *Lady Mary Wortley Montagu*, Oxford: Oxford University Press, 1999.

Grundy, Isobel, ' "The Barbarious Character We Give Them": White Women Travellers Report on Other Races', *Studies in Eighteenth Century Culture* 2 (1992), pp. 73–86.

Hackforth-Jones, Jos, and Roberts, Mary, eds, *Edges of Empire: Orientalism and Visual Culture*, Oxford: Blackwell, 2004.

Halsband, Robert, *The Life of Mary Wortley Montagu*, New York: Oxford University Press, 1960.

Hansen, Miriam, 'Pleasure, Ambivalence, Identification: Valentino and Female Spectatorship', *Cinema Journal* 25/4 (1986), 6–32.

Hanssen, Eirik, 'Symptoms of Desire: Colour, Costume, and Commodities in Fashion Newsreels of the 1910s and 1920s', *Film History* 21/2 (Special Issue: Early Colour Part 2, 2009), pp. 107–21.

Harlow, Barbara, and Carter, Mia, *Imperialism and Orientalism: A Documentary Sourcebook*, Oxford: Blackwell, 1999.

Hayms, Ronald, *Empire and Sexuality*, Manchester: Manchester University Press, 1990.

Head, Matthew, *Orientalism, Masquerade and Mozart's Turkish Music*, London: Royal Music Association, 2000.

Heath, Deborah, 'Fashion, Anti-Fashion, and Heteroglossia in Urban Senegal', *American Ethnologist* 19/1 (1992), 19–33.

Hebdidge, Dick, *Subculture: The Meaning of Style*, London: Routledge, 1979.

Herzig, Edmund, 'The Iranian Raw Silk Route and European Manufacture', in Maureen Fennel Marouzi, ed., *Textiles: Production, Trade and Demand*, Aldershot: Ashgate, 1998.

Hibberd, John, 'Paris Fashions in Kleist's "Berliner Abendblätter"', *The Modern Language Review* 94/1 (1999), pp. 122–31.

Highsmith, Patricia, 'Djemal's Revenge', *Selected Stories*, New York and London: Norton, 2001.

Hiner, Susan, *Accessories to Modernity: Fashion and the Feminine in Nineteenth-century France*, Philadelphia: University of Pennsylvania Press, 2010.

Holborn, Mark, *Issey Miyake*, Cologne: Taschen, 1995.

Hollander, Anne, *Feeding the Eye*, Berkeley: University of California Press, 1999.

Honour, Hugh *Chinoiserie: The Vision of Cathay*, London: John Murray, 1961.

Impey, Oliver, 'Japanese Export Art of the Edo Period and Its Influence on European Art', *Modern Asian Studies* 18/4 (Special Issue: Edo Culture and Its Modern Legacy, 1984), pp. 685–97.

Inankur, Zeynep, Lewis, Reina and Roberts, Mary, eds, *The Poetics and Politics of Place: Ottoman Istanbul and British Orientalism*, Istanbul: Pera Museum, 2011.

Irwin, John, *Shawls,* London: Victoria and Albert Museum, 1953.

Jacobson, Dawn, *Chinoiserie*, London: Phaidon, 1993.

Jarry, Madeliene, *Chinoiserie*, New York: Vendome Press, 1981.

Jasanoff, Maya, *Edge of Empire: Conquest and Collecting in the East, 1750–1850*, London: Harper, 2006.

Jerome, Jerome K., *Three Men in a Boat*, Harmondsworth: Penguin, [1889] 1957.

Jirousek, Charlotte, 'From "Traditional" to "Mass Fashion System" Dress Among Men in a Turkish Village', *Clothing and Textiles Research Journal* 15/4 (1997), pp. 203–15.

Jirousek, Charlotte, 'More than Oriental Splendour: European and Ottoman Headgear, 1380–1580', *Dress, the Annual Journal of the Costume Society of America* 21 (1995), pp. 22–33.

Charlotte Jirousek, 'Ottoman Influences on Western Dress', in S. Faroqhi and C. K. Neumann, eds, *Ottoman Costumes: From Textile to Identity*, Istanbul: Eren, 2004.

Jones, Jennifer, 'Repackaging Rousseau: Femininity and Fashion in Old Regime France', *French Historical Studies* 18/4 (1994), pp. 939–67.

Karabuda, Barbaro, *Good bye to the Fez: A Portrait of Modern Turkey*, Maurice Michael, trans., London: Denis Dobson, 1959.

Karaminas, Vicki, 'Imagining the Orient: Cultural Appropriation in the Florence Broadhurst Collection', *International Journal of Design* 1/2 (2007), pp. 11–20.

Karpinski, Caroline, 'Kashmir to Paisley', *The Metropolitan Museum of Art Bulletin*, New Series 22/3 (1963), pp. 116–23.

Kawamura, Yuniya, *The Japanese Revolution in Paris Fashion*, Oxford: Berg, 2004.

Kennedy, Alan, *Japanese Costume: History and Tradition*, Paris: Adam Biro, 1990.

Khan, Nasa, 'Asian Women's Dress: From Burqah to Blogs—Changing Clothes for Changing Times', in J. Ash and E. Wilson, eds, *Chic Thrills*, London: Pandora Press, 1992.

Kisch, Bruno, 'Europerien auf China-Porzellan', *Artibus Asiae* 6/3–4 (1937), pp. 272–82.

Knapton, Ernest John, *Empress Josephine*, Cambridge, MA: Harvard University Press, 1963.

Ko, Dorothy, *Teachers of the Inner Chambers: Women and Culture in Seventeenth-century China*, Stanford: Stanford University Press, 1994.

Ko, Dorothy, 'Jazzing into Modernity: High Heels, Platforms and Lotus Shoes', in Victoria Steele and John S. Major, *China Chic*, New Haven, CT: Yale University Press, 1999.

Kondo, Dorinne, *About Face: Performing Race in Fashion and Theatre*, London: Routledge, 1997.

Lamb, Charles, 'Old China', *The Collected Essays of Charles Lamb in Two Volumes*, vol. 1, London: J. M. Dent and Sons, [1823] 1929.

Lancaster, Clay, 'Oriental Contributions to Art Nouveau, *The Art Bulletin* 34/4 (1952), pp. 297–310.

Lant, Antonia, 'Haptical Cinema', *October* 74 (1995), pp. 45–73.

Laver, James, *Costume and Fashion: A Concise History*, 4th edn, London: Thames and Hudson, 2002.

Lawamura, Yuniya, *The Japanese Revolution in Paris Fashion*, Oxford: Berg, 2004.

Lemire, Beverly, *Dress, Culture and Commerce: The English Clothing Trade Before the Factory, 1600–1800*, London: Macmillan, 1997.

Lewis, Bernard, *The Emergence of Modern Turkey*, 3rd edn, Oxford: Oxford University Press, 2002.

Lewis, Reina, *Rethinking Orientalism: Women, Travel and the Ottoman Harem*, London: I. B. Tauris, 2004.

Lipovetsky, Gilles, *L'empire de léphémère*, Paris: Gallimard, 1987.

Longfield, Ada, 'Linen and Cotton Printing in the Eighteenth Century at Ballsbridge, Dublin', *The Burlington Magazine for Connoisseurs* 89/531 (1947), pp. 156–59.

Longfield, Ada, 'Some Eighteenth-Century Advertisements and the English Linen and Cotton Printing Industry', *The Burlington Magazine* 91/552 (Mar., 1949), pp. 70–3.

Lopez, Judith, and Farrell-Beck, Jane, 'What Colored the Transition from Madder to Alizarine?', *Clothing and Textiles Research Journal* 10 (1992), pp. 36–43.

Loughran, Kristyne, 'Jewelry, Fashion, and Identity: The Tuareg Example', *African Arts* 36/1 (Memorial to Roy Sieber, Part 1), pp. 52–65, 93.

Low, Gail Ching-Liang, *White Skins/Black Masks: Representation and Colonialism,* London: Routledge, 1996.

Lowenthal, Cynthia, 'The Veil of Romance: Lady Mary's Embassy Letters', *Eighteenth Century Life* 14 (1970), pp. 66–82.

Lurie, Alison, *The Language of Clothes*, London: Heinemann, 1981.

Lyotard, Jean-François, *La Condition Postmoderne*, Paris: Minuit, 1979.

McCabe, Ina Baghdiantz, *Orientalism in Early Modern France: Eurasian Trade, Exoticism, and the Ancien Régime*, Oxford: Berg, 2008.

MacFie, A. L., *Orientalism: A Reader*, Edinburgh: Edinburgh University Press.

MacKenzie, John, *Orientalism: History, Theory and the Arts*, Manchester: Manchester University Press, 1995.

Mackie, Erin, *Market à la Mode: Fashion, Commodity and Gender in* The Tatler *and* The Spectator, Baltimore: Johns Hopkins University Press, 1997.

MacLean, Gerald, *The Rise of Oriental Travel*, Basingstoke: Palgrave Macmillan, 2004.

Maeder, Edward, *An Elegant Art: Fashion and Fantasy in the Eighteenth Century*, exhibition catalogue, New York: Abrams Publishers and Los Angeles County Museum of Art, 1983.

Makdisi, Ussama, 'Ottoman Orientalism', *The American Historical Review* 107/3 (2005), pp. 768–796.

Mallarmé, Stéphane, *La Dernière Mode*, in Henri Mondor and G. Jean-Aubry, eds, *Œuvres complètes*, Paris: Gallimard Pléiade, [1874–5] 1945.

Mango, Andrew, *Turkey*, London: Thames and Hudson, 1968.

Mann, Thomas, *Der Zauberberg*, Fischer Verlag: Frankfurt am Main, [1924] 1977.

Martin, Richard, and Koda, Harold, *Orientalism: Visions of the East in Western Dress*, Museum of Modern Art exhibition catalogue, New York: Abrams, 1994.

Martin, Morag, *Selling Beauty: Cosmetics, Commerce, and French Society, 1750–1830*, Baltimore: Johns Hopkins University Press, 2009.

Maskiell, Michelle, 'Consuming Kashmir: Shawls and Empires, 1500–2000', *Journal of World History* 13/1 (Spring 2002), 27–65.

Mathur, Saloni, *India by Design: Colonial History and Cultural Display*, Berkeley: University of California Press, 2007.

Maynard, Margaret, 'Grassroots Style: Re-evaluating Australian Fashion and Aboriginal Art in the 1970s and 1980s', *Journal of Design History* 13/2 (2000), pp. 137–150.

Maxwell, Robyn, *Sari to Sarong: Five hundred years of Indian and Indonesian Textile Exchange*, exhibition catalogue, Canberra: National Gallery of Australia, 2003.

Mayor, A. Hyatt, 'Chinoiserie', *The Metropolitan Museum of Art Bulletin* 36/5 (May 1941), pp. 111–14.

Mazzaoui, Maureen Fennell, ed., *Textiles: Production, Trade and Demand*, Aldershot: Ashgate, 1998.

Mercier, Louis-Sébastien, *Tableau de Paris*, 2 vols., Jean-Claude Bonnet, ed., Paris: Mercure de France, [1781–9] 1994.

Meyer, Eve, 'Turquerie and Eighteenth-Century Music', *Eighteenth Century Studies*, 7 (1974), pp. 474–88.

Mikosch, Elizabeth, 'The Scent of Flowers: Kashmiri Shawls in the Collection of the Textile Museum', *Textile Museum Journal* 24 (1985), 6–54.

Mirzoeff, Nicholas, 'Disorientalism: Minority and Visuality in Imperial London', *The Drama Review* 50/2 (2006), pp. 52–69.

Molà, Luca, *The Silk Industry of Renaissance Venice*, Baltimore: Johns Hopkins University Press, 2000.

Montagu, Mary Wortley, *Complete Letters*, vol. 1, 1708–1720, Robert Halsband, ed., Oxford: Oxford University Press, 1965.

Montagu, Mary Wortley, *Turkish Embassy Letters*, Malcolm Jack, ed., London: William Pickering, 1993.

Montgomery, Florence, 'English Chintz and the Victoria and Albert', *The Burlington Magazine* 102/688 (1960), pp. 338–39.

Moon, Michael, 'Flaming Closets', *October* 51 (1989), 19–54.

Morris, Frances, 'Chinoiserie in Printed Fabrics', *The Metropolitan Museum of Art Bulletin* 22/7 (July 1927), pp. 194–96.

Na, Hyunshin, 'Echoes of the East: Patternworks International Best Solution to a Patternmaking Problem Award, 2004', *Clothing and Textiles Research Journal* 25/2 (2007), pp. 202–4.

Nakagawa, Keiichiro, and Rosovsky, Henry, 'The Case of the Dying Kimono: The Influence of Changing Fashions on the Development of the Japanese Woolen Industry', *The Business History Review* 37/1–2 (1963, Special Illustrated Fashion Issue), pp. 59–80.

Nerval, Gérard de), '*Voyage en Orient*,' in Jean Guillaume and Claude Pichois, eds*Œuvres complètes*, vol. 2, Paris: Gallimard Pléiade, [1851] 1984.

Nichols, Sarah, 'Lasenby Liberty: A Mere Adjective?', *The Journal of Decorative and Propaganda Arts* 13 (1989), pp. 76–93.

Niessen, Sandra, Jones, Carla, and Leshkowich, Ann Marie, eds, *Re-Orienting Fashion: The Globalization of Asian Dress*, Oxford: Berg, 2003.

Nordquist, Barbara, 'International Trade in Textiles and Clothing: Implications for the Future', *Clothing and Textiles Research Journal* 35/3 (1985), pp. 35–39.

Obelkevich, Mary, 'Turkish Affect in the Land of the Sun King', *The Musical Quarterly* 63/3 (July 1977), pp. 367–89.

Özdalga, Elisabeth, *The Veiling Issue: Official Secularism and Popular Islam in Modern Turkey*, Richmond, VA: Curzon, 1998.

Pavitt, Jane, *Fear and Fashion in the Cold War*, London: V&A Publishing, 2008.

Paxton, Robert, 'Can You Really Become French?', *New York Review of Books* (April 2009), 52–6.

Peltre, Christine, *Orientalism in Art*, John Goodman, trans., London: Abeville, 1997/8.

Perl, Benjamin, 'Mozart in Turkey', *Cambridge Opera Journal* 12/3 (2000), pp. 219–35.

Perry, Gill, and Rossington, Michael, eds, *Femininity and Masculinity in Eighteenth Century Art and Culture*, Manchester: Manchester University Press, 1994.

Phillips, John Goldsmith, 'An Exhibition of European Fans', *The Metropolitan Museum of Art Bulletin* 27/12 (Dec. 1932), pp. 252, 254.

Picardie, Justine, 'The Beautiful and the Damned', *Harper's Bazaar* Australia, November 2008.

Poiret, Paul, *En habillant l'epoque*, Paris: Grasset, 1930.

Polan, Brenda, and Tredre, Roger, *The Great Fashion Designers*, Oxford: Berg, 2009.

Price, Sally, *Primitive Art in Civilized Places,* Chicago: University of Chicago Press, 1989.

Prideaux, Tom, *The World of Delacroix, 1798–1863*, The Netherlands: Time-Life International, 1966.

Proust, Marcel, *A la recherché du temps perdu*, C. K. Scott Moncrieff and Terence Kilmartin, trans., Harmondsworth: Penguin, 1989

Puwar, Nirmal, 'Multicultural Fashion . . . Stirrings of Another Sense of Culture and Memory', *Feminist Review* 71 (2002), pp. 63–87.

Puwar, Nirmal, and Bhatia, Nandi, eds, *Fashion Theory* 7/3–4 (Special Double Issue on Fashion and Orientalism, 2003).

Rabine, Leslie, *The Global Circulation of African Fashion*, Oxford: Berg, 2002.

Raby, Julian, 'The Serenissima and the Sublime Porte: Art in the Art of Diplomacy, 1453–1600', in Stefano Carboni, ed., *Venice and the Islamic World*, exhibition catalogue, New York: Metropolitan Museum of Art, 2007.

Razek, Rula, *Dress Codes: Reading Nineteenth Century Fashion*, Stanford, CA: Stanford Honors Essay in Humanities, no. 43, 1999.

Ribeiro, Aileen, *The Dress Worn at Masquerades in England, 1730–1790, and its Relation to Fancy Dress in Portraiture*, New York: Garland, 1984.

Ribeiro, Aileen, *Ingres in Fashion*, New Haven: Yale University Press, 1999.

Ribeiro, Aileen, ' "The Whole Art of Dress': Costume in the Work of John Singleton Copley', in Carrie Rebora et al., eds, *John Singleton Copley*, New York: Metropolitan Museum of Art, 1995.

Richardson, Joanna, *Théophile Gautier: His Life and Times*, London: Max Reinhardt, 1958.

Riello, Giorgio, and Roy, Tirthankar, eds, *How India Clothed the World*, Leiden: Brill, 2009.

Rimsky-Korsakoff, Nikolay, *My Musical Life*, Judah A. Joffe, trans., Carl van Vechten, ed., New York: Tudor Publishing, 1935.

Roach-Higgins, Mary Ellen et al., eds, *Dress and Identity*, New York: Fairchild, 1995.

Robb, Graham, *Rimbaud*, New York: Norton, 2000.

Roche, Daniel, *The Culture of Clothing: Dress and Fashion in the Ancien Régime*, Jean Birrell, trans., Cambridge: Cambridge University Press, [1989] 1994.

Rolley, Katrina, and Ash, Caroline, *Fashion in Photographs, 1900–1920*, London, B.T. Batsford, 1992.

Rowbotham, Sheila, *Edward Carpenter: A Life of Liberty and Love*, New York: Verso, 2009.

Rubin, William, ed., *'Primitivism' in 20th Century Art: Affinity of the Tribal and the Modern*, New York: MOMA, 1984.

Said, Edward, *Culture and Imperialism*, London: Vintage, 1994.

Said, Edward, *Orientalism*, London: Vintage, 1978.

Sapin, Julia, 'Merchandising Art and Identity in Meiji Japan: Kyoto *Nihonga* Artists' Designs for Takashimaya Department Store, 1868–1912', *Journal of Design History* 17/4 (2004), pp. 317–36.

Sapori, Michelle, *Rose Bertin: Ministre des modes de Marie Antoinette*, Paris: Éditions de l'Institut Français de la Mode, 2003.

Sardar, Ziauddin, *Orientalism*, Buckingham: Open University Press, 1999.

Scarce, Jennifer, *Women's Costume of the Near and Middle East*, London: Unwin Hyman, 1987.

Scott, Katie, 'Playing Games with Otherness: Watteau's Chinese Cabinet at the Château de la Muette', *Journal of the Warburg and Courtauld Institutes* 66 (2003), pp. 189–248.

Scott, Philippa, *Turkish Delights*, London: Thames and Hudson, 2001.

Seni, Nora, 'Fashion and Women's Clothing in the Satirical Press of Istanbul at the End of the 19th Century', in Sirin Tekeli, ed., *Women in Modern Turkish Society*, London: Zed Books, 1995.

Sennett, Richard, *The Fall of Public Man*, Cambridge: Cambridge University Press, 1977.

Singh, Jyotsna G., *Colonial Narratives, Cultural Dialogues: 'Discoveries' of India in the Language of Colonialism*, London: Routledge, 1996.

Slade, Toby, *Japanese Fashion: A Cultural History*, Oxford: Berg, 2009.

Spate, Virginia, and Bromfield, David, 'A New and Strange Beauty: Monet and Japanese Art', in *Monet and Japan*, exhibition catalogue, Canberra: National Gallery of Australia, 2001.

Spivak, Gayatri Chakravorty, *A Critique of Postcolonial Reason: Toward a History of the Vanishing Present*, Cambridge, MA: Harvard University Press, 1999.

Spivak, Gayatri Chakravorty, *Nationalism and the Imagination*, London: Seagull Books, 2010.

Standen, Edith Appleton, 'Embroideries in the French and Chinese Taste', *The Metropolitan Museum of Art Bulletin* 13/4 (New Series, Dec., 1954), pp. 144–47.

Standen, Edith Appleton, 'English Tapestries "After the Indian Manner"', *Metropolitan Museum Journal* 15 (1980), pp. 119–142.

Steele, Valerie, *Fashion and Eroticism*, Oxford: Oxford University Press, 1985.

Steele, Valerie, *Paris Fashion*, 2nd edn, Oxford: Berg, 1998.

Steele, Valerie, and Major, John S., *China Chic: East Meets West*, New Haven, CT: Yale University Press, 1999.

Steensgaard, Niels, *The Asian Trade Revolution of the Seventeenth Century*, Chicago: University of Chicago Press, 1973.

Stein, Perrin, 'Amédée Van Loo's *Costume turc*: The French Sultana', *The Art Bulletin* 78/3 (Sept. 1996), pp. 417–38.

Stein, Perrin, 'Boucher's Chinoiseries: Some New Sources', *The Burlington Magazine* 138/1122 (1996), pp. 598–604.

Strathern, Paul, *Napoleon in Egypt*, London: Vintage, 2007

Sweetman, John, *The Oriental Obsession: Islamic Inspiration in British and American Art and Architecture, 1500–1920*, Cambridge: Cambridge University Press, 1988.

Tarlo, Emma, *Clothing Matters: Dress and Identity in India*, Chicago: University of Chicago Press, 1996.

Tarlo, Emma, *Visibly Muslim: Fashion, Politics, Faith*, Oxford: Berg, 2010.

'Three Chinoiserie Textiles', *Bulletin of the Pennsylvania Museum* 18/75 (1923), pp. 12–15.

Thurman, Christa, and Batty, Jessica, 'Long Shawl', *Art Institute of Chicago Museum Studies* 29/2, pp. 28–9, 94.

Troy, Nancy, *Couture Culture: A Study of Modern Art and Fashion*, Cambridge, MA: MIT Press, 2003.

Tsunoda, Ryusaku, et al., *Sources of Japanese Tradition*, New York: Columbia University Press, 1958.

Turner, Katherine, 'From Classical to Imperial: Changing Visions of Turkey in the Eighteenth Century', in Steve Turner, ed., *Travel Writing and Empire: Postcolonial Theory in Transit*, London: Zed Books, 1999.

'Turquerie', *The Metropolitan Museum of Art Bulletin* 26/5 (New Series, Jan. 1968), pp. 225–39.

Ulrich, Pamela, 'From Fustian to Merino: The Rise of Textiles Using Cotton Before and After the Gin', *Agricultural History* 68/2, Eli Whitney's Cotton Gin, 1793–1993: A Symposium (Spring 1994), pp. 219–231.

Venice and the Islamic World, exhibition catalogue, New York: Metropolitan Museum of Art and Yale University Press, 2007.

Walker, Hallam, 'Strength and Style in "Le Bourgeois Gentilhomme"', *The French Review* 37/3 (1964), pp. 282–87.

Wichmann, Siegfried, *Japonisme*, New York: Park Lane, 1985.

Williams, Patrick, and Chrisman, Laura, eds, *Colonial Discourse and Postcolonial Theory*, New York: Columbia University Press, 1994.

Wilson, Elizabeth, *Adorned in Dreams*, London: Virago, 1985.

Wilson, Elizabeth, *Bohemians: Glamorous Outcasts*, London: I. B. Tauris, 2000.

Wipper, Audrey, 'African Women, Fashion, and Scapegoating', *Canadian Journal of African Studies/Revue Canadienne des Études Africaines* 6/2 (Special Issue: The Roles of African Women: Past, Present and Future, 1972), pp. 329–49.

Wollen, Peter, *Reading the Icebox: Reflections on Twentieth Century Culture*, London: Verso, 1993.

Worth, Susannah, and Sibley, Lucy, 'Maja Dress and the Andalusian Image of Spain', *Clothing and Textiles Research Journal* 12 (1994), pp. 51–60.

Young, Robert, *White Mythologies: Writing History and the West*, London: Routledge, [1990] 2004.

Zhao, Steven, 'Analysis of Chinese Clothing Consumption in Market in 2007 and 2008', http://www.buzzle.com/articles/analysis-of-chinese-clothing-consumption-in-market-in-2007-and-2008.html

Zizek, Slavoj, *Welcome to the Desert of the Real*, London: Verso, 2002.

Zola, Émile, *Au Bonheur des dames*, Paris: Le Livre de Poche, [1883] 1980.

Zutshi, Chitralekha, '"Designed for Eternity": Kasmiri Shawls, Empire, and Cultures of Production and Consumption in Mid-Victorian Britain', *Journal of British Studies* 48 (2009), pp. 420–40.

WEB SITES AND OTHER INTERNET SOURCES

http://geniusbeauty.com/fashion-and-wear/paris-fashion-week-dior/

http://www.guerlain.com/int/en/base.html#/en/home-parfum/catalogue-parfums/men-fragrances/men-fragrances-habit-rouge/habit-rouge-eau-de-parfum.html

http://www.thehijabshop.com

www.tx.ncsu.edu/jtatm/volume3issue1/all%20docs/Ahp1.doc

http://www.religionandsociety.org.uk/publications/podcasts/show/mediating_modesty_reina_lewis

http://www.fashion.arts.ac.uk/research/projects-collaborations/modest-dressing.

Index

*Note that 'orient' and 'oriental' is not listed as they and related terms are on almost every page.